Lifting Techniques in Plastic Surgery

Won Lee • Kyu Hwa Jung

Lifting Techniques in Plastic Surgery

A Practical Guide on Thread Lifting, Mini-Lifting and Rhytidectomy

Springer

Won Lee
Yonsei E1 Plastic Surgery Clinic
Anyang, Korea (Republic of)

Kyu Hwa Jung
Liting Plastic Surgery Clinic
Seoul, Korea (Republic of)

ISBN 978-981-96-4819-1 ISBN 978-981-96-4820-7 (eBook)
https://doi.org/10.1007/978-981-96-4820-7

This Springer imprint is published by the registered company Springer Nature Singapore Pte Ltd.
The registered company address is: 152 Beach Road, #21-01/04 Gateway East, Singapore 189721, Singapore

Preface by Won Lee

Lifting is an essential surgical technique in the field of plastic surgery. The primary concern of patients we meet daily is antiaging, and surgeries around the eyes, such as upper and lower blepharoplasty, are among the most commonly performed procedures in plastic surgery in South Korea. Rhytidectomy is the most effective facial lifting surgery and has evolved over the years. However, due to concerns about the burden of surgery and fear of scarring, minimally invasive techniques have developed, with thread lifting being a representative procedure.

Thread lifting has also seen significant advancements with the development of various types of threads; however, there are many cases where the effectiveness is diminished or the duration of the results is short due to the patient's condition or the operator's inexperience. Personally, I believe that minimally invasive procedures such as botulinum toxin, fillers, thread lifting, and skin boosters have many undisclosed aspects because they are procedures that cannot be viewed internally. I think there is still much to uncover regarding filler injections, and I continue to experiment in this area. The reason deep plane surgical techniques, which actually visualize the Superficial Muscular Aponeurotic System (SMAS) layer or deeper layers, have advanced significantly is that they allow for direct observation. However, if we can apply this knowledge to achieve similar effects in a minimally invasive manner, I believe it would represent the optimal surgical method.

Therefore, I felt the need to comprehensively summarize lifting surgical techniques for comparison and to scientifically present better outcomes based on this application. While writing the paper on thread lifting, I encountered many reference papers, most of which reported good results using specific company threads or discussed the side effects of thread lifting. Additionally, I have noticed that my submissions on thread lifting are more readily accepted and published compared to other topics. This seems to indicate that there are still many scientifically unexplored areas regarding thread lifting.

Thus, in this book, I aimed to compile the techniques we have developed in our own papers and the surgical methods currently in practice. I also wrote this to provide readers with helpful information based on the summarized and scientific content. Throughout my 25 years as a plastic surgeon, I have always held one principle in mind: if the patient in front of me were my beloved daughter, it would be my duty as a plastic surgeon to present and perform the most ideal lifting technique scientifically.

I first met Dr. Kyu Hwa Jung at the Minimally Invasive Plastic Surgery Society. He is passionate about writing papers and, above all, values loyalty, which has led us to collaborate. We plan to continue writing papers together, filling in each other's gaps. This book has also been completed by addressing our shortcomings and including various photos and illustrations for the readers' convenience. I would like to express my gratitude to Lee Kyungjun, a junior from Sang Moon High School, CEO of N Finders Co., for assisting with the illustrations.

I would like to thank my two daughters, Seunghyun and Hyunji, who always support me, and express my love and gratitude to Jung Youn, who I cherish above all. I dedicate this book to the late Lee Hyang Ran, who will be commemorated on the first anniversary of her passing on November 26, 2023.

Anyang, South Korea
May 2025

Won Lee

Preface by Kyu Hwa Jung

Lifting is a procedure that reverses the changes brought about by time, akin to a journey through time. As seen in many films that deal with time travel, there are still many undisclosed aspects and imperfections. Sometimes, it can yield unexpected results.

For this reason, we must engage in further research and contemplation. We should strive to find methods that can produce effects in a more natural and healthy way, based on scientific evidence. The destiny of a physician performing lifting procedures is to discover the best path for those who wish to appear younger, building upon the knowledge that accumulates over time.

Through numerous experiences with antiaging procedures, from fillers and thread lifting to traditional facial incision facelifts, I have learned to view lifting procedures not just as individual trees but as a forest. It is important to recognize that not all problems can be solved by lifting alone; sometimes, even after an effective lifting procedure, unsatisfactory results occur because the lifting was viewed as a single tree rather than part of a larger ecosystem.

There may be times when the appropriate path is not visible, and in such cases, we must be able to analyze patient factors more clearly to find alternative routes. Ultimately, patients' desires are not merely for external youth but for beauty. The ultimate goal for patients is to regain the beauty they have lost and to find happiness through the paths we help them discover.

Establishing a clear concept of what lifting is and setting one's own standards is an essential element for absorbing the myriad of information available today and for maintaining a flexible approach. It is my hope that this book will assist you in understanding the broader picture of "lifting."

I would like to express my gratitude to president of Minimally Invasive Plastic Surgery Association (MIPS), Won Lee for solidly filling in my shortcomings and motivating me to keep going until this book was completed. I also want to thank my daughters, Ji-yul and Ji-a, who, despite not being able to spend much time together, always bring happiness, and to Bo-young, who quietly and steadfastly supports everyone from behind. Finally, I wish to extend my deep gratitude to my brother, Chang-hwa Jung who has been my mental mentor and guide in life for many years.

Seoul, South Korea
May 2025

Kyu Hwa Jung

Contents

About the Author: Won Lee

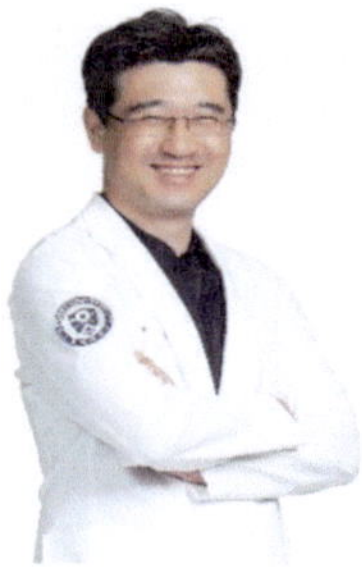

Won Lee MD, PhD, Board certified plastic surgeon, South Korea

Main Profiles

Director of Yonsei E1 Plastic Surgery Clinic
Graduated Yonsei University Medical College
Doctor of Phylosophy degree from the Graduate School of Dongguk University
President of MIPS, 2022 ~ 2025
Full Members of the Korean Society of Plastic and Reconstructive Surgeons
Scientific faculty, IMCAS 2020, 2024
Scientific committee, MAIS 2024

Books

1. [Korean] Advances lifting technique, thread lifting, minilifting and rhytidectomy
2. [English] Springer: Advances in hyaluronic acid filler injections 2024
3. [Korean] Advances in hyaluronic acid filler injection 2024
4. [English] Cambridge Scholars Publishing: A guide to aesthetic medicine and cosmetic surgery chapter 23 2023
5. [English] Springer: Minimally invasive aesthetic surgery techniques 2022
6. [Korean] Minimal Invasive plastic surgery 2022

7. [English] Springer: Safe filler injection technique 2021
8. [English] Springer: Video book: regional filler injection techniques 2021
9. [English] Springer: State of the art rhinoplasty techniques 2021
10. [Korean] Recent Safe injection technique 2021
11. [Korean] Writing Medical article 2020
12. [English] Springer: Filler complications 2019
13. [English] ICALA: Effective and safe filler injections English edition 2019
14. [Korean] Filler Complications and management 2018
15. [Korean] Atlas of minimally invasive facelift 2019 translation

Awards

2021 best paper award—PRS Atlanta
2024 best cosmetic book award—IMAAC

Articles

1.	Injectable "Skin Boosters" in Aging Skin Rejuvenation: A Current Overview	Archive PS 2024 Nov
2.	Double-Layer Cogged Thread Lifting Technique: A Superficial and Deep-Layer Lifting Method	APS 2024 Nov
3.	Structural Analysis of Hyaluronic Acid Fillers Using Nuclear Magnetic Resonance: Implications for Quality Control and Clinical Performance	Polymer 2024 Oct
4.	Minilifting: Short-scar rhytidectomy with thread lifting	Archive PS 2024 Sept
5.	Deliberations of the Safety Task Force: Risk factors and treatment of adverse events associated with aesthetic injectables	JCD 2024 Aug
6.	Mapping high-risk arteries using doppler ultrasound for forehead contouring in Korean patients	DS 2024 July
7.	Sonographic observation of the paradoxical masseteric bulging and clinical implication of functional compartment	Anat Cell Biol 2024 Mar
8.	"Cohesiveness of Hyaluronic Acid Fillers": Evaluation Using Multiple Cohesion Tests	Archives PS 2024 Feb
9.	Unilateral platysma muscle rupture as an effect of using a hard wooden block for facial massage.	Archives PS 2024 Feb
10.	Etiology of Delayed Inflammatory Reaction Induced by Hyaluronic Acid Filler	Archives PS 2024 Feb
11.	Comparative Analysis of Temperature-Responsive Hydrogel (PF72) for Postoperative Pain After Bimaxillary Surgery: A Retrospective Study	APS 2024 Feb
12.	Transumbilical Silicone Breast Augmentation: A 13-Year Experience and 5-Year Analysis	APS 2024 Feb
13.	Needle-Free Jet Injection of Poly-(Lactic Acid) for Atrophic Acne Scars: Literature Review and Report of Clinical Cases	JCM 2024 Jan

14.	Effectiveness of a Novel Temperature-Responsive Hydrogel (PF72) for Postoperative Pain Relief in Breast Augmentation	JCM 2023 Dec
15.	Ultrasound-guided thread lifting for the prevention of parotid gland and diagnosing parotid duct complications	Skin Res Technol. 2023 Dec
16.	Assessing the Practical Application of Rheological Properties of Hyaluronic Acid Fillers: A 1-Year Follow-Up Photographic Analysis	APS 2023 Sept
17.	Endoscopically Assisted Correction of Malpositioned Breast Implants Using Absorbable Barbed Sutures	APS 2023 August
18.	Hyaluronic acid filler injection guided by doppler	Archive PS 2023 July
19.	Dynamic evaluation of skin displacement by the frontalis muscle contraction using 3D skin displacement vector analysis	YMJ 2023 June
20.	A Novel Method Using the Petal Pattern for Contouring a Domed Nipple in Tuberous Breasts	PRS 2023 June
21.	Use of LetibotulinumtoxinA for Aesthetic Treatment of Asians: A Consensus DOI: 10.1093/asj/sjad151 ASJ 2023 June 50. Eyebrow lifting using multidirectional absorbable thread	JCD 2023 April
22.	Determination of Hyaluronic Acid Dermal Filler Impurities Using SEM/EDS Analysis	Polymers 2023 March
23.	Comparative study of the penetration force between the superficial and deep temporal fascia for easier temple augmentation technique using hyaluronic acid filler	JPRAS 2022 Dec
24.	Five Factors to Consider before Treatment of a Hyaluronic Acid Filler-Induced Vascular Complications	APS 2022 June
25.	Comments on "Hyaluronic Acid Filler Injection Technique in Multiple Layers of the Nasolabial Fold"	PRS GO 2022 May
26.	Temple augmentation by injecting a hyaluronic acid filler between the superficial and deep temporal fasciae	JCD 2022 April
27.	Reply: Use of Autologous Adipose-Derived Stromal Vascular Fractions in Revision Rhinoplasty for Severe Contractures in Asian Patients	PRS 2020 Jan
28.	Pre-injection ultrasound scanning for treating temporal hollowing	JCD 2021 Sep
29.	The Osteogenic Differentiation of Human Dental Pulp Stem Cells through G0/G1 Arrest and the p-ERK/Runx-2 Pathway by Sonic Vibration	international journal of molecular sciences 2021 Sep
30.	Dynamic evaluation of facial muscles: 3D skin displacement vector analysis using a facial painting model	Laryngoscope Investigative Otolaryngology 2021 July
31.	Aspiration Before Filler Injection: Rethinking the Paradigm?	ASJ 2021 June
32.	Unexpected Bone Resorption in Mentum Induced by the Soft-Tissue Filler Hyaluronic Acid: A Preliminary Retrospective Cohort Study of Asian Patients	PRS 2021 May
33.	Gluteal Soft-Tissue Repositioning Using Polydioxane Threads	DS 2021 May
34.	Usefulness of Ultrasound Devices in Facial Plastic Surgery	Aesthetic 2021 April

35.	Aspiration revisited: Prospective evaluation of a physiologically pressurized model with animal correlation and broader applicability to filler complications	ASJ 2021 April
36.	Soft Tissue Filler Injections along the Nose: On-line Survey	Aesthetic 2021 March
37.	Comparison of hyaluronic acid filler ejection pressure with injection force for safe filler injection	JCD 2021 March
38.	Use of Autologous Adipose-derived Stromal Vascular Fraction for Revision Rhinoplasty for Severe Contractures in Asian Patients	PRS 2021 March
39.	Comments on "Hyaluronidase: an overview of its properties, applications, and side effects"	Archive PS 2020 November
40.	Identification of a suitable layer for injecting calcium hydroxyapatite fillers in the hands	JPRAS 2020 October
41.	Doppler Ultrasonographic Anatomy of the Midline Nasal Dorsum	APS 2020 October
42.	Non-Surgical Rhinoplasty with Polydioxanone Threads and Hyaluronic Acid Filler to Treat a Widened Nose after Repeated Injections of Hyaluronic Acid Filler	Aesthetic 2020 April
43.	ABCs in the Prevention of Filler-induced Ocular Complications	Aesthetic 2020 April
44.	Development and Usability of a Virtual Reality-Based Filler Injection Training System	APS 2020 July
45.	Safe Glabellar Wrinkle Correction With Soft Tissue Filler Using Doppler Ultrasound	ASJ 2020 July
46.	Comments on "Filler rhinoplasty based on anatomy: The dual plane technique"	JPRAS 2020 June
47.	Comparative analysis of botulinum toxin injection after corrective rhinoplasty for deviated nose and alar asymmetry	JCD 2020
48.	Prevention of hyaluronic acid filler-induced blindness,	Dermatologic therapy 2020
49.	Safe Doppler ultrasound-guided method for nasolabial fold correction with hyaluronic acid filler	ASJ 2020
50.	Reply: Infraorbital groove correction by microfat injection after lower blepharoplasty	JPRAS 2020
51.	Short-term Treatment Outcomes of Facial Rejuvenation Using the Mint Lift Fine	PRS global 2020
52.	Comparative Effectiveness of Different Interventions of Perivascular Hyaluronidase	PRS 2020
53.	Comments on "Update on Avoiding and Treating Blindness From Fillers: A Recent Review of the World Literature"	Aesthetic Surgery Journal 2020
54.	Reply: Effectiveness of Retrobulbar Hyaluronidase Injection in an Iatrogenic Blindness Rabbit Model Using Hyaluronic Acid Filler Injection	PRS 2020
55.	Novel technique for infraorbital groove correction using multiple twisted polydioxanone thread	JCD 2019
56.	Doppler ultrasound-guided thread lifting	JCD 2019
57.	Infraorbital groove correction by microfat injection after lower blepharoplasty	JPRAS 2019
58.	Ocular complications of soft tissue filler injections: A review of literature	JCD 2019

59.	Soft tissue properties can be altered by a small diameter	DS 2019
60.	Nasal dorsum augmentation using soft tissue filler injection.	JCD 2019 Jun
61.	Effectiveness of retrobulbar hyaluronidase injection in an iatrogenic blindness rabbit model using hyaluronic acid filler injection.	2019 PRS Jul;144(1): 137–143
62.	Staged mosaic punching excision of a kissing nevus on the eyelid 2019 Jun;43(3):652–657	Aesthetic plastic surgery
63.	Practical Guidelines for Hyaluronic Acid Soft-Tissue Filler Use in Facial Rejuvenation.	Dermatol Surg 2019;00:1–9
64.	Novel technique of filler injection in the temple area using the vein detection device.	J Plast Reconstr Aesthet Surg. 2019
65.	Clinical application of a new hyaluronic acid filler based on its rheological properties and the anatomical site of injection.	Biomedical dermatology 2018 2:22
66.	Is injury to the inferior alveolar nerve still common during orthognathic surgery? Manual twist technique for sagittal split ramus osteotomy.	2018 The British Association of Oral and Maxillofacial Surgeons.
67.	Modified Rotational Anterior Segmental Osteotomy for Prevention of Common Complication (Aged Appearance).	J Craniofac Surg. 2018 Jul;29(5):e517-e518
68.	Correction of sunken upper eyelid with orbital fat transposition flap and dermofat graft.	J Plast Reconstr Aesthet Surg. 2017 Dec;70(12):1768–1775.
69.	Augmentation mammoplasty with silicone implant using transumbilical approach at a subpectoral level.	Lee Won, Choi BK, Bang SI, Yang EJ Ann Plast Surg. 2014 Sep;73(3):268
70.	Glomus tumor of the hand. Lee Won, Kwon SB, Cho SH, EoSR	Arch Plast Surg 2014 May

Speaker

2024, Oct, 25th, IMAAC, Shenzhen, China
2024, Oct, 4th 5th, Injectable summit, Marbella, Spain
2024, Sept, 24th, Allergan Aesthetic Asia Journal Club, zoom
2024, Sept, 8th, Samyang Cadaver international symposium, Seoul, Korea
2024, July, 20th, Keblyn launching symposium, Seoul, Korea
2024, June 29th, book ceremony conference, Seoul, Korea
2024, June 23, imcas asia, Bangkok, Thailand
2024, May 19th MIPS, Seoul, Korea
2024, April 7th, AestheticPS, Seoul, Korea
2024, Feb 1st, IMCAS, Paris, France
2023, Dec 10th, MIPS, Korea
2023, Dec 2nd , ISWAM, Jakarta, Indonesia
2023, Oct 5–8th, Holistic Aesthetics Congress, Istanbul, Turkiye
2023, July 30th, HELF, Korea
2023, July 15th, AMSC, Kuala Lumpur, Malaysia
2023, June 25th, Koreaderma, Korea
2023, June 25th, Severance symposium, Korea

2023, June 11th, CyAsia
2023, April 30th, MIPS, Korea
2023, Mar 23rd, GLAM, Korea
2023, Mar 1st , Dubai Derma, Dubai, UAE
2022, Dec 11th , MIPS, Korea
2022, Dec 4th, KALDAT, Korea
2022, Nov 13th, KPRAS
2022, Oct 30th, HELF, Korea "Update rheology"
2022, Oct 16th, KPRS, Korea "COVID 19 and filler"
2022, Oct 1st, LMSTW, Taiwan, online, eyebrow lifting,
2022, Sep 30th, IMCAS Asia, Bangkok, Thailand, "ultrasound, pf72, dynamic botox"
2022, Sep 18th, Demire, Korea
2022, Aug 20th, AMSC, Kuala Lumpur, Malaysia "filler impurities, ultrasound guided filler injection"
2022, July 1st, APEM, Kuwait, "Safe filler injection"
2022, May 29th, MIPS, Korea
2022, May 22th, KALDAT, Korea
2022, May, 22th, Aesthetic Plastic Surgery Association,
2022, Mar, 31st, AMWC, Monaco, Online "how to avoid complications in HA filler injection"
2022, Mar 12th, LMSTW, Spring meeting, Taiwan, Online
2022, Feb 20th, Justmake conference, Taiwan, Online
2022, Jan 9th, Mint conference, Taiwan, Online
2021, Dec 12th, LiftingAss, Korea
2021, Dec 5th, KALDAT, Korea
2021, Dec 2nd, Jetema Uzbekistan Webinar Online
2021, Oct 27th, MGR, Yonsei University, Korea
2021, Oct 24th, HELF, Korea,
2021, Oct 21th, Allergan, Asia journal club
2021, Oct 2nd, TAPS, Taiwan, Online, PDO thread technique
2021, Sep, 21th, MIPS, International webinar
2021, Sep 11th, ICLAS, Korea, current global consensus about treatment and prevention of IRVC
2021, Sep 2nd, Allergan, Korea
2021, July 11th, APS, Korea
2021, May 22th, JAM, Korea
2021, April 25th, KALDAT, Korea
2021, April 18th, MIPS, Korea
2020, Dec 6th, KALDAT, Korea, prevention of IRVC
2020, Oct, 18th, MIPS, Korea
2020, Sep 12th, Oct 24th, Allergan IRVC meeting, Online
2020, Sep 20th, IMSA, Online
2020, July, 6th, KALDAT, Korea, comparison of current filler
2020, April 21th, HELF, Korea
2020, Jan 31th, IMCAS, Paris, France
2019, Oct, 28th, GAIN, Korea
2019, Oct 13th, HELF, Korea

2018, Nov 11th, PRS Korea, PRS Korea, Ocular complication by soft tissue filler

2018, Oct, 28th, HELF, Korea

2018, May 6th, AMWC Taiwan, current injection trend using Neuronox and neuramis

2018, April 7th, Aesthetic Plastic Surgery Korea, proper use of fillers for volume restoration

2018, Feb 3rd, GALAA, Thailand, Filler rheology

2017, Nov, 11th, PRS Korea, Filler property

2017, Sept, 10th, MIPS, Korea, Filler rheology

2017, July 11th, ITCAM, Bangkok, Thailand, Essential anatomy of faces

2017, April 23th, MIPS, Korea, Fibroblast

2016, Oct 2nd, Taiwan, Justmake conference

2016, May 14th, OSAPS, Taiwan, TUBA, Filler

2015, Aug, 15th, TAAMS, Taiwan, Filler A ~ Z

2014, Oct 19th, TAAMS, Taiwan, TUBA

2014, June 7th, Instructional course of oculoplasty, Taipei, Taiwan, Sunken eyelid correction

2012, Oct 7th, OSAPS, Korea, TUBA

About the Author: Kyu Hwa Jung

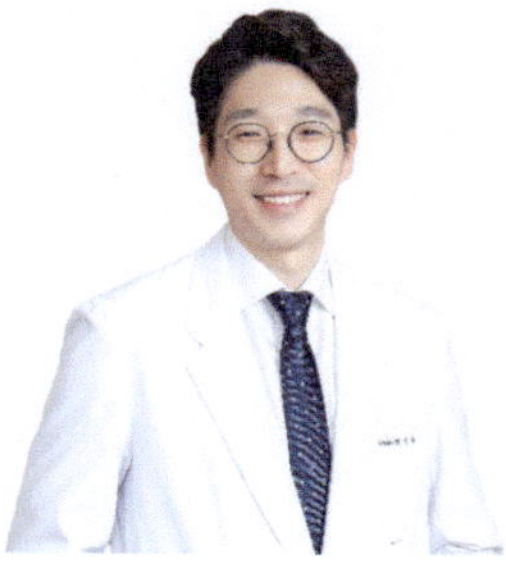

Kyu Hwa Jung, MD, MS, Board certified Plastic Surgeon, South Korea
Graduated Soonchunhyang University Medical College

Master of Medical science from Soonchunhyang University Medical College

Full Members of the Korean Society of Plastic and Reconstructive Surgeons

Scientific faculty, IMCAS 2022, 2024

Books

1. [Korean] Advances lifting technique, thread lifting, minilifting and rhytidectomy
2. [English] Springer: Minimally invasive aesthetic surgery techniques 2022
3. [Korean] Minimal Invasive plastic surgery 2022

Articles

1.	Double-Layer Cogged Thread Lifting Technique: A Superficial and Deep-Layer Lifting Method	APS 2024 Nov
2.	Minilifting: Short-scar rhytidectomy with thread lifting	Archive PS 2024 Sept
3.	Unilateral platysma muscle rupture as an effect of using a hard wooden block for facial massage.	Archives PS 2024 Feb
4.	Various applications of deep temporal fascia in rhinoplasty	Yonsei Med J. 2015 Jan

5.	Pathologic Patency Analysis of the Descending Branch of the Lateral Femoral Circumflex Artery in Head and Neck reconstruction	J craniofacial 2016 Jun
6.	Clinical Analysis of risk factors of patency of the descending branch of the lateral circumflex femoral artery	J Plast Surg Hand Surg 2014 Dec
7.	Nodular fasciitis on temple area resulting in surgical trauma	J Craniofacial Surg. 2014. 2014
8.	Characteristics of Dermoid Cyst of the Auricle	Arch Craniofacial Surg. 2014 Apr
9.	Leiomyoma on nasal dorsum	Arch Plast Surg. 2015 Jan

Speaker

2024, Sept, 8th, Samyang Cadaver international symposium, Seoul, Korea
2024, Aug 28–29th IFAAS "Deep plane facelift live surgery"
2024, June 29th, Book ceremony conference, Seoul, Korea
2024, June 23rd, IMCAS Asia, Bangkok, Thailand "eyebrow thread lifting"
2024, April 7th, AestheticPS, Seoul, Korea
2023, Dec 2nd , ISWAM, Jakarta, Indonesia
2023, Nov 12th KPRS, Korea
2023, Dec 10th, MIPS, Korea
2023, Oct 8th BAPS, Korea "Mini-lift video session"
2023, Sep 2nd, Demire, Korea
2023, Aug 20th KAAD, Korea
2023, July 15th, AMSC, Kuala Lumpur, Malaysia
2023, April 30th, MIPS, Korea
2023, April 1st APS, Korea
2022, Nov. 13th KAFC, Korea
2022, Dec 11th, MIPS, Korea
2022, Sep 30th, IMCAS Asia, Bangkok, Thailand

About the Author

Won Lee is a plastic surgeon. He received his MD from Yonsei University Medical College and PhD from College of Medicine, Dongguk University, Seoul, South Korea. Currently, he is the Director of Yonsei E1 Plastic Surgery Clinic, Anyang. Dr. Lee is a member of the Korean Society of Plastic and Reconstructive Surgeons and he is the president of Minimal Invasive Plastic Surgery association from 2022 to 2025. His books include: *Filler Complications* (Springer 2019), *Safe Filler Injection Techniques* (Springer 2022), *Minimally Invasive Aesthetic Surgery Techniques* (Springer 2022), *Advances in Hyaluronic Acid Filler Injections* (Springer 2024), and *Lifting Techniques in Plastic Surgery* (Springer 2025). He has published 73 articles about plastic surgery fields until 2025 and has received the "best paper ward" from Plastic and reconstructive surgery in 2021.

Kyu Hwa Jung is a plastic surgeon specializing in antiaging procedures, including thread lifting, facelift surgery, and injectables. He actively shares his expertise at international conferences and contributes to the development of new medical products. He has published several papers and two books on lifting procedures, recently released in both local and global editions.

Beyond his clinical practice, Dr. Jung has hosted live surgery sessions for international doctors, providing a training in advanced techniques. At overseas conferences, he has delivered thought-provoking presentations, encouraging a new perspective on antiaging. By integrating innovative approaches with practical surgical expertise, he continues to shape the future of aesthetic medicine.

Basic Anatomy for Lifting

1

Contents

The facial region consists of multiple layers depending on the area, and the primary target layer varies according to the different lifting methods. Energy-based devices (EBD), such as radiofrequency and ultrasound devices, generate heat from the dermal layer of the face to the superficial musculo-aponeurotic system (SMAS) layer, causing contraction. In the case of thread lifting, the subcu-

W. Lee, K. H. Jung, *Lifting Techniques in Plastic Surgery*,
https://doi.org/10.1007/978-981-96-4820-7_1

taneous fat layer and SMAS layer are mechanically pulled to create a lifting effect. Surgical facelift procedures primarily involve lifting the subcutaneous fat layer, the SMAS layer, and the deeper sub-SMAS layer. Of course, excess skin is excised after the overall lifting procedure. Therefore, it is essential for the surgeon to be well aware of which layer is the primary surgical site according to the method of lifting being performed, and understanding the corresponding anatomical structures is crucial. This chapter will examine the layers of the face, the main anatomical structures located in the face, and the ultrasound detected structures.

1.1 Facial Layers

The most fundamental aspect of all lifting techniques is the layers of the face. In both thread lifting and surgical lifting, the proper movement of soft tissues is a crucial factor in evaluating the initial effects and enhancing patient satisfaction. Therefore, understanding each layer of the face is the foundation of lifting.

While the layers of the face are often described in five parts, there can be more layers depending on the specific area. The primary divisions are the skin, subcutaneous fat, SMAS, sub-SMAS, and the periosteal layer, starting from the outermost layer (Fig. 1.1). Different layers and terminologies exist depending on the area (Table 1.1). The superficial fascia of the face, known as the SMAS, is the most important structure for lifting. The SMAS is thick near the parotid gland but gradually becomes thinner as it moves medially, connecting to the broad platysma muscle in neck region and forming layers with the superficial temporal fascia in the upper temporal region. The relatively deeper fascia consists of structures known as the parotid masseteric fascia, which envelops the masseter muscle and parotid gland, and it continues as the deep temporal fascia in the temporal region.

Generally, there are various layers of the skin, and to apply a range of lifting techniques—from procedures that deliver energy to the dermis layer to induce contraction, to techniques that involve inserting threads into the subcutaneous fat layer to create tension, to procedures that place threads into the SMAS layer for lifting, and to facelifts

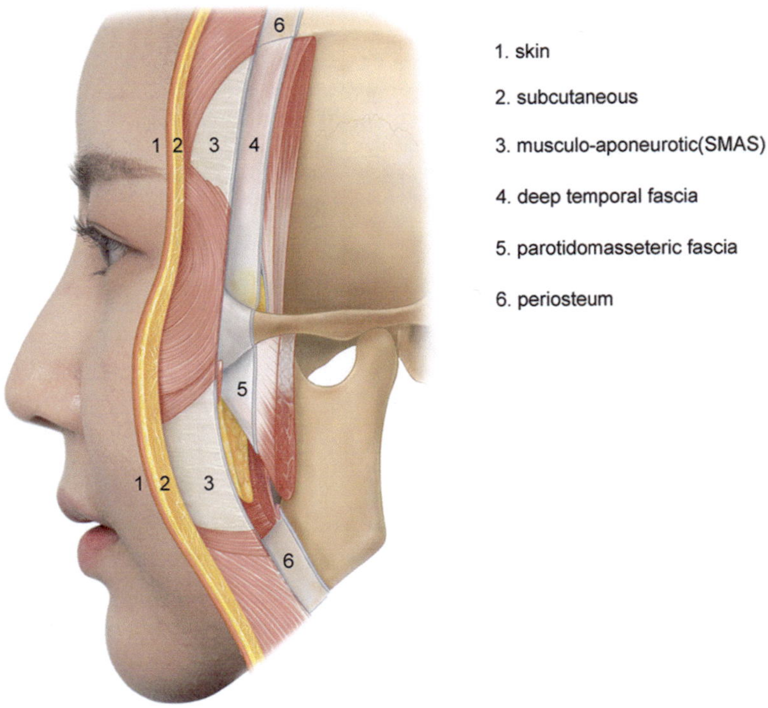

Fig. 1.1 Facial layers

Table 1.1 Facial layers

Layer	Scalp	Forehead	Temple	Cheek (lateral)	Cheek (medial)
1	Skin	Skin	Skin	Skin	Skin
2	Connective tissue	Superficial fat layer	Superficial fat layer lateral temporal cheek compartment	Superficial fat layer	Superficial fat layer
3	Aponeurotica	Frontalis muscle	Superficial temporal fascia	SMAS Platysma	Mimetic muscle
4	Loose areolar tissue	Subgaleal space ROOF Galeal fat pad	Loose areolar tissue Innominate fascia / Parotid temporal fascia	SubSMAS plane Premasseteric space	Deep fat layer Prezygomatic& premaxillary space
5	Periosteum	Periosteum	Deep temporal fascia Temporal fat pad	Parotid masseteric fascia	
6			Temporalis muscle	Parotid gland Masseter muscle Buccal fat	

that involve dissecting the sub-SMAS layer—anatomical knowledge is essential.

1.2 Histological Anatomy

As mentioned above, the facial layers are divided into the skin, subcutaneous fat, SMAS, and sub-SMAS. The skin is divided into the epidermis and dermis, with the epidermal layer further divided into four (or five) layers: stratum corneum, stratum granulosum, stratum spinosum, and stratum basale. The outermost layer, the stratum corneum, consists of 15–20 layers of soft keratin filaments with a squamous (flattened appearance) structure.

The dermis is composed of cells such as macrophages, mast cells, and fibroblasts, as well as an extracellular matrix (ECM) made up of collagen, elastin, and various other components. Collagen is the primary element of the extracellular matrix, accounting for 70% of the dry weight of the dermis, and it forms a network with elastin. The amount and ratio of these components determine the tensile strength of collagen, while elastin contributes to flexibility and resilience.

Collagen can be further categorized based on its location and function, with type I collagen being the most abundant and primarily responsible for determining tensile strength due to its rigid properties. In contrast, type III collagen forms a relatively elastic network. It is known that the ratio of type I to type III collagen increases with age, which is believed to contribute to skin firmness and the formation of wrinkles (Table 1.2 [1]).

Other components of the extracellular matrix, such as amorphous glycosaminoglycans (GAGs) and glycoproteins, account for only 0.1–0.3% of the weight but play very important roles. GAGs, also known as natural moisturizing factors (NMFs), are involved in hydration, with hyaluronic acid having the greatest impact on water binding capacity. Additionally, hair follicles, sebaceous glands, and sweat glands are distributed throughout the dermal layer depending on the area.

Moreover, glycoproteins such as laminin, which stabilizes the epidermal layer at the epidermis-dermis junction, and fibronectin, which provides structural support through interactions with collagen and facilitates cell adhesion, are also components of the dermal layer.

The dermis is broadly divided into the papillary dermis and the reticular dermis. The papillary dermis consists of loose connective tissue and contains a plexus of blood vessels and lymphatic vessels, making it thinner and softer compared to the reticular dermis. In contrast, the reticular dermis is characterized by a relatively acellular, thick, and dense mesh network of collagen and elastic fibers.

At the very bottom of the dermis lies a layer of adipocytes known as dermal white adipose tissue

Table 1.2 Dermal extracellular matrix components localization and function. *GAG* glycoaminoglycan, *HS* heparan sulfate, *BM* basement membrane, *TSP-1* thrombospondin1, *FACIT* fibril-associated collagens with interrupted triple helices

Collagen	Localization within skin	Function
Type 1	Interstitial matrix, dermis	Most common support, tensile strength, fibrillary
Type 3	Interstitial matrix, dermis	1/3 of fibrillary collagen, support, tensile strength, fibrillary
Type 4	Basement membrane	Network-forming structure, highly flexible
Type 5	Interstitial matrix, dermis	Minor type
Type 6	Papillary dermis, Interstitial matrix	Links collagen 4 to fibrillary collagen 1 and 3 in papillary dermis, binds fibronectin, builds beaded microfibrils
Type 7	Basement membrane Papillary dermis	Assembles into anchoring fibrils that anchor BM to papillary dermis
Type 12	Papillary dermis Interface between BM	Fibril associated interacts with TSP-1, FACIT
Type 13	Keratinocyte surface	Transmembrane, ectodomain release by cleavage
Type 14	Papillary dermis Interface between BM	Fibril associated interacts with TSP-1, FACIT
Type 17	Keratinocyte surface	Transmembrane release by cleavage, attached keratinocyte to basement membrane, regulates keratinocyte proliferation, maintains stem cells in hair follicles

Elastic fibers	Localization within skin	Function
Elastin	Interstitial matrix, dermis, vessel	Elasticity and resilience
Fibrillin-1	Interstitial matrix, dermis	Elasticity and flexibility assist in BM anchorage to interstitial matrix, regulates TGF-β bioavailability, mechanosensor
Fibrillin-2	Interstitial matrix, dermis	Present during development and wound healing, similar functions as Fibrillin-1

Glycoproteins, matricellular proteins	Localization within skin	Function
Laminin	Epidermal basement membrane	Stabilize epidermal adhesion, mediate epidermal-dermal communication
Fibronectin	Interstitial matrix, dermis	Interacts with collagen, provide adhesion cues for cells
Nidogen/ entactin	Basement membrane	Bridging molecules, helps maintain epidermal integrity
TSP-1	Basement membrane, papillary dermis,	Would healing, stimulates cell proliferation and tissue homeostasis, stimulates ECM synthesis
Periostin	Papillary dermis	Wound healing, stimulates cell proliferation, involved in collagen deposition and scar formation
Tenascin C	Interstitial matrix, dermis, wound edges	Upregulated in wound healing, stimulates cell proliferation

Proteoglycans (PG)	Localization within skin	Function
Biglycan	Interstitial matrix, dermis	Collagen-interacting protein, highly abundant in papillary dermis, regulates collagen fibril formation
Decorin	Interstitial matrix, dermis	Collagen-interacting protein, highly abundant in papillary dermis, regulates collagen fibril formation, stabilizes tissue
Perlecan	Basement membrane	Aids laminin-collagen4 linkage, signals via integrin binding, and supports keratinocyte proliferation
Versican	Reticular dermis	Promotes stability via interaction with elastic fibers and matricellular proteins, stimulate fibroblast proliferation

(continued)

Table 1.2 (continued)

Proteoglycans (PG)	Localization within skin	Function
Fibromodulin	Interstitial matrix, dermis	Uncertain
Lumican	Interstitial matrix, dermis	Uncertain
Agrin	Basement membrane	Not fully understood

GAG	Localization within skin	Function
Heparan sulfate	Basement membrane	Involved in Wnt signaling pathway, development, angiogenesis, attachment site for virus
Hyaluronan/ hyaluronic acid	Interstitial matrix, dermis	Tissue repair, regulates tissue hydrodynamics by water binding, interacts with CD44
Dermatan sulfate	Interstitial matrix, dermis	Involved in wound repair, infection, fibrosis

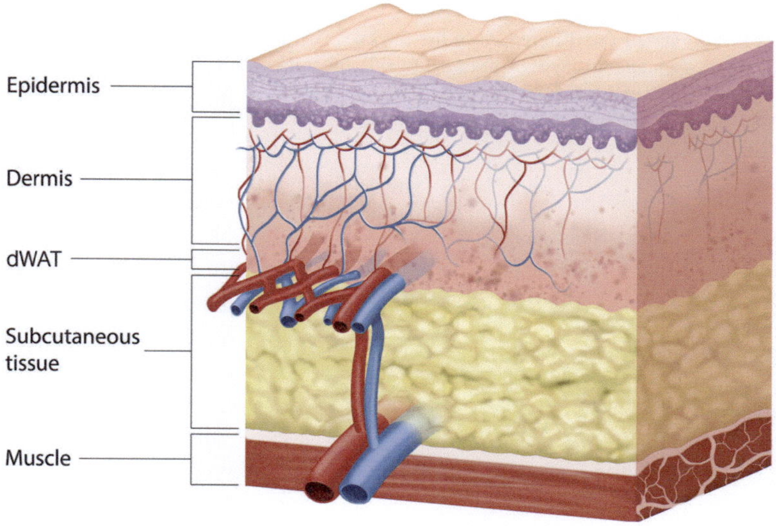

Fig. 1.2 Facial histological anatomy

(dWAT), which is the only layer of fat cells embedded in the reticular dermis and has a cone-shaped geometric structure. This layer is primarily distributed around hair follicles, sebaceous glands, and perilymphatic muscles and is distinct from subcutaneous white adipose tissue (sWAT). Consequently, some literature refers to the dWAT fat layer as the hypodermis and the sWAT as the subcutaneous layer (Fig. 1.2) [2].

Changes in the ratio and quantity of dermal components due to aging cannot be easily resolved by lifting procedures alone. However, this suggests that enhancing the components of the dermis through additional skin treatments may yield better results when combined with lifting procedures.

The hypodermis is a layer composed of subcutaneous white adipose tissue (sWAT), where large spherical adipocytes are densely distributed. This layer is organized into an egg-crate-like structure or honeycomb pattern by vertical retinacula between the surface and deep fascia, with nerve neurons and blood vessels passing through the connective septa. In the face, this layer belongs to the superficial musculoaponeurotic system (SMAS) and is divided into regions by retaining ligaments, which constitute the superficial fat compartment.

The SMAS contains a slightly lower but similar proportion of collagen (38.7 ± 5.9) and elastin (4.71 ± 1.2) compared to the skin, along with muscular cells and hypodermal fat cells [3] (Fig. 1.3).

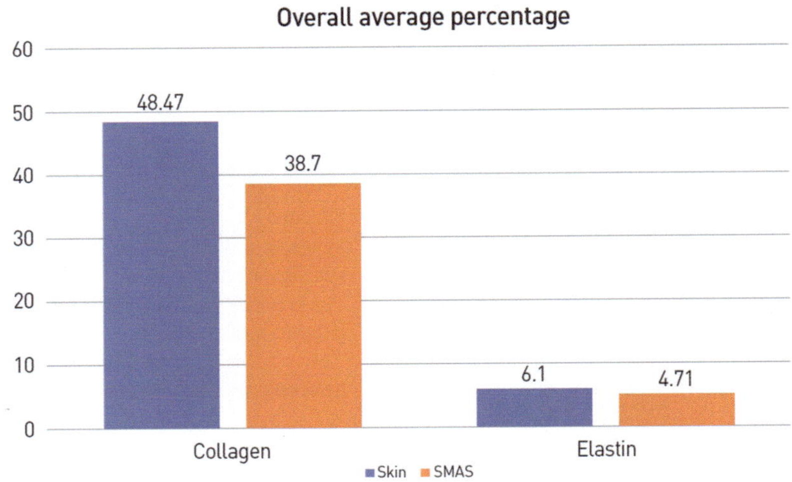

Fig. 1.3 The ratio of collagen and elastin in the skin layer and the SMAS layer. The proportions of collagen and elastin in the skin and fascia are shown. In the skin, collagen accounts for an average of 48.47 ± 6.96%, while elastin accounts for 6.1 ± 1.8%. In contrast, the SMAS contains a relatively lower proportion of collagen at 38.7 ± 5.9% and elastin at 4.71 ± 1.2%

Table 1.3 shows the differences in the thickness of the skin and subcutaneous layer by region. Overall, the thickness of the skin and subcutaneous layer in the middle and lower facial areas is greater than that in the upper facial area

Regions	Skin (mm)	Hypodermis (subcutaneous fat, mm)
Forehead	1.70 ± 0.71	1.99 ± 1.21
Radix and dorsum	1.51 ± 0.55	1.61 ± 1.07
Supraorbital	1.67 ± 0.83	1.82 ± 1.22
Infraorbital	1.97 ± 0.84	4.93 ± 2.98
Perioral	1.82 ± 0.83	5.14 ± 3.31
Temple	1.65 ± 0.91	2.58 ± 1.68
Cheek	1.85 ± 1.03	4.54 ± 2.71

The thickness of the skin and hypodermis (subcutaneous fat layer) varies depending on the facial region. The skin is generally thinner than 2 mm on average, showing no significant clinical differences. In contrast, the hypodermis is thicker in the middle and lower facial areas compared to the forehead, with the perioral area exhibiting the thickest layer of subcutaneous fat (Table 1.3) [4].

Additionally, the subcutaneous fat layer contains fibromuscular septa composed of collagen, elastin, and muscular cells, which connect the skin to the SMAS (superficial musculoaponeurotic system).

By region, the parotid region and preparotid region exhibit distinct characteristics (Fig. 1.4). In the parotid region, transverse fibromuscular septa run parallel to the skin layer in areas close to the skin. Lymph nodes are also observed in this region. In contrast, the preparotid region features fibromuscular septa in a vertical orientation. In this area, the vertical septa penetrate through a layer resembling muscle located in the middle of the SMAS. After penetrating, they again take on a transverse orientation at deeper levels. There are no nerve cells present in this lower layer [5]. This suggests that during facelift surgery, even with extensive sub-SMAS dissection, there is minimal risk of sensory damage in this area due to the absence of nerve cells.

The importance of the above histological findings lies in the fact that in the preparotid region, the vertical fibrous septa tightly anchor the dermis to the SMAS (superficial musculoaponeurotic system). This allows for a composite rhytidectomy to achieve significant lifting effects even with minimal subcutaneous dissection, as lifting the SMAS layer alone can also elevate the skin layer. This is also the reason why, during thread lifting, a lifting effect can be observed without the threads needing to directly approach the corners of the mouth.

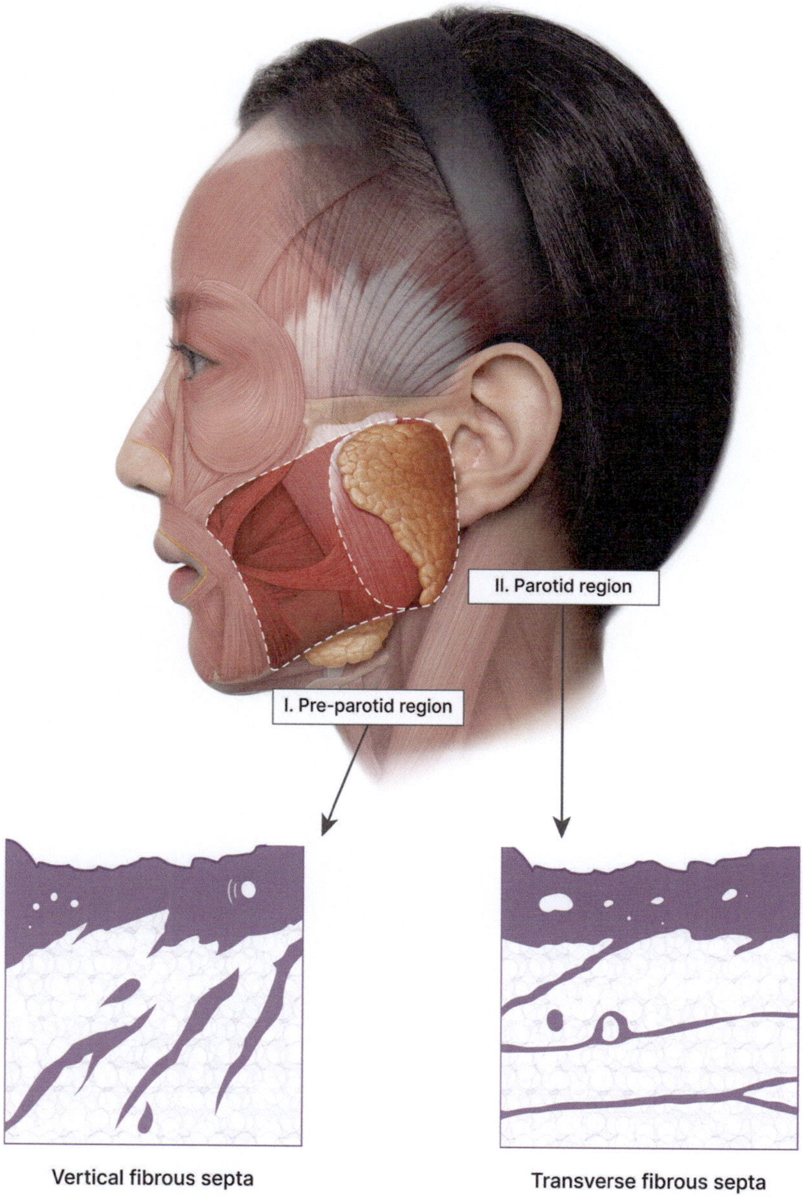

Fig. 1.4 Different shape of fibromuscular septa

1.3 Considerations for Vessels During Lifting

Understanding the main vessels anatomically is essential during thread lifting and facelift procedures. The important arteries in the facial region are as follows (Fig. 1.5). Among these, we will examine in detail the relatively significant vessels involved in lifting.

1.3.1 Superficial Temporal Artery

The superficial temporal artery is a vessel that is easily damaged by needles during thread lifting procedures, making it essential to have a thorough understanding of its anatomical structure. As the final branch of the external carotid artery, the superficial temporal artery is generally located laterally to the mandibular condyle at the

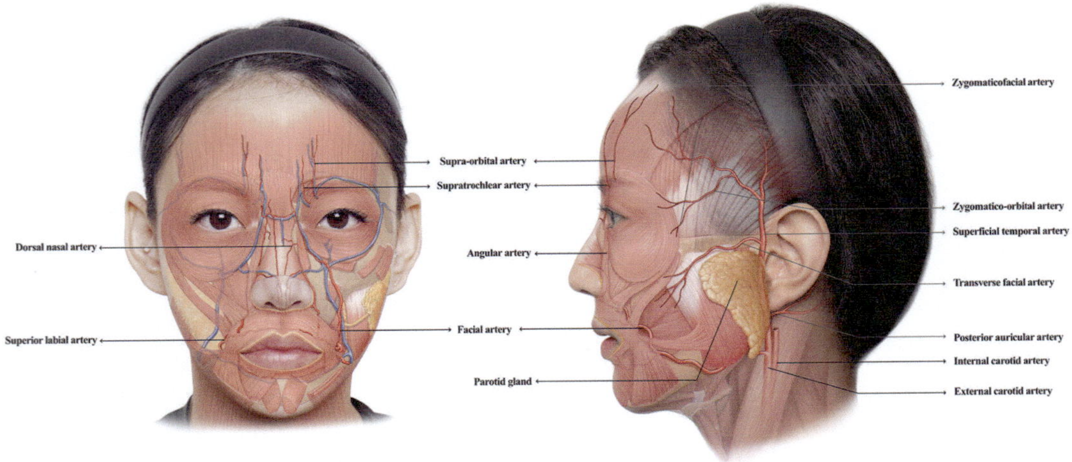

Fig. 1.5 Arteries of the face

Fig. 1.6 Frontal and posterior branch of superficial temporal artery

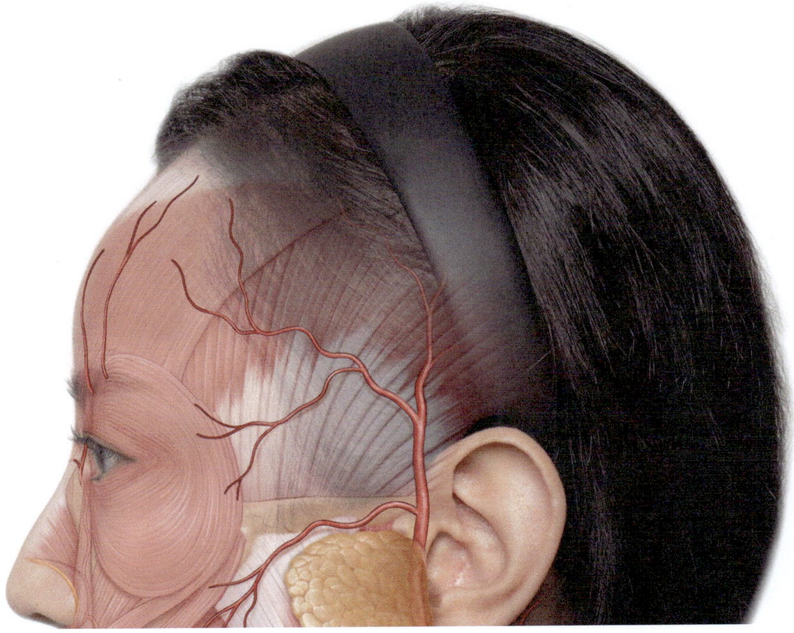

level of the zygomatic arch and bifurcates into the frontal branch and posterior branch above the zygomatic arch (Figs. 1.6 and 1.7). At the level of the temple, it runs within the superficial temporal fascia [6].

In cases where the skin is thin, the pulsation of the frontal branch can be felt by hand. The artery may be located at the level of the hairline or further medially. Therefore, to ensure a safer approach, the use of Doppler ultrasound is sometimes employed (Fig. 1.8). Confirming the location of the superficial temporal artery before performing lifting procedures can lead to a safer intervention [7].

1.3.2 Superficial Temporal Vein

The superficial temporal vein follows a path similar to that of the artery in front of the ear, but diverges from this pattern at the point where it splits into the frontal and parietal branches. While the artery consistently divides into two branches, the vein exhibits a variety of variations, ranging from one to three branches. The superficial temporal vein (STV) is located above the deep temporal fascia on its lateral side, but as it branches, it becomes more superficial, which is why it is more clearly distinguished as the superficial temporal cutaneous vein. This main vessel is connected to many small ascending veins that contribute to the venous network of the scalp. These veins contain valves to prevent reflux, but they do not possess strong resistance.

Further along the temporal region, the middle temporal vein is located (Fig. 1.9 [8]), which facilitates the movement of blood from the sentinel vein (zygomaticotemporal vein) toward the forehead. When observing the vein via ultrasound, the probe can cause the vein to disappear from the screen. Therefore, it is more effective to visualize the vein using a near-infrared device, which allows for the observation of superficial veins (Fig. 1.10).

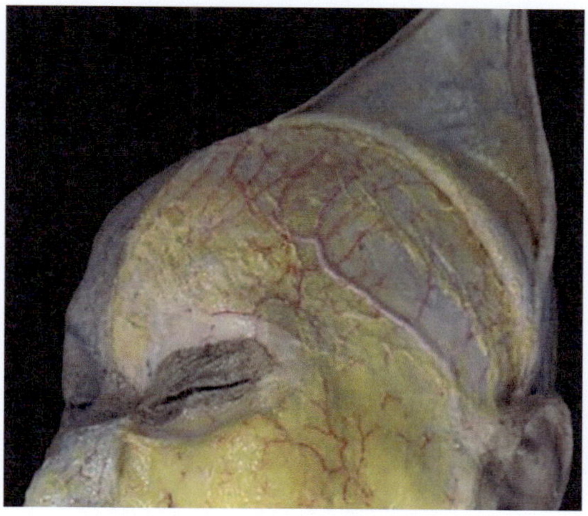

Fig. 1.7 Cadaveric findings of the superficial temporal artery

1.3.3 Transverse Facial Artery

The transverse facial artery branches from the external carotid artery approximately 1.7 cm below the zygomatic arch before the superficial temporal artery divides into two branches. It runs parallel to the zygomatic arch on the surface of the deep fascia, which is deeper than the SMAS (superficial muscular aponeurotic system) (Fig. 1.5). This artery gives rise to one to three perforator arteries (TFPA) at a distance of 3.1 cm laterally and 3.8 cm inferiorly from the lateral

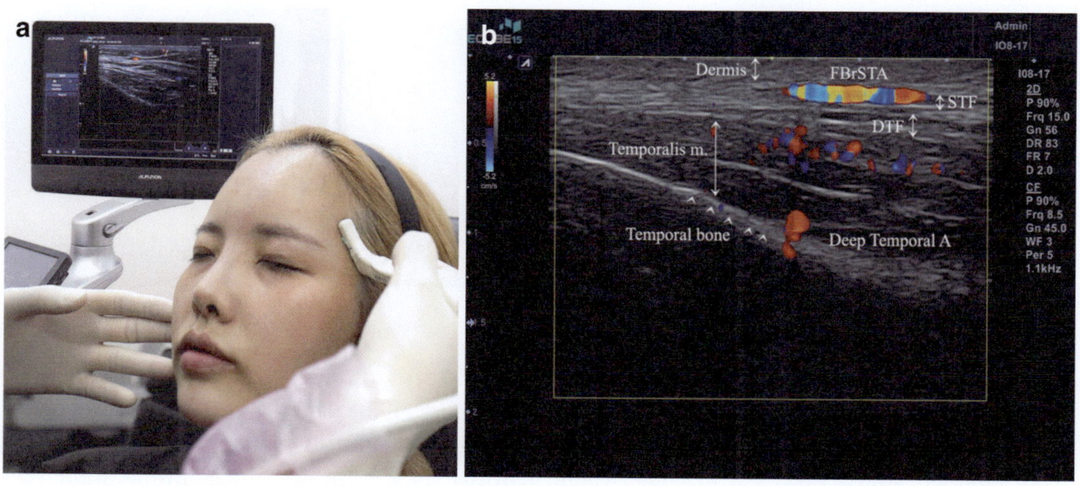

Fig. 1.8 Ultrasound findings of the superficial temporal artery. (**a**) Ultrasound procedure of the temporal region. (**b**) Frontal branch of the superficial temporal artery and anterior branch of deep temporal artery

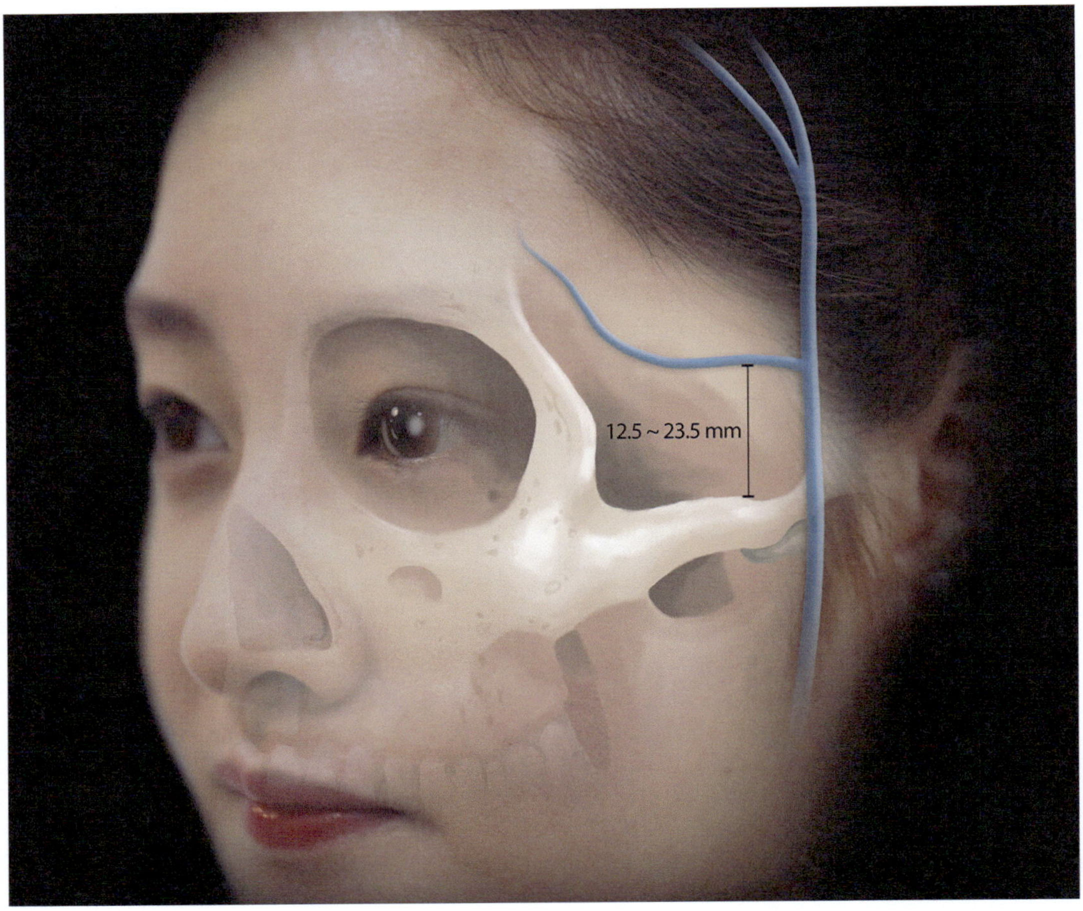

Fig. 1.9 Middle temporal vein pathway

Fig. 1.10 Vein detection by near infrared device

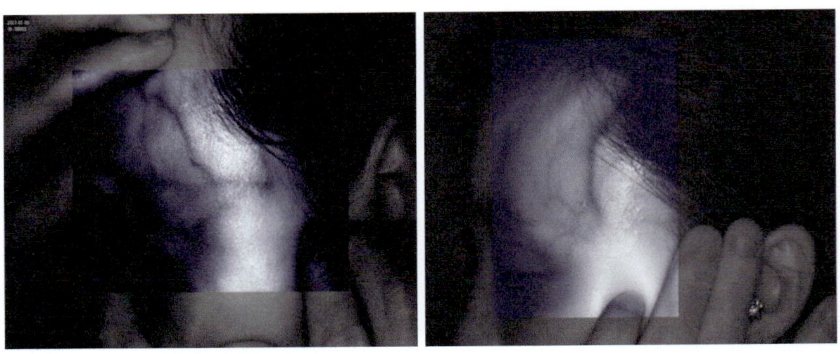

canthus, and it is responsible for the circulation of the lateral cheek [9]. In most cases (75%), it anastomoses with the facial artery and the superficial temporal artery; however, in cases where this anastomosis does not occur, vascular damage during sub-SMAS dissection may lead to circulation issues in the skin flap (see Chap. 8). Therefore, it becomes a particularly important vessel during facelift operations compared to less invasive procedures like thread lifting. If the vessel is damaged during surgery, serious hematomas may develop in the cheek area.

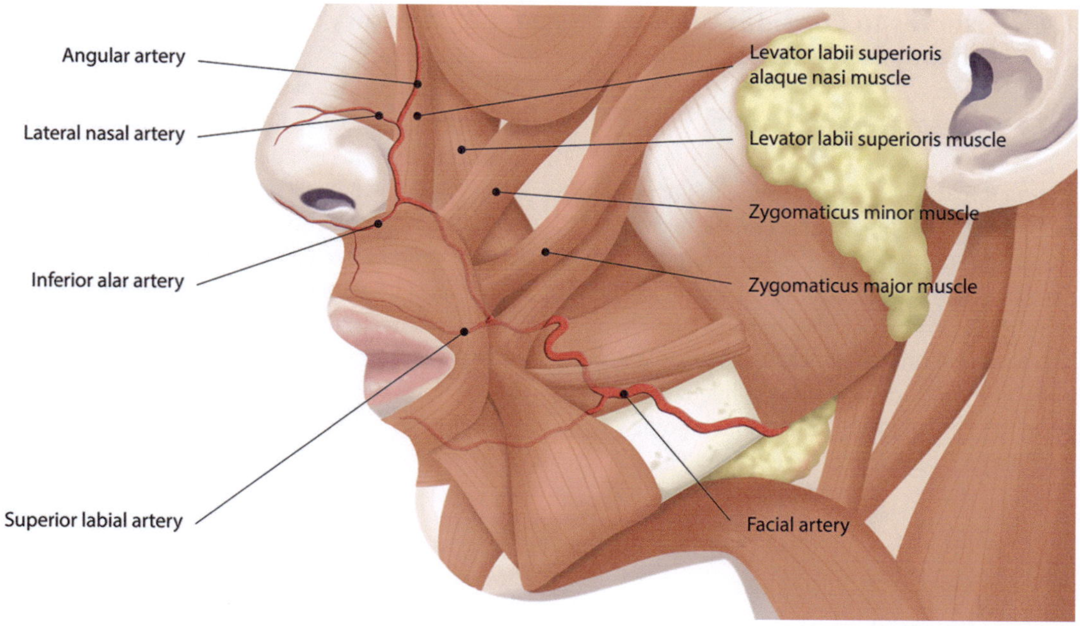

Fig. 1.11 Facial artery pathway

1.3.4 Facial Artery

The facial artery runs beneath the zygomaticus major and zygomaticus minor muscles, then ascends above the levator labii superioris and levator labii superioris alaeque nasi muscles to travel within the subcutaneous layer [10]. Consequently, the lateral nasal artery is located within the subcutaneous layer (Fig. 1.11).

Of course, statistically, not all vessels follow this course, and this can be confirmed with ultrasound prior to the procedure. The facial artery is primarily found within the subcutaneous fat layer (Fig. 1.12) [11].

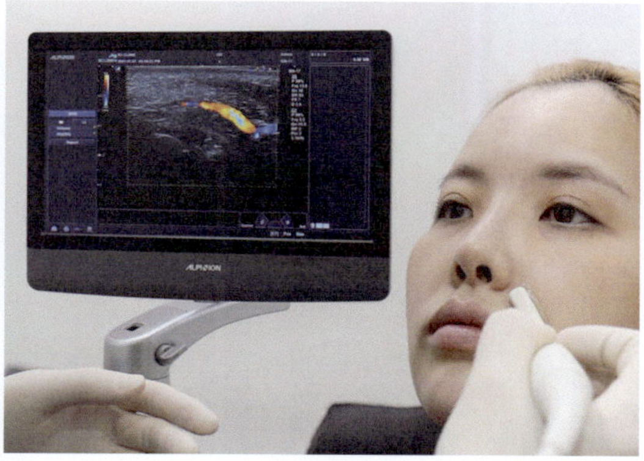

Fig. 1.12 Ultrasound findings of the facial artery

1.3.5 Posterior Auricular Artery

The posterior auricular artery, a branch of the external carotid artery, branches off above the posterior belly of the digastric muscle and ascends between the auricle and the mastoid process, passing beneath the parotid gland. It then divides into two branches (mastoid and auricular), with the mastoid (posterior) branch anastomosing with the superficial temporal artery (STA) and the occipital artery in the parietal region [12]. Care should be taken with the small branches of this vessel, as they can cause posterior auricular hematomas during facelift operations.

1.4 Nerves to Consider During Lifting Procedures

1.4.1 Motor Nerves

During thread lifting, blunt cannulas are primarily used, which minimizes the risk of nerve injury. However, during facelift surgery, temporary paralysis may occur, making anatomical knowledge of the course of the facial nerve essential. The temporal branch of the facial nerve is known to be primarily located along a line connecting a point 0.5 cm below the tragus and a point 1.5 cm lateral to the outer eyebrow (Fig. 1.13).

1.4.2 Sensory Nerves

After thread lifting, patients may experience pain due to stimulation of the sensory nerves during facial expressions such as opening the mouth. Additionally, when performing lifting in the neck area, it is important to be aware of the course of the great auricular nerve. The zygomaticofacial nerve, auriculotemporal nerve, and greater auricular nerve are significant sensory nerves that can be stimulated by the projections of the threads during the procedure (Fig. 1.14).

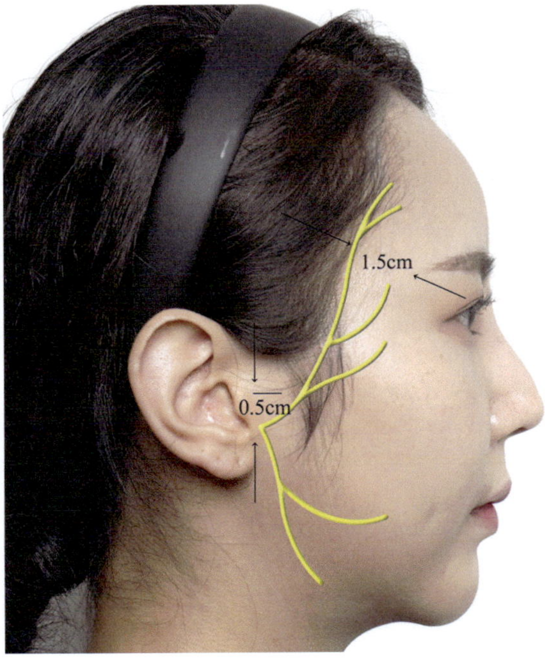

Fig. 1.13 Facial nerve temporal branch

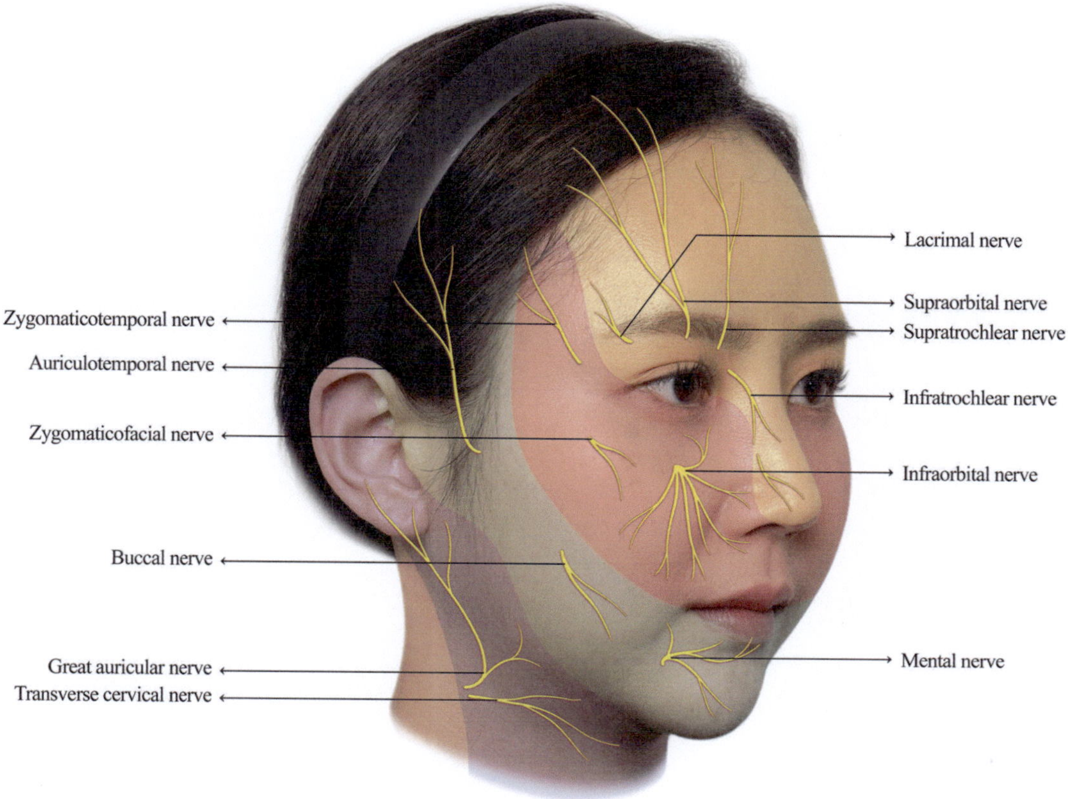

Fig. 1.14 Sensory nerves of the facial region

1.5 Muscles to Consider During Lifting Procedures

The muscles that should be considered during facial lifting include the muscles of expression and the masticatory muscles. In forehead lifting, the position of the forehead muscles laterally can affect the outcome, while in facial lifting, the strength and positioning of the muscles that act in the opposite direction of the lift can also influence the results. This section aims to explore the important muscles involved in lifting (Fig. 1.15).

The muscles of the facial region vary slightly from person to person and change according to facial expressions (Fig. 1.16). However, the layers are clearly defined, and understanding each muscle's function, as well as their origins and insertions, plays a crucial role in lifting surgery.

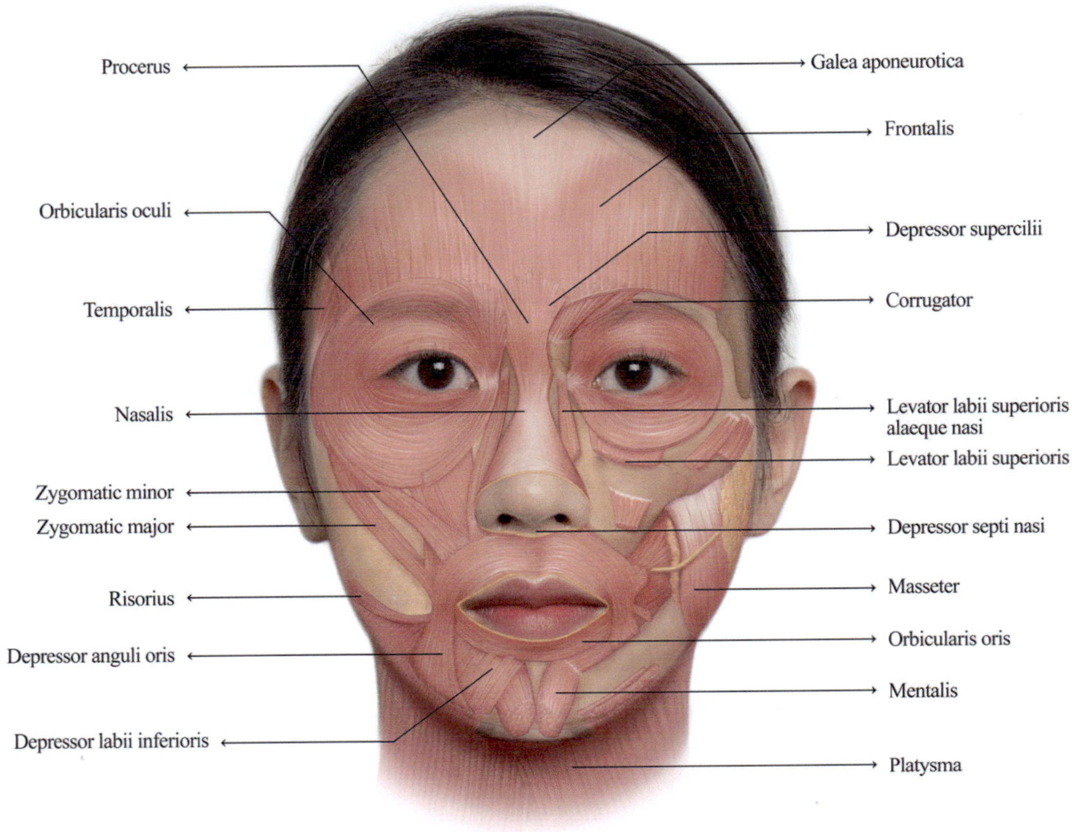

Fig. 1.15 Muscles of the face

1.5.1 Masseter Muscle

The masseter muscle, commonly known as the square jaw muscle, is primarily divided into three parts: the superficial layer, the deep layer, and the deep inferior tendon (DIT), which serves as the fascial structure that separates the two layers (Fig. 1.17) [13]. Based on the DIT, the superficial part of the masseter muscle originates from the maxillary process of the zygomatic arch and attaches to the angle of the mandible, thereby moving the subcutaneous tissue and skin in a superomedial direction. Consequently, the lifting vector should also be directed superomedially. Additionally, it is important to understand the relationship between the masseter muscle and the parotid gland, which lies in a more superficial layer, during thread lifting procedures.

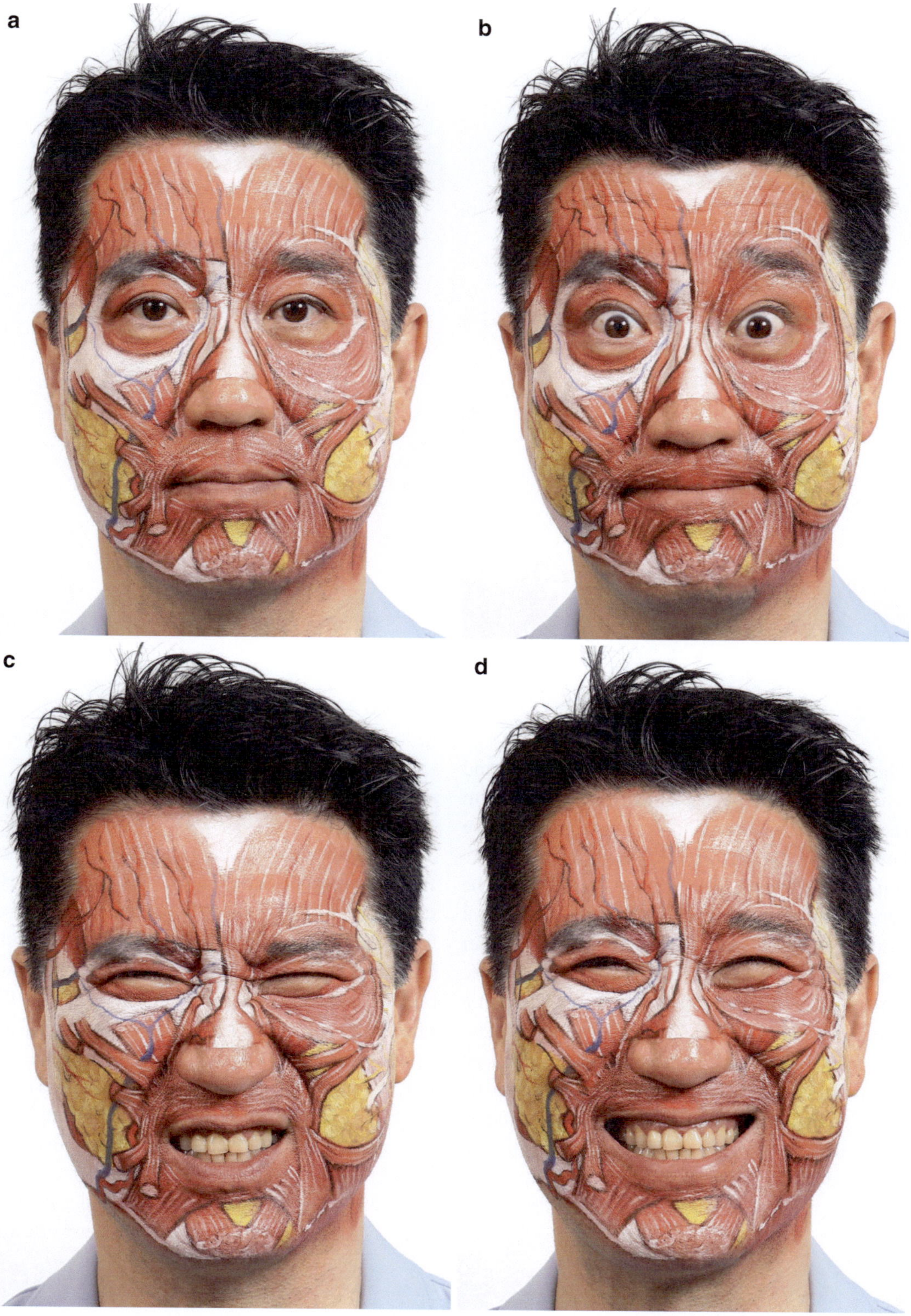

Fig. 1.16 Changes in facial muscles according to expression

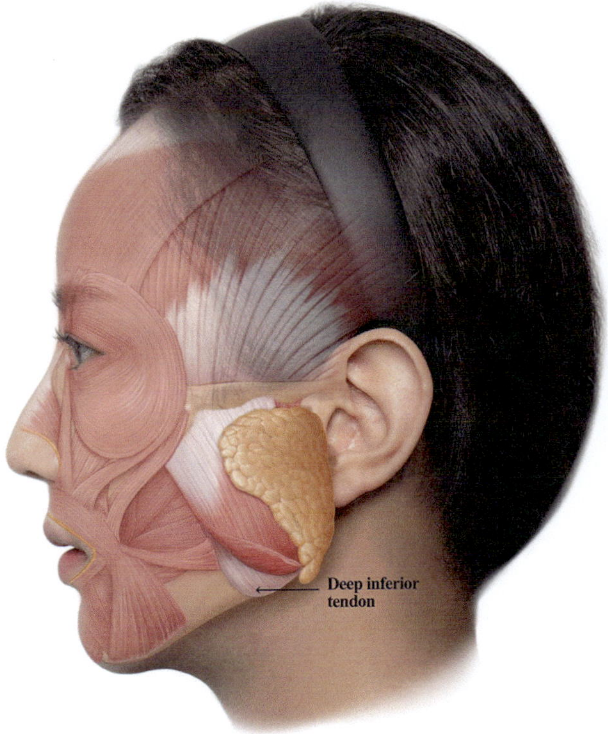

Fig. 1.17 Deep inferior tendon

1.5.2 Temporalis Muscle

The temporal region contains various layers, and when using fixed-type threads, procedures to secure them to the deep temporal fascia have been commonly performed. Therefore, the layers primarily involved in lifting are classified as the superficial temporal fascia and the deep temporal fascia. The temporalis muscle, located deeper than these layers, is a broad, fan-shaped muscle situated deeper than other facial muscles and, like the masseter muscle, belongs to the masticatory muscles. The temporalis muscle is a muscle that is strongly attached to the temporal bone and lacks a periosteum. It is one of the muscles that is most clearly visible on ultrasound, with the deep temporal artery located in its lower part, which can also be observed using Doppler ultrasound [14].

1.5.3 Levator Labii Superioris Alaque Nasi (LLSAN) and Levator Labii Superioris (LLS) Muscle

The LLSAN muscle is located on the surface of the LLS muscle and follows a path that nearly coincides with the outer boundary of the nose. The muscle originates from a position slightly lateral to the midline between the two eyebrows and descends along the boundary between the nose and cheek, attaching near the center of the upper lip (Fig. 1.18). The levator labii superioris (LLS) muscle originates from the lower part of the arcus marginalis, located at the midpupillary line, and extends to the area above the midsection of the lip, positioned relatively deeper than the orbicularis oris muscle. The zygomaticus minor and zygomaticus major muscles are located

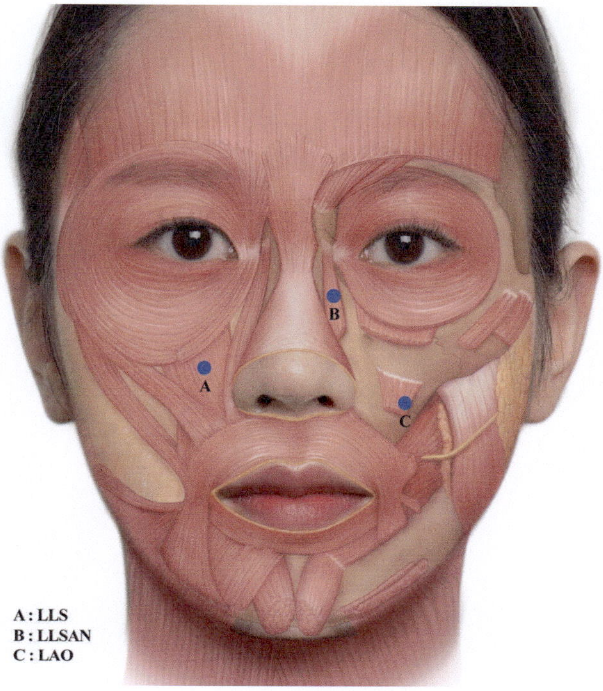

Fig. 1.18 Lip elevator muscles (medial)

sequentially outside this muscle. Clinically, this muscle, along with the depressor septi nasi muscle, elevates the inner part of the upper lip, which can induce a gummy smile upon contraction.

1.5.4 Zygomatic Major and Minor Muscle

The zygomaticus major muscle (Zmj) and zygomaticus minor muscle (Zmi) are the primary muscles responsible for elevating the corners of the mouth outward and upward. The Zmi is located along a line connecting the outer corner of the eye to the corner of the mouth, while the Zmj is positioned at the intersection of a vertical line drawn from the outer corner of the eye and a line that meets the base of the alar (Fig. 1.19). These two muscles play a crucial role in smiling and facial expressions, making them important considerations during surgical lifting procedures or thread lifting. Typically, if one side of the muscles on either side is overly active, this should be taken into account during surgery. Lifting should be performed with a vertical vector against gravity above the LLSAN and LLS muscles, while lifting above the Zmj and Zmi muscles should be done in a superolateral direction.

1.5.5 Orbicularis Oculi Muscle

The orbicularis oculi muscle is divided into three parts from the outer to the inner: the orbital, preseptal, and pretarsal parts. Clinically, it functions to close the eyelids and plays an important role in facial expressions (Fig. 1.20). Contraction of the orbicularis oculi muscle leads to the formation of crow’s feet, which are often treated with botulinum toxin injections for correction. It is known that the orbicularis oculi muscle does not degenerate easily with the aging process and tends to

Fig. 1.19 Lip elevator muscles (lateral)

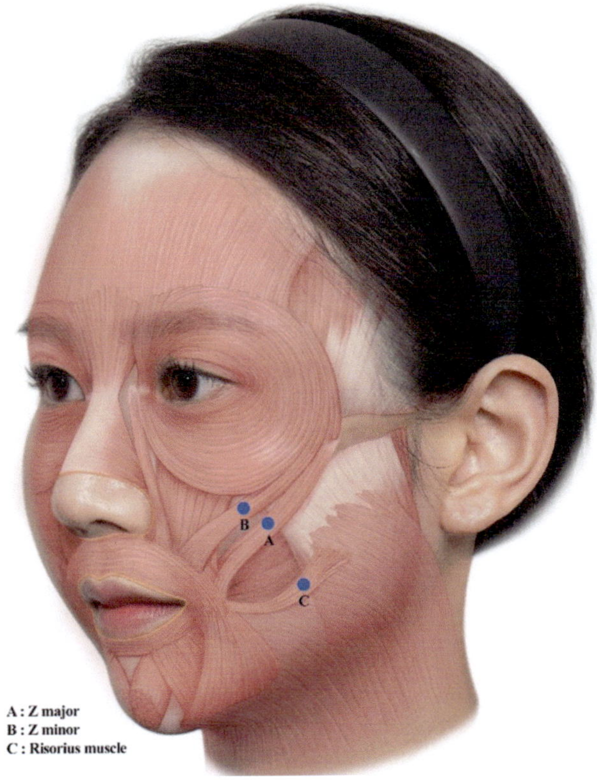

Fig. 1.20 Orbicularis oculi muscle: three divisions

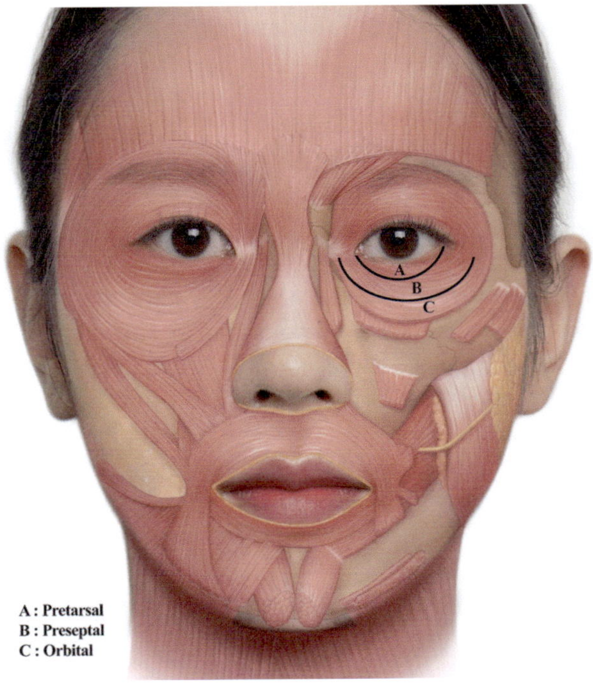

maintain its strength. As a result, the contraction intensity that lowers the eyebrows is often strong, leading to drooping of the outer eyebrows. Additionally, there is a region where the medial muscular band protrudes, and also there is a region where the lateral muscular band exists, which runs shallower than the zygomaticus major.

1.5.6 Risorius Muscle

The risorius muscle is responsible for pulling the corners of the mouth outward. The location of this muscle relative to the cheilion varies by ethnicity. When it attaches relatively higher on the corners of the mouth, it can create a more smiling appearance, whereas if it attaches lower, contraction may result in a more frowning look (Fig. 1.19). The muscle originates from the fascia of the parotid gland and attaches to the corners of the mouth, which can lead to clinical complications such as paralysis when botulinum toxin is injected into the masseter area.

1.5.7 Depressor Anguli Oris (DAO) Muscle

The depressor anguli oris (DAO) muscle originates from the mandible and attaches to the corners of the mouth, functioning to pull the corners of the mouth downward and outward upon contraction (Fig. 1.21). The area where the DAO attaches to the skin plays a crucial role in forming the labiomandibular fold, along with the zygomaticus major muscle and the platysma muscle. Since the DAO pulls downward in conjunction with the mentalis muscle, weakening these muscles can be beneficial during lifting procedures.

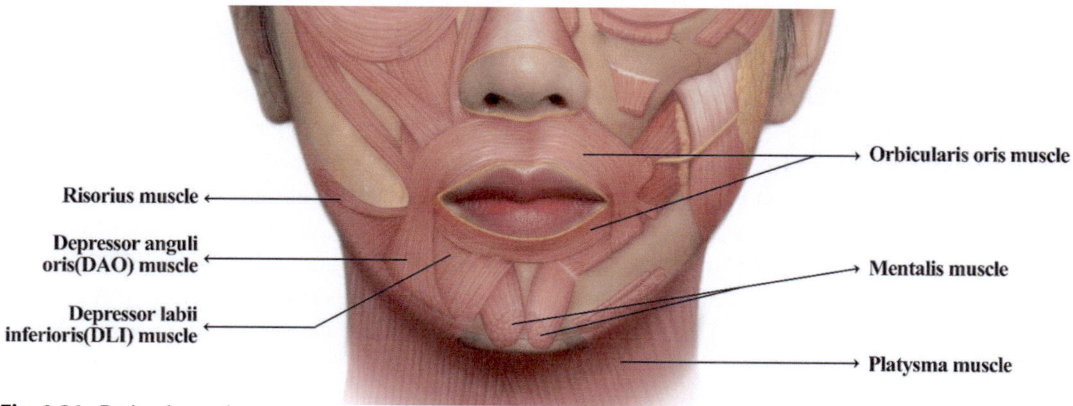

Fig. 1.21 Perioral muscles

1.6 Ligaments to Consider During Lifting Procedures

Plastic surgeons who perform facial surgeries and anatomists who conduct dissections cadavers have historically referred to the tissues that anchor the skin to the underlying structures by various names. As a result, many terms have been generated and used interchangeably, leading to confusion. Structures such as the Lore's fascia (temporoparietal fascia), platysma-auricular fascia, McGregor's patch, platysma-auricular ligament, parotid cutaneous ligament, and anterior platysma-cutaneous ligament refer to retaining ligaments that maintain various anatomical structures. This section will examine two structures that can be used as fixation points during facelift or thread lifting procedures.

Lore's fascia, also known as temporoparotid fascia or tympanoparotid fascia, is located anterior to the tragus and is firmly attached to the superficial fascia of the parotid gland (Fig. 1.22). Due to its strength, which is similar to that of the sternocleidomastoid fascia, Lore's fascia can be utilized as a fixation point during thread lifting or facelift procedures [15]. The platysma-auricular ligament is a structure that extends approximately 2 cm in width from the inferior border of the auricular cartilage downward for about 5–6 cm, and can be considered a retaining ligament of the neck. Therefore, during rhytidectomy, it is essential to adequately release this ligament to achieve lifting effects on both the jawline and neck, and it can also serve as a fixation point during thread neck lifting.

Retaining ligaments in the facial region have also been referred to by many different names, including orbicularis retaining ligament, lateral orbital thickening, superior temporal septum, masseteric cutaneous ligament, and anterior platysma cutaneous ligament. These various terms have been used in different contexts. However, it is crucial to understand that these tissues anchor the skin and compartmentalize the facial area, which is a significant factor in facelift surgery.

Retaining ligaments are generally classified into true and false categories. True ligaments originate from the bone and extend to the skin, representing strong ligaments, such as the orbital retaining ligament, zygomatic ligament, maxillary ligament, and mandibular ligament (Fig. 1.23). These retaining ligaments primarily serve to hold the skin and soft tissues in place, preventing sagging. However, it is more accurate to understand them as tissues that anchor softer areas that need to move for facial expressions and mouth opening, rather than as rigid structures like other ligaments in the body. Proper utilization of these ligaments can enhance the effectiveness of thread lifting, and adequate release of these ligaments can improve the outcomes of facelift surgery.

The important retaining ligaments during thread lifting are the zygomatic ligament and masseteric cutaneous ligaments. These two ligaments intersect in a T-shape, providing strong support to the skin and soft tissues. Therefore, even when using floating-type threads instead of fixed-type threads, once the threads are anchored to these strong ligamentous tissues and the soft tissues below are lifted, the threads will create a supportive effect without needing additional fixation from above. Conversely, if the threads are excessively anchored to these retaining ligaments, side effects such as dimpling may occur. In such cases, it is crucial to perform early massage to alleviate the tension.

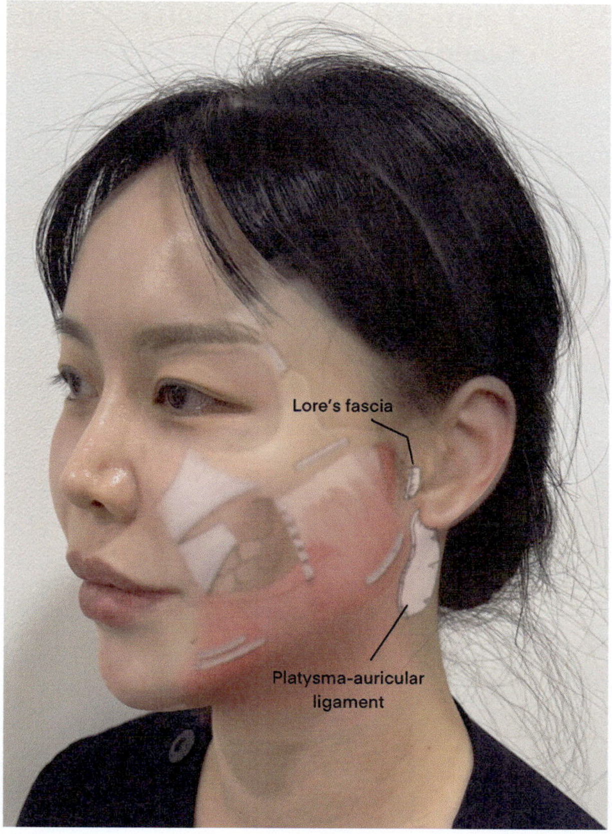

Fig. 1.22 Lore's fascia and platysma-auricular ligament

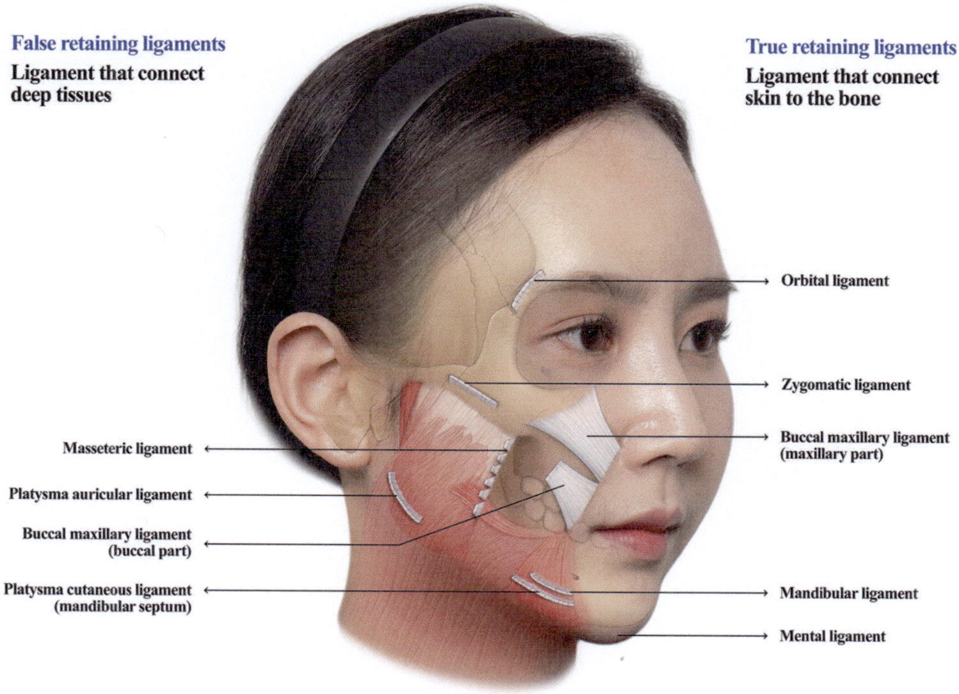

Fig. 1.23 Facial ligaments

1.7 Parotid and Submandibular Glands

One of the structures to be cautious of during thread lifting is the parotid gland and submandibular gland. Generally, complications are rare; however, in cases where threads are inserted deeply or in patients with benign parotid gland hypertrophy, the threads may penetrate internally and cause inflammation. Detailed information will be discussed in the section on the side effects of thread lifting (Chap. 6).

The parotid gland is primarily located with its upper boundary at the zygomatic arch, posterior boundary at the earlobe, and lower boundary at the mandibular border. In cases of hypertrophy, the posterior boundary may extend beyond this, causing a bulging appearance beneath the ear. Additionally, the facial nerve passes between the superficial and deep lobes of the parotid gland, and there may be an accessory parotid gland located near the parotid duct. Although it is encapsulated below the facial SMAS layer, it can still be damaged during thread lifting (Fig. 1.24). Furthermore, when performing thread lifting in the neck area, there is a risk of damaging the submandibular gland.

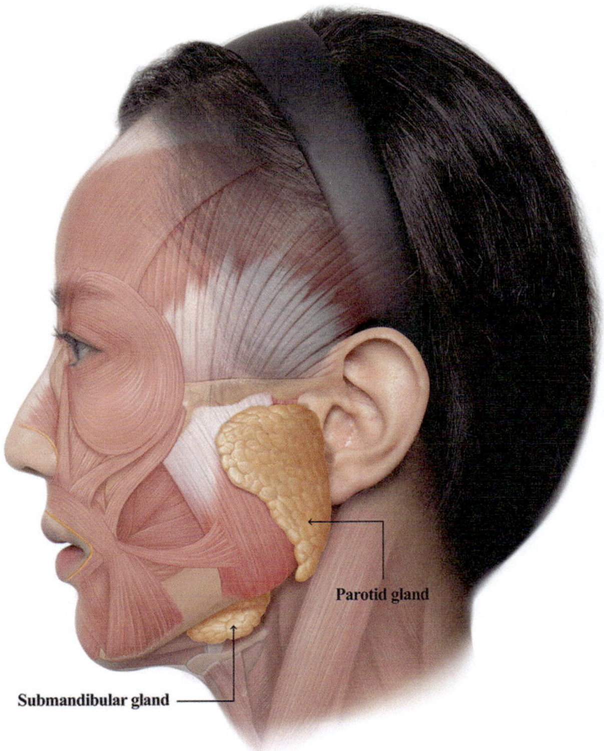

Fig. 1.24 Parotid gland and submandibular gland

1.8 Conclusion

Lifting procedures can be performed using various methods, including techniques utilizing EBD, thread lifting, and surgical facelifts, each of which should target specific anatomical layers to achieve optimal results. The face consists of various layers, and different regions may be referred to by different names. Therefore, it is essential to understand that the superficial layer of the face connects to the SMAS, the superficial temporal fascia connects to the temporal region, and the deep layer connects the parotid masseteric fascia to the deep temporal fascia in the temporal region.

Understanding the retaining ligaments that connect these layers is crucial, as they can be utilized during thread lifting, and releasing these ligaments during facelift surgery can yield better results. Additionally, a thorough understanding of the dermal layer and subcutaneous fat layer is necessary to determine the appropriate thickness for creating and elevating flaps during facelift procedures, which involves understanding the concepts of dWAT and sWAT.

A comprehensive understanding of the various components of the dermal layer is essential for grasping the aging process. While performing lifting procedures is important, understanding this aging process and combining it with other treatments will also be a significant task. The face contains various expression muscles, and understanding these muscles is crucial not only for addressing aging due to gravity but also for performing lifting procedures against the opposing vector of muscle action to achieve better lifting results.

Therefore, understanding the anatomical structures that form the basis of various procedures and applying this knowledge during lifting is of utmost importance.

References

1. Pfisterer K, Shaw LE, Symmank D, Weninger W. The extracellular matrix in skin inflammation and infection. Front Cell Dev Biol. 2021;9:682414.
2. Li Y, Long J, Zhang Z, Yin W. Insights into the unique roles of dermal white adipose tissue (dWAT) in wound healing. Front Physiol. 2024;15:1346612.
3. Har-Shai Y, Sela E, Rubinstien I, Lindenbaum ES, Mitz V, Hirshowitz B. Computerized morphometric quantitation of elastin and collagen in SMAS and facial skin and the possible role of fat cells in SMAS viscoelastic properties. Plast Reconstr Surg. 1998;102(7):2466–70. https://doi.org/10.1097/00006534-199812000-00033.
4. Kim YS, Lee KW, Kim JS, Gil YC, Tanvaa T, Shin DH, Kim HJ. Regional thickness of facial skin and superficial fat: application to the minimally invasive procedures. Clin Anat. 2019;32(8):1008–18. https://doi.org/10.1002/ca.23331.
5. Sandulescu T, Buechner H, Rauscher D, Naumova EA, Arnold WH. Histological, SEM and three-dimensional analysis of the midfacial SMAS – new morphological insights. Ann Anat. 2019;222:70–8. https://doi.org/10.1016/j.aanat.2018.11.004.
6. Lee JG, Yang HM, Hu KS, Lee YI, Lee HJ, Choi YJ, et al. Frontal branch of the superficial temporal artery: anatomical study and clinical implications regarding injectable treatments. Surg Radiol Anat. 2015;37(1):61–8.
7. Lee W, Moon HJ, Kim JS, Chan BL, Yang EJ. Doppler ultrasound-guided thread lifting. J Cosmet Dermatol. 2020;19(8):1921–7. https://doi.org/10.1111/jocd.13240.
8. Jung W, Youn KH, Won SY, Park JT, Hu KS, Kim HJ. Clinical implications of the middle temporal vein with regard to temporal fossa augmentation. Dermatol Surg. 2014;40(6):618–23.
9. Pierrefeu A, Brosset S, Lahon M, Guerid S, Shipkov H, Boucher F, Breton P, Sigaux N, Mojallal A. Transverse facial artery perforators: anatomical, two- and three-dimensional radiographic study. Plast Reconstr Surg. 2019;143(4):820e–8e. https://doi.org/10.1097/PRS.0000000000005421.
10. Lee JG, Yang HM, Choi YJ, Favero V, Kim YS, Hu KS, et al. Facial arterial depth and relationship with the facial musculature layer. Plast Reconstr Surg. 2015;135(2):437–44.
11. Lee W, Kim JS, Moon HJ, Yang EJ. A safe Doppler ultrasound-guided method for nasolabial fold

correction with hyaluronic acid filler. Aesthet Surg J. 2021;41(6):NP486–92. https://doi.org/10.1093/asj/sjaa153.
12. Nguyen JD, Duong H. Anatomy, head and neck, posterior auricular artery. 2023 June 5. In: StatPearls [Internet]. Treasure Island (FL): StatPearls Publishing; 2024 Jan–.
13. Yi KH, Bae H, Kim SB, Kim WR, Lee W, Kim JS, Kim HJ. Sonographic observation of the paradoxical masseteric bulging and clinical implication of functional compartment. Anat Cell Biol. 2024;57(1):13–7. https://doi.org/10.5115/acb.23.234.
14. Lee W, Moon HJ, Kim MS, Cheon GW, Yang EJ. Pre-injection ultrasound scanning for treating temporal hollowing. J Cosmet Dermatol. 2022;21(6):2420–5. https://doi.org/10.1111/jocd.14471.
15. O'Brien JX, Rozen WM, Whitaker IS, Ashton MW. Lore's fascia and the platysma-auricular ligament are distinct structures. J Plast Reconstr Aesthet Surg. 2012;65(9):e241–5. https://doi.org/10.1016/j.bjps.2012.03.007.

Changes in the Face Related to Aging Process

2

Contents

Patients seeking lifting procedures for antiaging share a common belief: as they age, their tissues sag, making them look older, and they think that lifting can rejuvenate them or restore their youthful appearance. This belief is partially correct and partially incorrect. The changes in the face due to aging result from a complex interplay of various factors. It is not just the sagging of tissues; the reduction of fat volume and bone resorption also contribute to changes in the facial framework, which organically affects facial aging. Lifting can only achieve the effect of elevating sagging tissues. Therefore, it is important to understand in detail the changes that occur in the face as one ages to know what effects can be achieved through lifting, what limitations exist, and what additional procedures can lead to better results (Fig. 2.1).

W. Lee, K. H. Jung, *Lifting Techniques in Plastic Surgery*,
https://doi.org/10.1007/978-981-96-4820-7_2

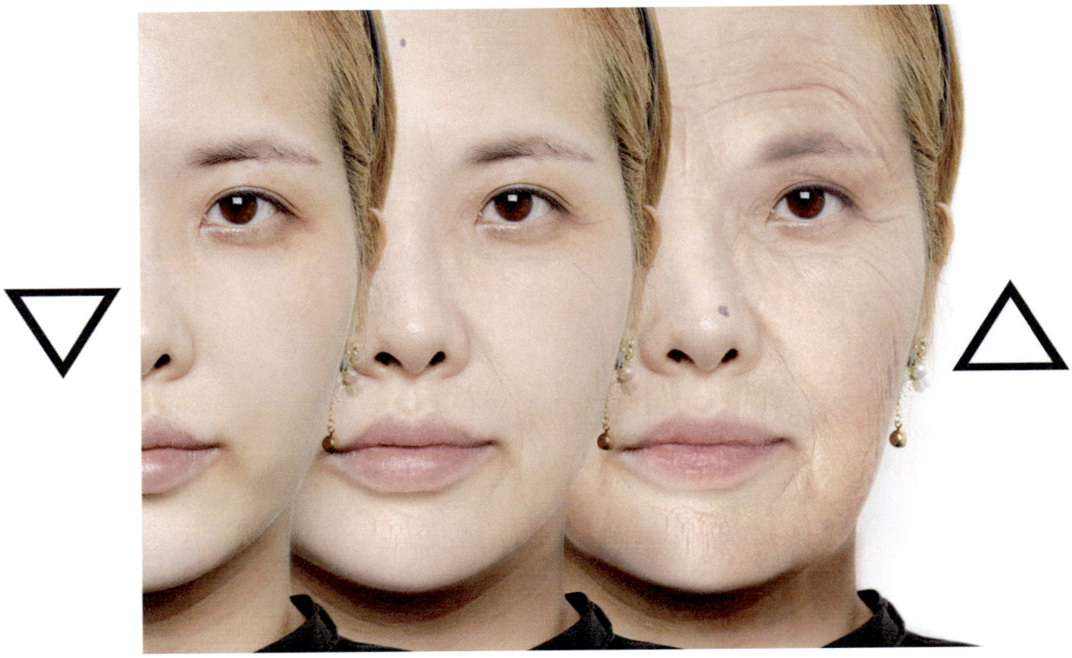

Fig. 2.1 Changes in facial shape with age

2.1 Bone Resorption

Bone resorption occurs with aging, and since the rate of resorption varies by region, the shape of the face changes, accelerating the visibility of certain wrinkle lines. In the orbital bone, the superomedial and inferolateral areas tend to experience relatively more resorption, leading to medial fat bulging above the eyes and worsening the medial parts of the tear trough and mid-cheek groove (Fig. 2.2). Among the maxilla and zygoma that comprise the midface, the maxilla experiences relatively more resorption than the zygoma, particularly due to the retrusion of the pyriform and anterior aspect of the maxilla, which makes the nasolabial fold appear deeper. Additionally, the mid-cheek groove becomes longer and more pronounced, and the zygomatic arch appears wider.

The mandible undergoes an overall reduction in size with age, resulting in a larger mandible angle and decreased height of the ramus and body. Medially, resorption in the pre-jowl area exacerbates the appearance of jowls.

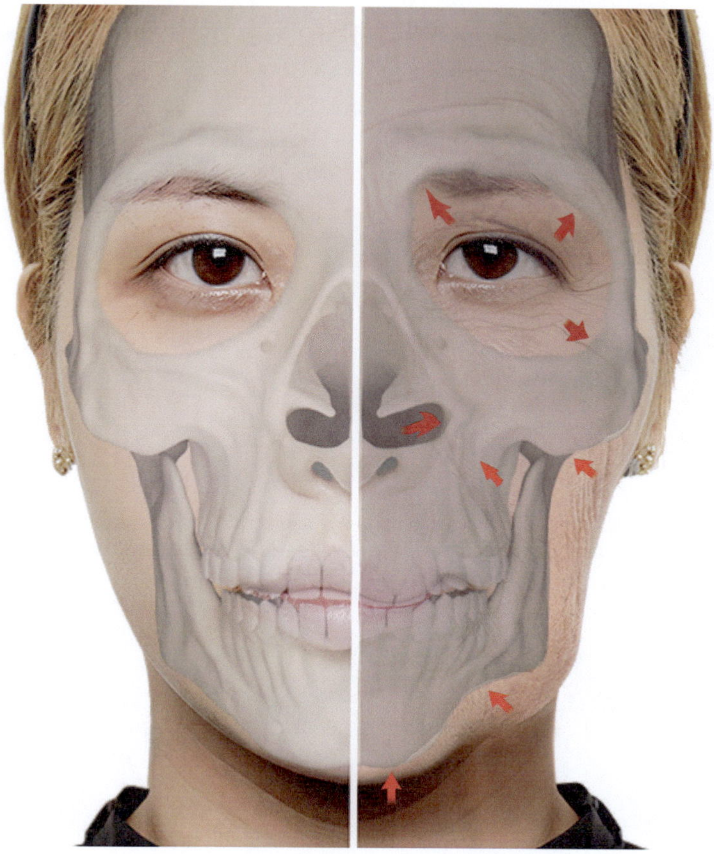

Fig. 2.2 Changes in bone resorption due to aging

2.2 Fat Deflation

Fat deflation is one of the important factors in the aging process because the surface shell of the area where fat is absorbed, that is, the skin, becomes crumpled. This crumpling leads to fine wrinkles, and the skin layer that loses tension descends under the influence of gravity, accumulating along the retaining ligaments. As a result, the face becomes divided into multi-units, leading to an uneven appearance (Fig. 2.3).

Fat deflation tends to occur sequentially, starting with medial cheek deflation in the 30s, lateral cheek deflation in the 40s, and malar deflation in the 50s, while nasolabial fat shows little to no deflation (Fig. 2.4 [1]). The signs of aging on the surface manifest differently depending on the deflation of deep and superficial fat compartments, making it important to set appropriate targets for lifting procedures. In some cases, the use of fillers may be necessary to achieve better results.

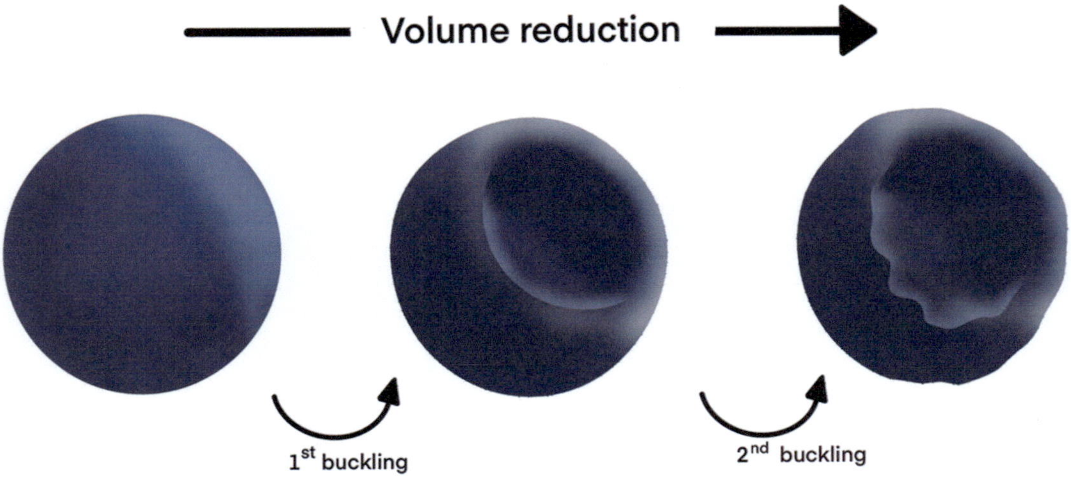

Fig. 2.3 Fat deflation. When deflation occurs in an elastic object, it initially buckles in an axis-symmetric shape, and the second buckling that appears subsequently progresses into a polygonal shape

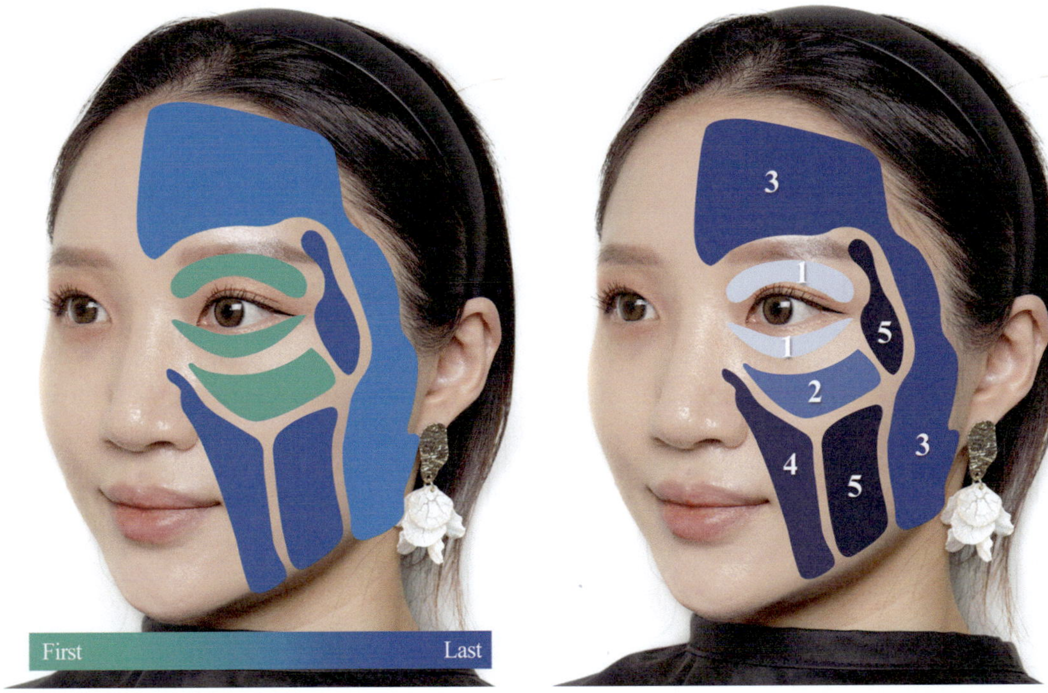

Fig. 2.4 Changes in fat deflation by age

2.3 Skin Loosening

As the aging process progresses, the shortening of telomeres in skin cells, including fibroblasts, negatively impacts cell proliferation. Additionally, the activity of matrix metalloproteinases increases, leading to a reduction in collagen and elastin levels. The decrease in collagen is accompanied by an increase in crosslinking, resulting in stiffer skin. Changes in other extracellular matrix components, such as glycosaminoglycans and proteoglycans, reduce functional components, while the volume of hyaluronic acid decreases, impairing its water-binding capacity and leading to reduced moisture levels. Furthermore, the reduction of dermal white adipose tissue (dWAT) is also known to be related to the aging of the skin, as it contributes to adipocyte-myofibroblast transition and a decrease in dermal volume (Fig. 2.5).

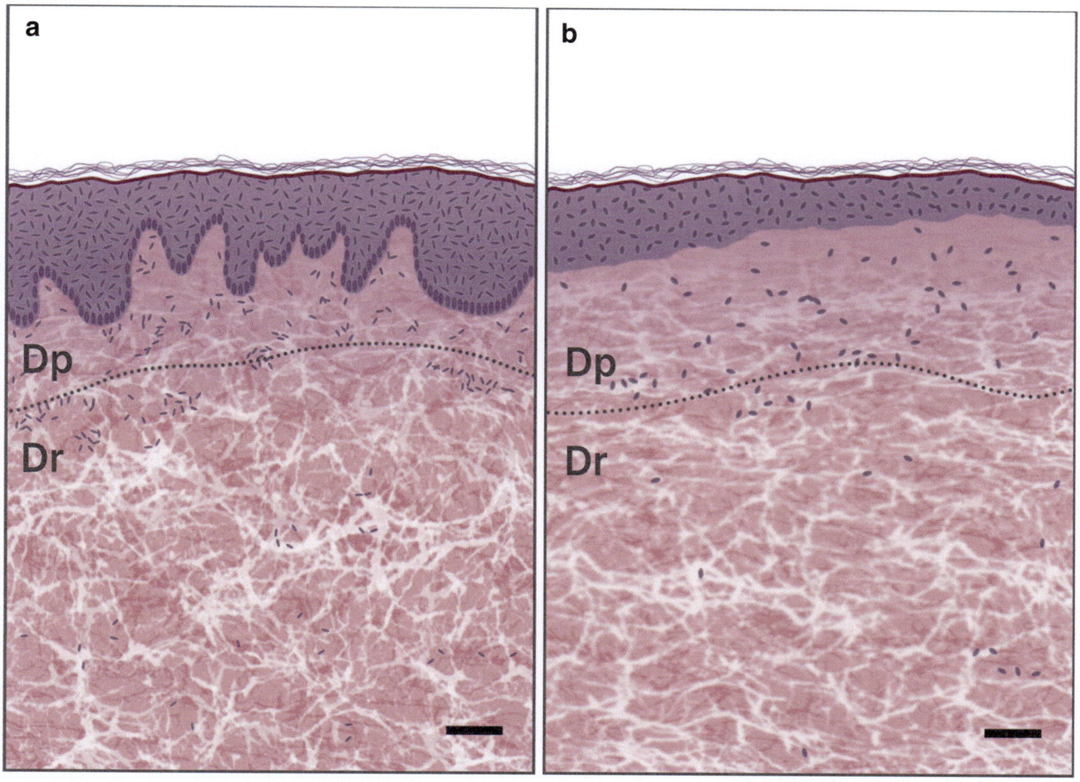

Fig. 2.5 Difference between young (**a**) and old human skin (**b**). Dp papillary dermis, Dr reticular dermis

2.4 Wrinkling

Changes in keratinocytes in the epidermis, reduced fibroblast function in the dermal layer, decreased collagen and elastin, particularly the reduction of type III collagen in the papillary dermis, all contribute to the formation of wrinkles. Additionally, biological and physiological changes, such as fluctuations in the composition of extracellular matrix (ECM) components that predominantly occupy the dermal layer, along with mechanical changes, determine the shape, length, and depth of wrinkles. The altered mechanical changes are clinically manifested as distinct wrinkles, primarily influenced by the facial expression muscles.

Facial wrinkles can be broadly categorized into those that occur in the skin located in the middle of the expression muscles and those that occur at the insertion points of the expression muscles.

2.4.1 Wrinkles on the Expression Muscle

Wrinkles ultimately manifest on the surface, which is the stratum corneum, and are determined by the interrelationship of the various layers of the facial region, each with different characteristics. All facial layers are subjected to repeated compression and band energy from the expression muscles as a single unit. In youth, not only the dermis and subcutaneous fat layer but also the viable epidermis (the epidermal layers excluding the stratum corneum) can act as a "cushion" that absorbs kinetic energy. As a result, wrinkling occurs only in the stratum corneum, presenting as fine and shallow wrinkles that are not easily noticeable. However, with aging, the composition of each facial layer changes, leading to a decline in mechanical properties that increasingly affect deeper layers. Consequently, wrinkling occurs throughout the entire epidermis and invades the dermis, resulting in more pronounced and deeper wrinkles, making the wrinkle lines more visible [2]. This transition is described as a switch from Skin Mode 1 to Mode 2, and it is at this point that patients begin to feel that "there are wrinkles on the face," typically starting in their 30s (Fig. 2.6).

2.4.2 Wrinkles at the End of the Expression Muscle

Among the wrinkles, there are areas that develop due to causes other than compression and band energy, specifically the nasolabial fold and marionette line. The nasolabial fold is the point where the muscles responsible for elevating the lips, including the levator labii superioris alaeque nasi (LLSAN), levator labii superioris (LLS), zygomatic major (Zmj), and zygomatic minor (Zmi), insert into the dermal layer (Fig. 2.7). The Zmj and Zmi, which are activated when smiling, and the LLSAN and LLS, which are activated during expressions of disgust, all originate from the bone. Therefore, when making facial expressions, the insertion site of the nasolabial fold deepens, forming an acute angle.

In youth, the presence of sufficient dermal fat and subcutaneous fat tissue buffers the energy exerted on the skin when the muscles contract. The skin's high elasticity allows for temporary wrinkles that disappear quickly. However, with aging, the reduction of dermal fat tissue and subcutaneous fat leads to the expression muscles pulling directly on the dermis, making the lines more pronounced. Additionally, the deflation of the deep medial cheek fat (DMCF) in the anterior cheek reduces the expansion of the tissue above the nasolabial fold, causing the tissue that has lost tension to sag under gravity. This sagging results in bulging above the nasolabial fold, making the nasolabial fold appear more distinct and deeper.

The marionette line is a line that extends from the medial border of the depressor anguli oris (DAO) along the modiolus to the border of the mandible. The upper third of this line runs from

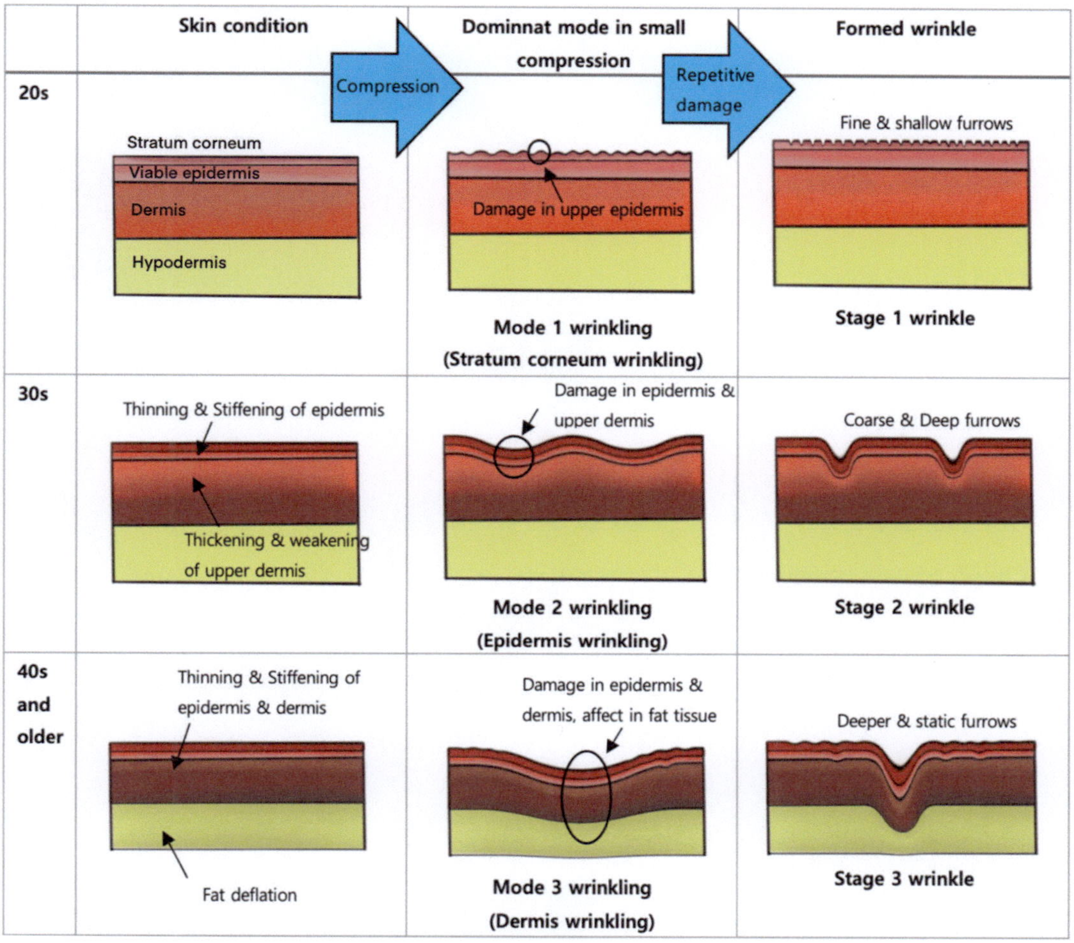

Fig. 2.6 Wrinkling formation mechanism based on multistage wrinkling theory [3]

the corners of the mouth to the modiolus, while the lower two-thirds is formed by the medial border of the DAO (Fig. 2.8). The modiolus is a tendinous structure formed by the convergence of fibers from nine facial expression muscles. With aging, the support of the expression muscles that constitute the modiolus weakens, and fat atrophy occurs, causing the upper third of the marionette line to deepen.

The lower two-thirds corresponds to the area where the medial border of the DAO inserts. The DAO originates at the mental tubercle and inserts into the dermis. When activated to express negative emotions such as depression and sadness, the medial border of the DAO is pulled posteriorly, deepening the line. As with the nasolabial fold, this line becomes deeper and more static with age (Fig. 2.9). The descending superficial fat tissue and skin accumulate above the static marionette line, resulting in a sharper and deeper appearance of the line.

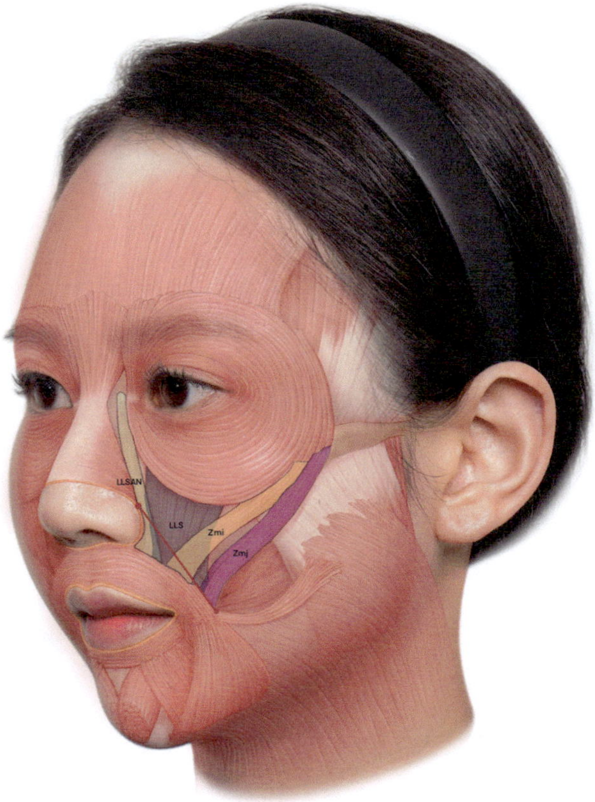

Fig. 2.7 Correlation between the nasolabial fold and the lip elevating muscles (LLSAN, LLS, Zmj, Zmi)

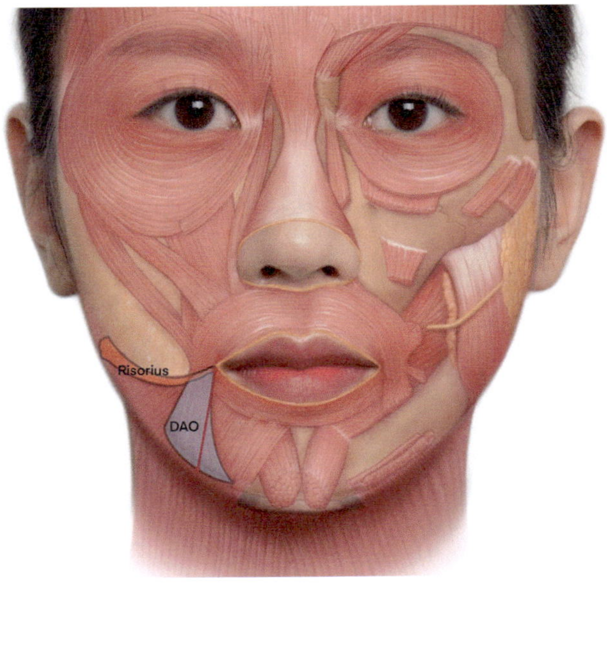

Fig. 2.8 Correlation between the marionette line and the depressor anguli oris muscle, risorius muscle

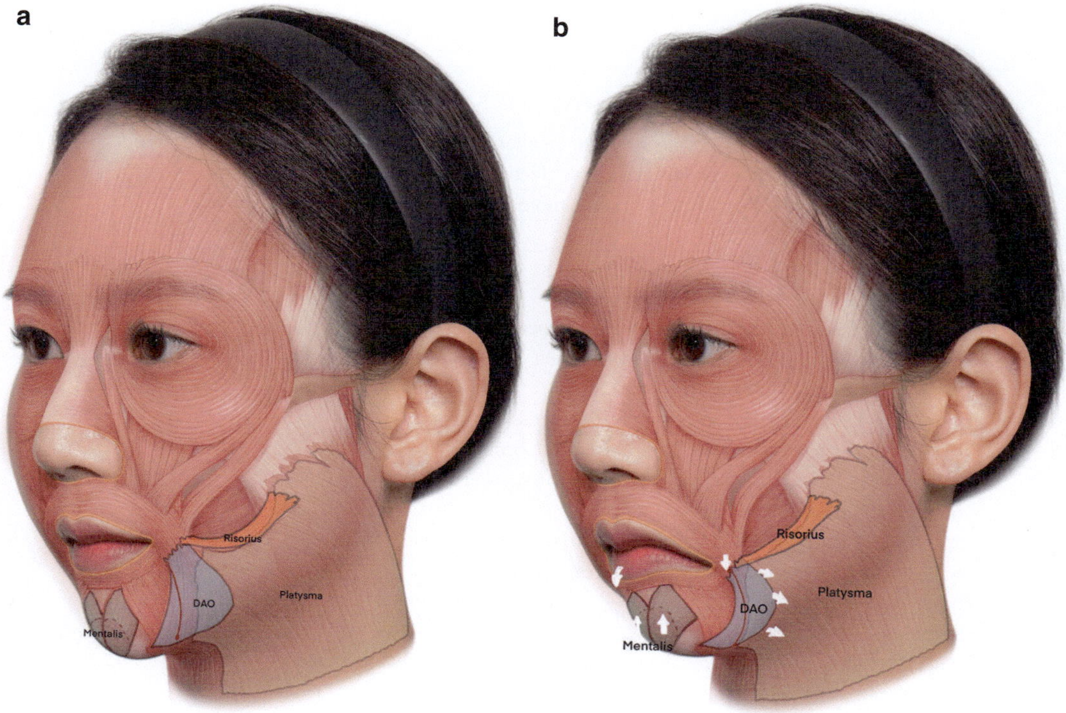

Fig. 2.9 Marionette line and the dynamic state of the DAO muscle, risorius muscle, and mentalis muscle action. (**a**) Static state. (**b**) Dynamic state

2.5 Conclusion

The aging process is a complex phenomenon that includes interrelated changes in bone, muscle, fat, and skin. Various manifestations of aging occur with age, including changes in skin tone, texture degradation, loss of skin elasticity, bone loss, fat loss, loss of muscle tone, and the loss of balance among interacting muscles (Table 2.1). However, clinicians sometimes attempt to treat these aging processes without understanding them. Understanding the aging process of patients and recognizing anatomical changes is believed to enable a more accurate and effective approach to procedures or surgeries such as lifting.

Table 2.1 Changes in the facial region by age [4]

Age(y)	Changes
30s	Forehead and glabellar lines appear
	Eyebrows may begin to descend
	Upper eyelid skin increases, and eyes appear smaller
	Fine lines around the lower eyelids and crows' feet emerge
	Tear trough lines and infraorbital fat become more prominent
	Midface aging begins
	Nasolabial folds form
	Lip thinning begins
	Alterations in skin texture and pigmentation appear
40s	Forehead, glabellar, and crow's feet lines deepen
	Eyebrows may continue to descend
	Upper eyelid skin increases in laxity and descends
	Tear trough elongates and the inferior orbital rim becomes visible
	Midface loses projection, hollows, and appears to descend
	Nasolabial folds deepen
	Lips thin and perioral lines develop
	Oral commissure and marionette lines become noticeable
	Chin begins to rotate/elongate
	Jawline loses definition
50s	Dynamic glabellar and forehead lines deepen and remain noticeable in repose
	Upper eyelid drooping increases
	Tear trough and lower eyelid scleral show worsens
	Nose begins to droop
	Midface structures noticeably descend
	If tooth loss occurs, the cheeks may appear hollow
	Nasolabial folds are increasingly prominent
	Jawline has diminished firmness and jowls may develop
60s and older	Eyes appear small and round
	Nose elongates
	Jowls are increasingly prominent
	Skin thins, loses elasticity, and sags significantly
	All previously noted changes are exaggerated

References

1. Stuzin JM, Rohrich RJ, Dayan E. The facial fat compartments revisited: clinical relevance to subcutaneous dissection and facial deflation in face lifting. Plast Reconstr Surg. 2019;144(5):1070–8.
2. Kuwazuru O, Saothong J, Yoshikawa N. Mechanical approach to aging and wrinkling of human facial skin based on the multistage buckling theory. Med Eng Phys. 2008;30(4):516–22.
3. Kuwazuru O, Miyamoto K, Yoshikawa N, et al. Skin wrinkling morphology changes suddenly in the early 30s. Skin Res Technol. 2012;18(4):495–503.
4. Swift A, Liew S, Weinkle S, Garcia JK, Silberberg MB. The facial aging process from the "inside out". Aesthet Surg J. 2021;41(10):1107–19. https://doi.org/10.1093/asj/sjaa339.

Patient Evaluation for Lifting

3

Contents

The changes in the face due to aging result from a complex interplay of various factors. It is not advisable to simply think that aging leads to sagging and that one can regain their youthful appearance solely through lifting procedures. In fact, inappropriate lifting techniques can eliminate the attractive features that a patient possesses, potentially leading to unwanted complications or results that do not meet expectations. Therefore, it is crucial to conduct a thorough evaluation and analysis of the patient before surgery to determine which lifting procedure is appropriate and to identify any areas that cannot be addressed by lifting alone, which may require complementary treatments. Additionally, sharing this medical analysis process with the patient enhances satisfaction with the procedure and helps to establish a good relationship with the patient.

3.1 Skin Quality

Skin quality is a key factor in selecting the appropriate treatment method, predicting surgical outcomes, and determining the need for additional procedures to achieve better and more lasting effects (Table 3.1).

In cases of pigmentation, roughness, and dryness, the aging-related factors in the skin do not disappear even after lifting procedures, leading to a tendency for lower satisfaction with the lifting results. When fine lines are present, it is essential to restore fullness through volume restoration, which can help alleviate wrinkles while improving radiance (Fig. 3.1). For coarse lines, different strategies may be required depending on the area, which will be explained in more detail below.

When skin laxity is moderate to severe, the effects achievable through minimally invasive procedures are limited. Therefore, it may be

W. Lee, K. H. Jung, *Lifting Techniques in Plastic Surgery*,
https://doi.org/10.1007/978-981-96-4820-7_3

advisable to consider more invasive lifting techniques or to insert thinner threads closer to the dermal layer to achieve skin tightening effects. Ultimately, the reduction in collagen and elastin in the dermis, along with a decrease in hyaluronic acid, leads to a loss of elasticity, causing the skin to sag and deepening wrinkles [1].

Table 3.1 Skin quality attributes and their definitions

Attribute	Definition
Uneven pigmentation	Variation in melanin
Redness	Erythema or visible hemoglobin
Dullness/shallowness	Absence of glow; yellow or grayish undertone
Radiance	Ability of skin to "glow" or reflect light
Oiliness/shine	Excess sebum on the skin surfaces
Dryness	Lack of moisture; dehydration
Roughness	Uneven, not level texture
Fine lines	Light wrinkles
Coarse lines	Deep wrinkles
Pores	Surface landmark of pilosebaceous unit
Crepiness	Fine cigarette paper wrinkling of skin
Hydration	Water content; moisturization
Laxity	Loose skin
Elasticity/pliability	Ability to recoil with manipulation
Firmness	Relative ability to be stretched
Thickness	Density of the epidermis and dermis

In cases where the skin is firm, there may appear to be little change when manipulating the tissue by hand before surgery; however, this indicates less loosening, which can result in better outcomes from lifting procedures. Conversely, if the skin is too thin or shows signs of telangiectasia, such as redness, there is a higher risk of the threads being visible or dimpling during thread lifting, necessitating caution. Among these concerns, crepiness, which is a symptom (crepey skin) caused by severe laxity in thin skin, should be explained to the patient as a reason why more invasive surgery may be more effective.

The thickness of the skin is primarily determined by the thickness of the dermis, which dictates the skin's mechanical properties. Thinner skin is more prone to deep and multiple wrinkles. Skin thickness is influenced by genetic factors and BMI, so assessing the condition of the eyelids, which have the thinnest skin on the face, or the neck can provide insight into the overall skin thickness of the patient's face. This is because, if the eyelid skin is considered as a baseline of 1, it can be inferred that the skin in other areas is thicker (Fig. 3.2 [2]). In patients with thin skin, even if tightening is achieved through lifting procedures, there is a tendency for quicker relaxation, resulting in shorter-lasting effects. Therefore, it is essential to emphasize to these patients that post-lifting skin management using energy-based devices (EBD) or skin boosters is necessary for prolonged results.

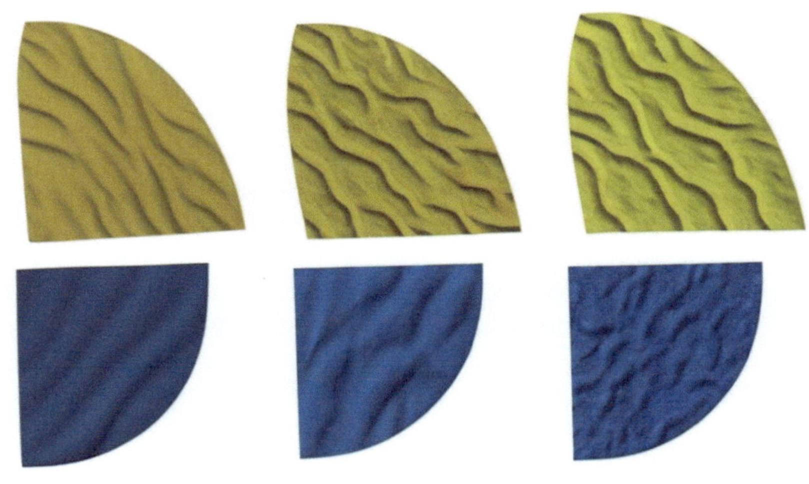

Fig. 3.1 Surface pattern morphology during the release of compressive pressure. Even with volume deflation, the pressure applied to the surface can decrease, leading to the formation of wrinkles on the surface, with the pattern and depth of the wrinkles varying according to the degree of pressure reduction

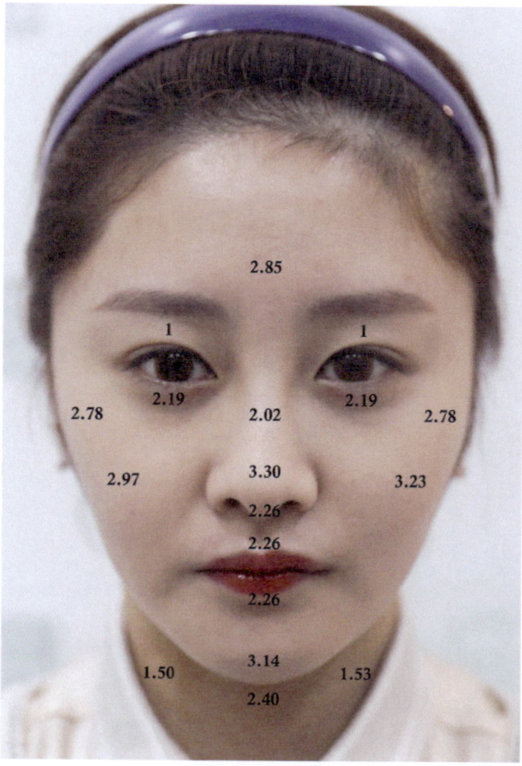

Fig. 3.2 Average skin thickness (relative skin thickness with eyelid skin as 1)

3.2 Patient Evaluation in the Midface

When evaluating patients for lifting procedures, it is important to first assess changes in the midface, lower face, and the upper face, which includes the forehead (Fig. 3.3).

The changes to be assessed in the midface can be categorized into three main areas: the mid-cheek groove, submalar hollowness, and nasolabial fold. Understanding the position of the retaining ligaments in the facial area is crucial for each of these wrinkles (Fig. 3.4). The retaining ligaments strongly influence the formation of wrinkles in the skin, and sufficient release of these ligaments during facelift surgery is necessary to achieve better results.

The mid-cheek groove is a wrinkle caused by the medial zygomatic cutaneous ligament, which can appear prominently regardless of age if it is genetically strong [3]. This is often referred to as the "Indian wrinkle." The gradual emergence of this groove with aging is primarily due to the deflation of the deep medial cheek fat (DMCF), which leads to changes in the morphology of the

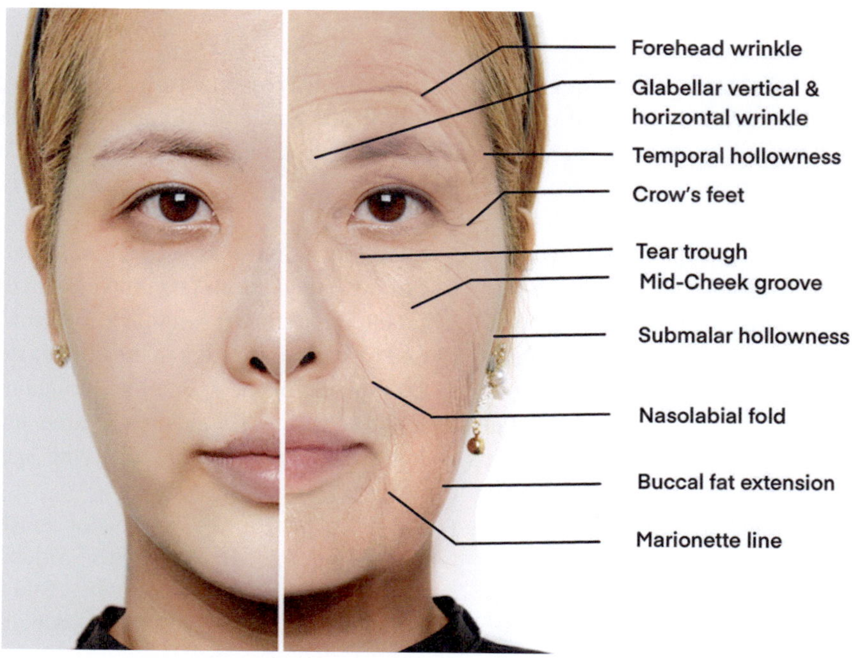

Fig. 3.3 Surface anatomy of the aging face

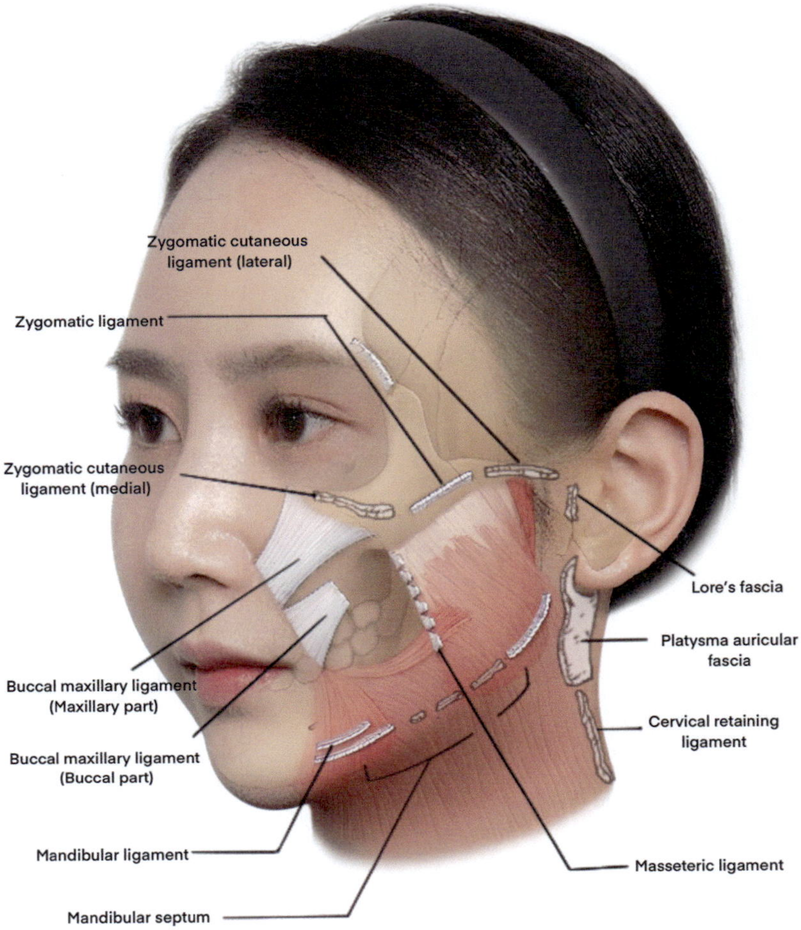

Fig. 3.4 Retaining ligaments of the facial area

superficial fat and skin. The superficial fat compartment is divided into two areas based on the medial zygomatic cutaneous ligament: the superficial medial cheek fat (SMCF) and nasolabial fat. Under the influence of gravity, the SMCF accumulates only above the mid-cheek groove, causing flattening near the arcus marginalis, while the area closer to the mid-cheek groove bulges, making the mid-cheek groove appear deeper (Fig. 3.5).

In this context, the separated nasolabial fat compartment also appears to bulge above the nasolabial fold due to the same underlying causes, making the nasolabial fold appear deeper. The mid-cheek groove can exhibit dynamic characteristics; for instance, when the inferolateral fibers of the orbital part of the orbicularis oculi muscle are strongly interconnected with the zygomatic cutaneous ligament, the groove becomes more pronounced when the eyes are closed. In such patients, if appropriate treatment is not administered, the groove may appear deeper after lifting, necessitating caution (Fig. 3.6).

Submalar hollowness occurs due to the deflation of the lateral cheek fat compartment and the reduction in intermolar width and vertical height caused by bone absorption in the maxilla, leading to a shrinkage of the frame that maintains fullness. In contrast, the zygomatic arch tends to maintain its shape relatively well with age, contributing to this condition.

The nasolabial fold is one of the most common wrinkles reported by patients worldwide. A detailed description of the nasolabial fold is provided in Chap. 2. Compared to the nasolabial fat adjacent to the nasolabial fold, there is minimal superficial fat, making it more noticeable; a small

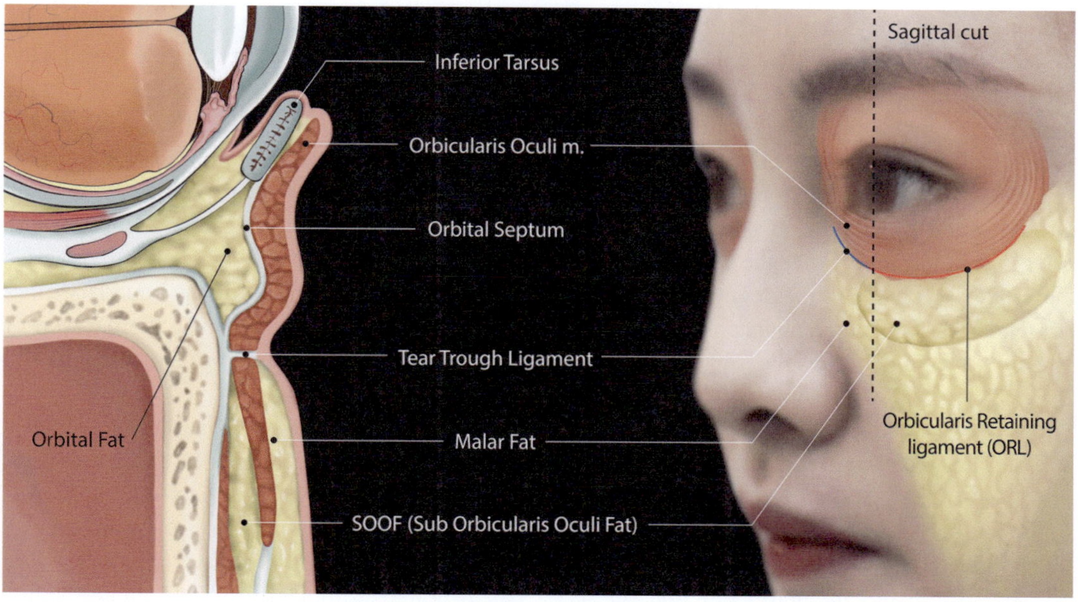

Fig. 3.5 Evaluation of the mid-cheek groove

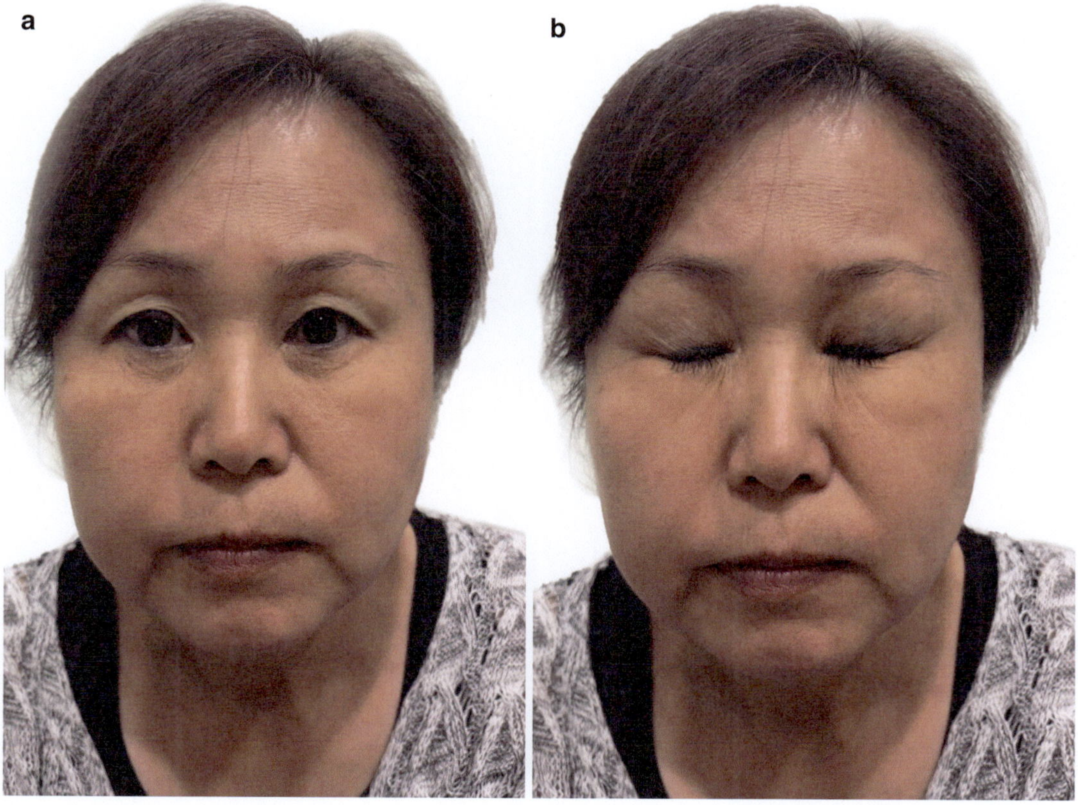

Fig. 3.6 Dynamic characteristics of the mid-cheek groove. (**a**) Static state. (**b**) When the eyes are closed

amount of hyaluronic acid filler can be beneficial in such cases. Additionally, the deeper layers of fat also undergo deflation with age, making volume replacement with fillers important. However, nasolabial folds that are more pronounced due to sagging midface fat or the repetitive action of lip elevator muscles may not respond adequately to filler injections alone. Since the causes of nasolabial folds involve multiple complex factors, a combination of volume enhancement and lifting is likely to yield better results.

3.3 Patient Evaluation in the Lower Face

In the lower face, three key areas must be assessed. The first is the marionette line, the second is the risorius line, and the third is the clarity of the jawline. The causes of marionette lines are varied. Hyperactivity of the depressor anguli oris (DAO) leads to the descent of jowl tissue, which, combined with midface fat loss and skin laxity, exacerbates the bulging of the descended tissue outside the marionette line. Furthermore, the reduction of subcutaneous fat tissue eliminates the cushioning effect that previously masked muscle movement, resulting in a strong adhesion between the hyperactivated inner border of the DAO and the dermis, making the boundary more pronounced [4]. Simultaneously, the position of the modiolus descends with age, deepening the marionette line (Fig. 3.7).

The second area to assess in the lower face is the risorius line, which must be evaluated prior to lifting procedures. The fibers of the risorius muscle can vary in pattern and layer among patients. When positioned superficially, the line can become prominently visible on the skin's surface, and during lifting procedures, this line may appear longer and more pronounced (Fig. 3.8).

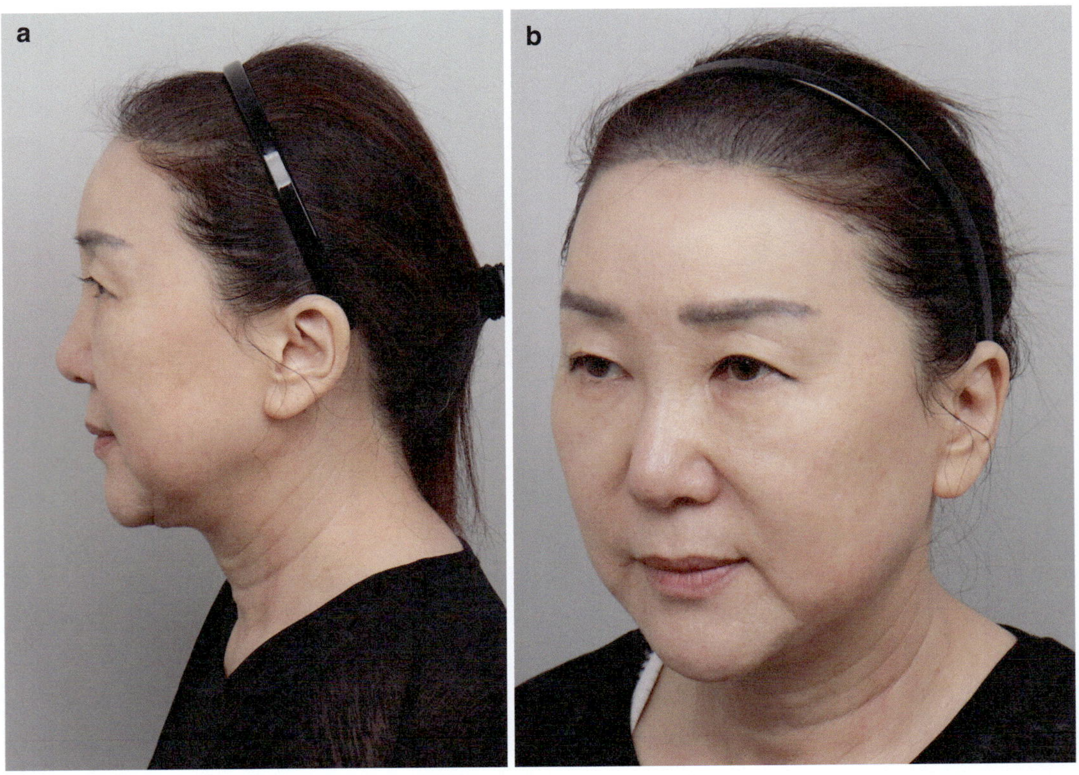

Fig. 3.7 Evaluation of the marionette line. A 50-year-old female patient exhibits a noticeably deep marionette line due to DAO hyperactivation and tissue sagging. (**a**) Lateral view. (**b**) Three-quarter view

Jawline clarity refers to the straightness of the lower border line of the mandible body (Menton-Gonion). With aging, bony atrophy in the prejowl region occurs, and the extension of buccal fat descends, creating bulging and convexity. In patients with DAO hyperactivation, this bulging becomes more pronounced. In patients with a strong masseteric retaining ligament, a distinct boundary forms along the anterior border of the masseter, resulting in a more irregular appearance of the lower face (Fig. 3.9). In cases where excessive botulinum toxin is injected into the jaw or where inappropriate indications are present, the supporting frame of the lower facial tissue may diminish, causing fat tissue and skin to shift inferomedially, which can iatrogenically worsen bulging and obscure the mandible angle, leading to a loss of jawline clarity (Fig. 3.10).

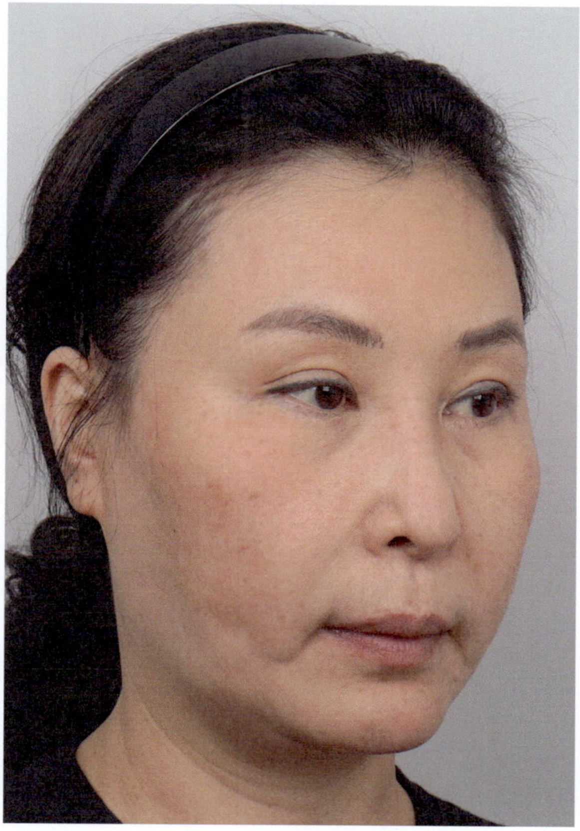

Fig. 3.8 Evaluation of the risorius line. A 54-year-old female patient shows a line caused by the risorius, which is strongly adhered to the dermis and has descended below the modiolus

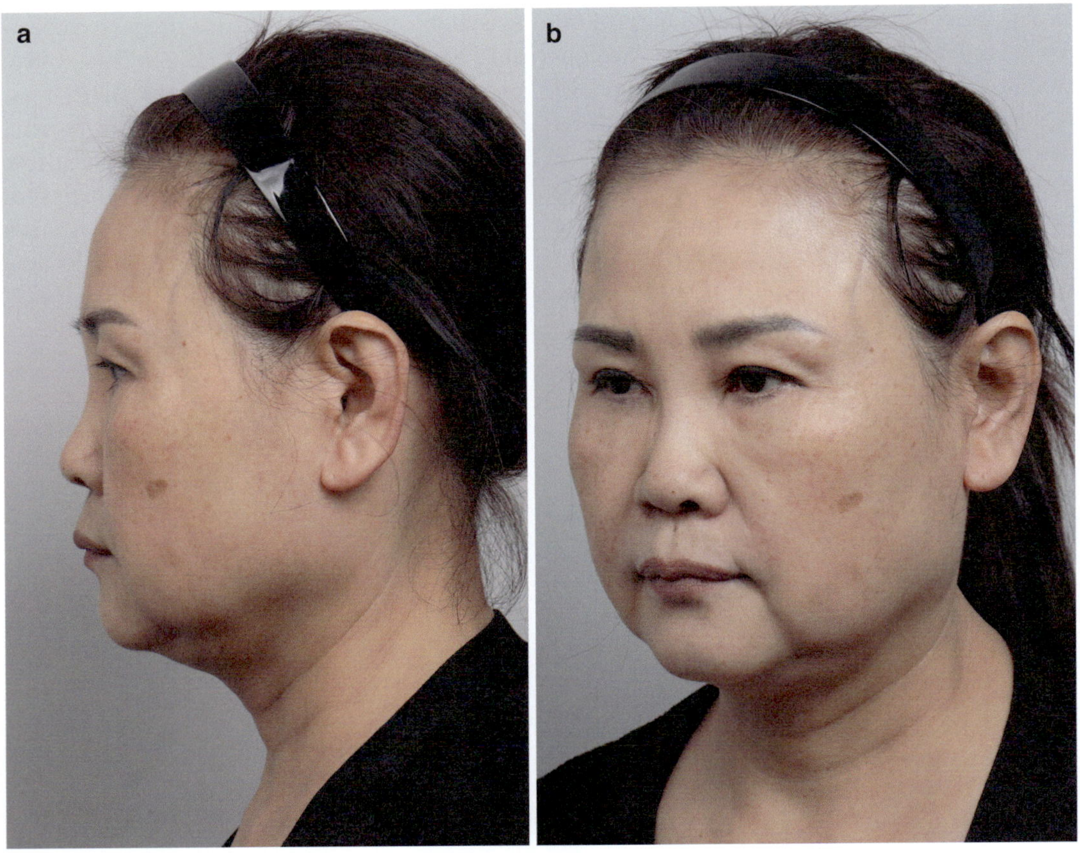

Fig. 3.9 Evaluation of jawline clarity. A 56-year-old female patient shows bone absorption in the prejowl region and buccal fat extension, with an irregular jawline due to the boundary of the masseteric retaining ligament. (**a**) Lateral view, (**b**) three-quarter view

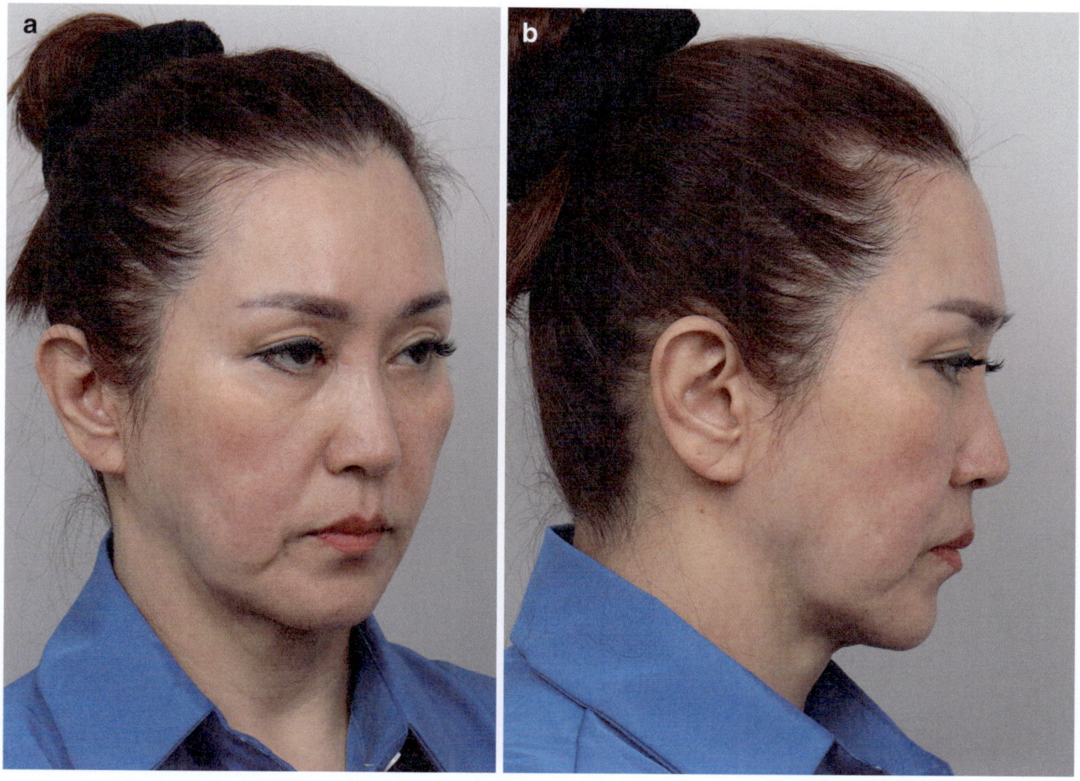

Fig. 3.10 Evaluation of jawline clarity. A 54-year-old female patient exhibits noticeable prominence in the jowl area and a loss of jawline clarity due to inferomedial movement of tissue following excessive botulinum toxin injection into the masseter muscle. (**a**) Three-quarter view, (**b**) lateral view

3.4 Patient Evaluation in the Upper Face

In the upper face, the depth of wrinkles, the degree of brow ptosis (brow ptosis grade), and the superior temporal line are important elements to assess. Generally, changes in the forehead due to aging are caused by blepharochalasia and blepharoptosis, which lead to a narrowed field of vision. To alleviate discomfort in the visual field, the frontalis muscle is excessively used, resulting in repeated folding and unfolding, which creates horizontal forehead wrinkles and leads to skin laxity over time. When soft tissue and skin loosen to the extent that compensation by the frontalis muscle is insufficient, droopy eyebrows can occur. Therefore, it is essential to first assess the brow ptosis grade. The perpendicular distance from the Frankfurt line to the end of the eyebrow is measured; if it is less than 1.8 cm, brow ptosis can be diagnosed (Fig. 3.11, Table 3.2 [5]). However, the degree of compensation by the frown muscle and frontalis varies among patients, and eyebrow shape can change, resulting in different degrees of droop at the center, medial, and lateral points of the eyebrow.

Clinically, if there are dynamic multiple horizontal wrinkles on the forehead in a neutral expression and the change in eyebrow height exceeds 4 mm upon relaxation of the frontalis muscle, brow ptosis can be diagnosed, indicating the need for brow lift and forehead lift surgery. In cases where the wrinkles are very deep and static, severe brow ptosis may be masked, and satisfactory improvement is often only achievable through invasive procedures.

Generally, the area between the superior temporal line and the zygomatic arch is referred to as the temple. The temple area is divided into several layers; in the subcutaneous fat layer, it is

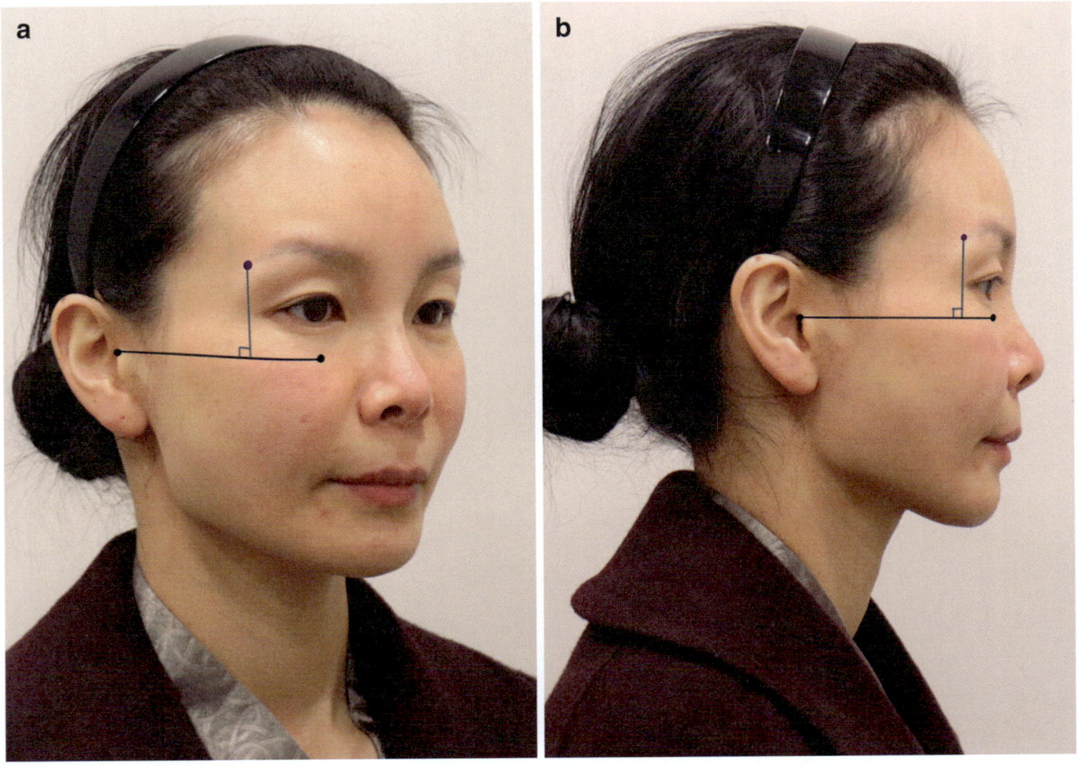

Fig. 3.11 Measurement method for brow ptosis grade. The measurement method is based on the vertical distance from the Frankfurt line (black horizontal line, the line passing through the orbitale and porion) to the outermost point of the eyebrow. (**a**) Three quarter view. (**b**) Lateral view

Table 3.2 Classification of brow ptosis vs. surgical indication. This classification is based on the vertical distance from the Frankfurt line to the outermost point of the eyebrow. A distance of less than 1.8 cm can be diagnosed as brow ptosis, and surgical indications are considered for grades II and above

Distance (cm)	Degree of ptosis	Surgical indication
≥1.8	Normal	No
1.7–1.5	I	No
1.4–1.2	II	Yes
1.1–0.9	III	Yes
≤0.8	IV	Yes

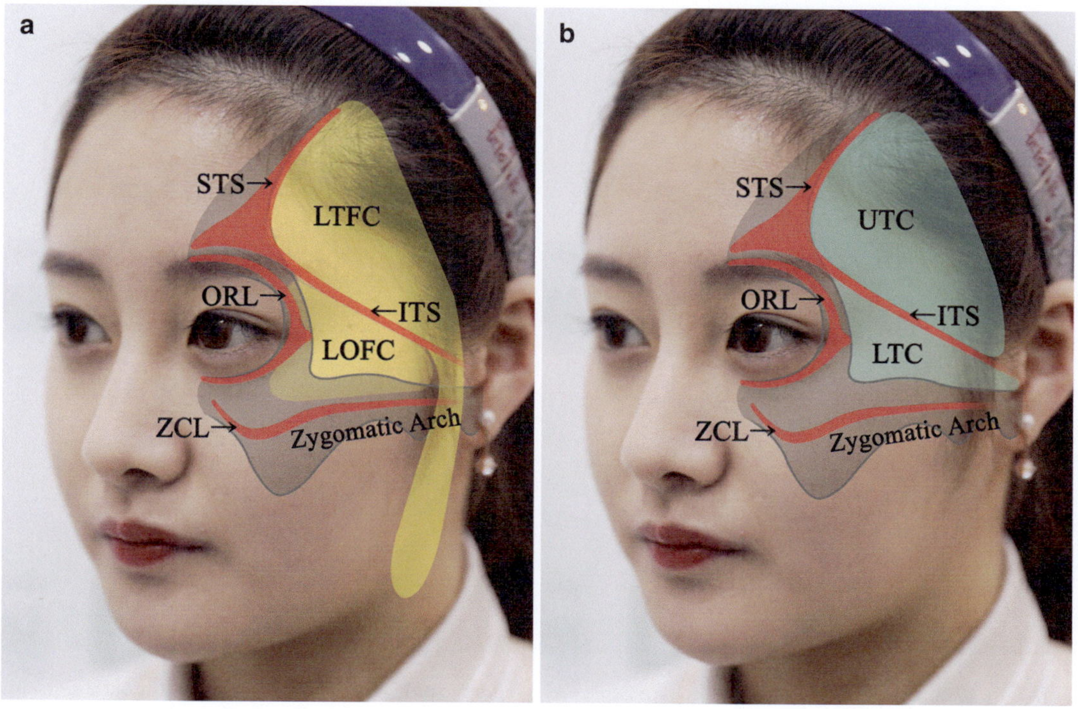

Fig. 3.12 Distribution of fat compartment in the temple area. (**a**) In the subcutaneous fat layer, it is divided into LTFC and LOFC. (**b**) In the deeper layer beyond the superficial temporal fascia, it is divided into UTC and LTC

divided into the lateral temporal cheek fat compartment (LTFC) and the lateral orbital fat compartment (LOFC). Deeper than the superficial temporal fascia, it is further divided into the upper temporal compartment (UTC) and lower temporal compartment (LTC) (Fig. 3.12) [6].

The superior temporal line becomes prominent due to atrophy associated with aging in the temple area. The degree of atrophy in the temple is assessed based on the depth of the most depressed point relative to the outer eyebrow area. In patients with severe atrophy, defined as more than 3 mm deeper than the outer eyebrow area, even after invasive forehead lift surgery, the boundary may still appear prominent. Therefore, it is necessary to address volume loss in the temple area as well (Fig. 3.13).

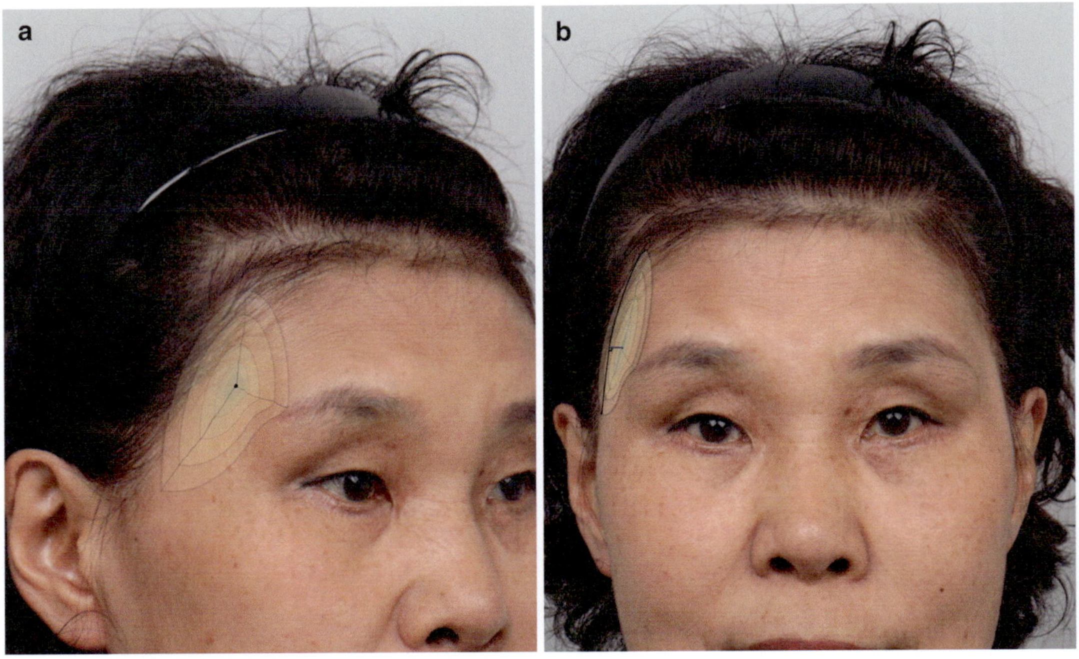

Fig. 3.13 Evaluation of the superior temporal line. A 63-year-old female patient shows temporal fossa atrophy assessed by the depth of the most depressed point, with the boundary of the superior temporal crest (STC) becoming more pronounced as temporal fossa atrophy worsens. (**a**) Three quarter view with the deepest point marked. (**b**) Frontal view

3.5 Conclusion

Patients seeking lifting procedures present various symptoms related to their age. Accurately assessing the skin condition, midface, lower face, and upper face aging phenomena, along with the patient's overall status, is essential for performing the most appropriate surgery, which is likely to yield better outcomes (Table 3.3).

Table 3.3 Patient evaluation elements for lifting procedures

Evaluation area	Evaluation elements
Skin quality	Pigmentation Wrinkle Laxity Skin thickness
Midface	Mid cheek groove Submalar hollowness Nasolabial fold
Lower face	Marionette line Risorius line Jawline clarity
Upper face	Wrinkle depth (horizontal forehead wrinkle, glabellar frown line) Brow ptosis grade Superior temporal line

References

1. Karim PL, Aryani IA. Anatomy and histologic of intrinsic aging skin. Bioscientia Medicina: J Biomed Transl Res. 2021;5(11):1065–77.
2. Ha RY, Nojima K, Adams WP Jr, Brown SA. Analysis of facial skin thickness: defining the relative thickness index. Plast Reconstr Surg. 2005;115(6):1769–73. https://doi.org/10.1097/01.prs.0000161682.63535.9b.
3. Wong CH, Mendelson B. Facial soft-tissue spaces and retaining ligaments of the midcheek: defining the premaxillary space. Plast Reconstr Surg. 2013;132(1):49–56. https://doi.org/10.1097/PRS.0b013e3182910a57.
4. Gierloff M, Stöhring C, Buder T, Wiltfang J. The subcutaneous fat compartments in relation to aesthetically important facial folds and rhytides. J Plast Reconstr Aesthet Surg. 2012;65(10):1292–7. https://doi.org/10.1016/j.bjps.2012.04.047.
5. Real DSS, et al. Classificação clínica de ptose da cauda do supercílio. Rev Bras Cir Plást. 2016;31(3):354–61.
6. Huang RL, Xie Y, Wang W, Herrler T, Zhou J, Zhao P, et al. Anatomical study of temporal fat compartments and its clinical application for temporal fat grafting. Aesthet Surg J. 2017;37(8):855–62.

Understanding Lifting Threads 4

Contents

A lot of medical sutures are materials made from synthetic biodegradable polymers that allow for use within the body. A commonly used suture, Trisorb®, is made from polyglycolic acid (PGA). To address the shortcomings of PGA, Vicryl™ is made from polylactic-co-glycolic acid (PLGA). PDS™ is produced using polydioxanone (PDO), while Prolene™ is made from polypropylene (PP). Lifting threads are also made from synthetic biodegradable polymers and are classified as medical devices manufactured for lifting purposes. Depending on their components and manufacturing methods, these threads exhibit different characteristics and properties. Since these various types of threads are inserted into the human body, a fundamental understanding of biomaterials is essential, particularly an understanding of polymers, to comprehend the threads used for lifting.

4.1 Understanding Biomaterials

A biomaterial is defined as a substance that replaces the function of living tissues or organs and is an inert material that does not elicit

W. Lee, K. H. Jung, *Lifting Techniques in Plastic Surgery*,
https://doi.org/10.1007/978-981-96-4820-7_4

Table 4.1 Biomaterial classification

Classification		Examples
Material	Polymers	Polyamide (Nylon), acryl polymers, fluorocarbon polymer (Teflon), polyester (Dacron), silicon rubber, polyurethane, hydrogels
	Steel	Stainless steel, cobalt-chrome alloys, titanium alloys
	Ceramic	Alumina, titanium oxides, carbons, hydroxyapatite, calcium phosphate
	Complex material	Carbon-carbon, ceramic-coated metal, carbon coated material
Raw	Natural	Natural rubber, proteins (collagen, gelatin, fibrinogen), polysaccharides (alginate, chitosan, hyaluronate, cellulose, heparin)
	Synthetic	Polyamide (Nylon), acryl polymers, fluorocarbon polymer (Teflon), polyester (Dacron), silicone rubber, polyurethane
Degradation	Nonabsorbable	Polyamide (Nylon), acryl polymers, fluorocarbon polymer (Teflon), polyester (Dacron), silicone rubber, polyurethane
	Absorbable	Polylactic acid, polyglycolic acid, polycaprolactone, polydioxanone, calcium phosphate

histological or pharmacological responses. Additionally, it must be a nonviable substance that possesses biocompatibility, meaning it does not induce a biological rejection response or toxic reaction when in contact with biological tissues, blood, or body fluids.

In the field of plastic surgery, various biomaterials are used, including implants, as well as artificial joints used in orthopedics. Among these, the polymers used in thread lifting are also considered biomaterials. It is important to recognize which classifications the polymers used in thread lifting fall under among the various biomaterials (Table 4.1).

Biomaterials can be categorized based on their types, such as polymeric materials like nylon or silicone, and metallic materials like titanium. They can also be classified according to whether their raw materials are natural or synthetic. As will be discussed later, the threads commonly used for lifting primarily fall into the categories of degradable and non-degradable polymers.

4.2 Manufacturing Process of Lifting Threads

Before lifting threads reach the hands of consumers and medical practitioners, such as physicians, they undergo numerous processes. After selecting the raw materials, polymerization is performed, followed by extrusion, spinning, and annealing processes to produce long threads (Fig. 4.1). These threads are produced in roll lengths of either 300 m or 500 m and are then used as sutures for incisional surgeries or laceration repairs.

The raw threads, packaged in roll form, are manufactured in a controlled environment that maintains appropriate standards (GMP regulations: temperature 20–30 °C, humidity 40–75%—2020 KFDA guidelines) to ensure they are suitable for tissue lifting in the form of cogged threads. Depending on the manufacturing method, they can be categorized as cutting type, molding type, or pressing type. Once the threads are produced in the desired shape, they are cut to the appropriate length and inserted into a cannula. After packaging and sterilization, they are labeled for management.

Throughout this series of processes, cogged threads are exposed to moisture in the air, and hydrolysis gradually occurs. Therefore, the maintenance of temperature and humidity in the manufacturing environment, the duration from manufacturing to storage, and the conditions under which they are stored after all processes are completed will determine the shelf life (effectiveness) and expiration date (performance) of the threads.

4.2.1 Characteristics of Raw Materials and Polymerization

Threads designed for lifting purposes can also be classified based on their raw materials, which can be broadly categorized into polydioxanone (PDO), poly-L-lactic acid (PLLA), polycaprolactone (PCL), and polypropylene (PP). The most commonly encountered thread in the South Korean lifting market is the one made from PDO. PDO is a polymer composed of multiple repeating ether-ester units, obtained through the ring-opening polymerization of the monomer p-dioxanone (Fig. 4.2). PDO typically exhibits about 55% crystallinity and has the advantage of relatively high strength, although it may vary slightly depending on the manufacturing process. Additionally, it is known for its excellent biocompatibility and low toxicity. The melting point of PDO is reported to be around 110 °C, which is lower than that of PGA and PLLA but higher than that of PCL (Table 4.2). However, PDO has a degradation period of 4–6 months, with strength retention lasting approximately 1.5 months; after this period, about 60% of its strength remains, gradually decreasing thereafter, which is a limitation in its durability.

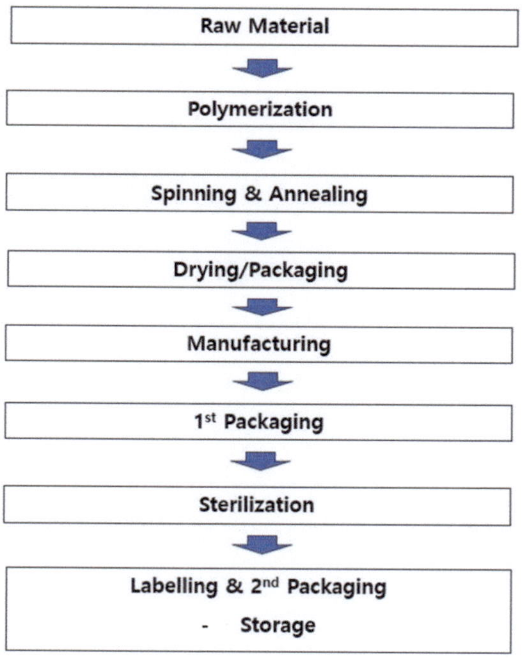

Fig. 4.1 Manufacturing process of threads

Polylactic acid (PLA) is a polymer composed of lactic acid, which occurs naturally. Lactic acid can be obtained through the fermentation of glucose derived from corn starch, a cheap and abundant natural resource (Fig. 4.3). The lactic acid obtained in this manner can be converted into PLA either through direct condensation polymerization or through the ring-opening polymerization of the cyclic intermediate lactide. Currently, the majority of PLA is produced using the ring-opening polymerization method (Fig. 4.4).

Lactic acid is divided into two types based on optical activity: L-type and D-type. Poly-L-lactic acid (PLLA), which is a polymer made from L-type lactic acid, possesses high crystallinity and high strength. Its degradation period is relatively long, ranging from 18 to 24 months, and it retains strength for 6 to 12 months, providing the advantage of long-term effectiveness (Table 4.2). However, paradoxically, the high strength results in reduced flexibility, leading to brittleness at certain stress levels, which may cause discomfort when applied to patients.

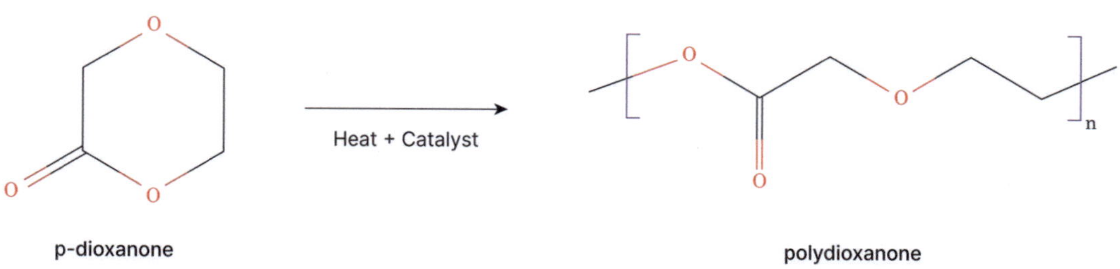

Fig. 4.2 Polymerization of PDO thread

Table 4.2 Properties of synthetic biodegradable polymers

Polymer	Structure	Melting point (°C)	Modulus (Gpa)	Mass degradation (months)	Strength retention (months)
PGA	-O-CH_2-CO-	225	7.0	3	1
PLLA	-O-$CHCH_3$-CO-	175	2.7	18–24	6–12
PDLLA	-O-$CHCH_3$-CO-	None	1.9	12–16	3–10
PCL	-O-$(CH_2)_5$-CO-	60	0.4	>24	>24
PDO	-O-CH_2CH_2-O-CH_2-O	110	1.5	4–6	1.5

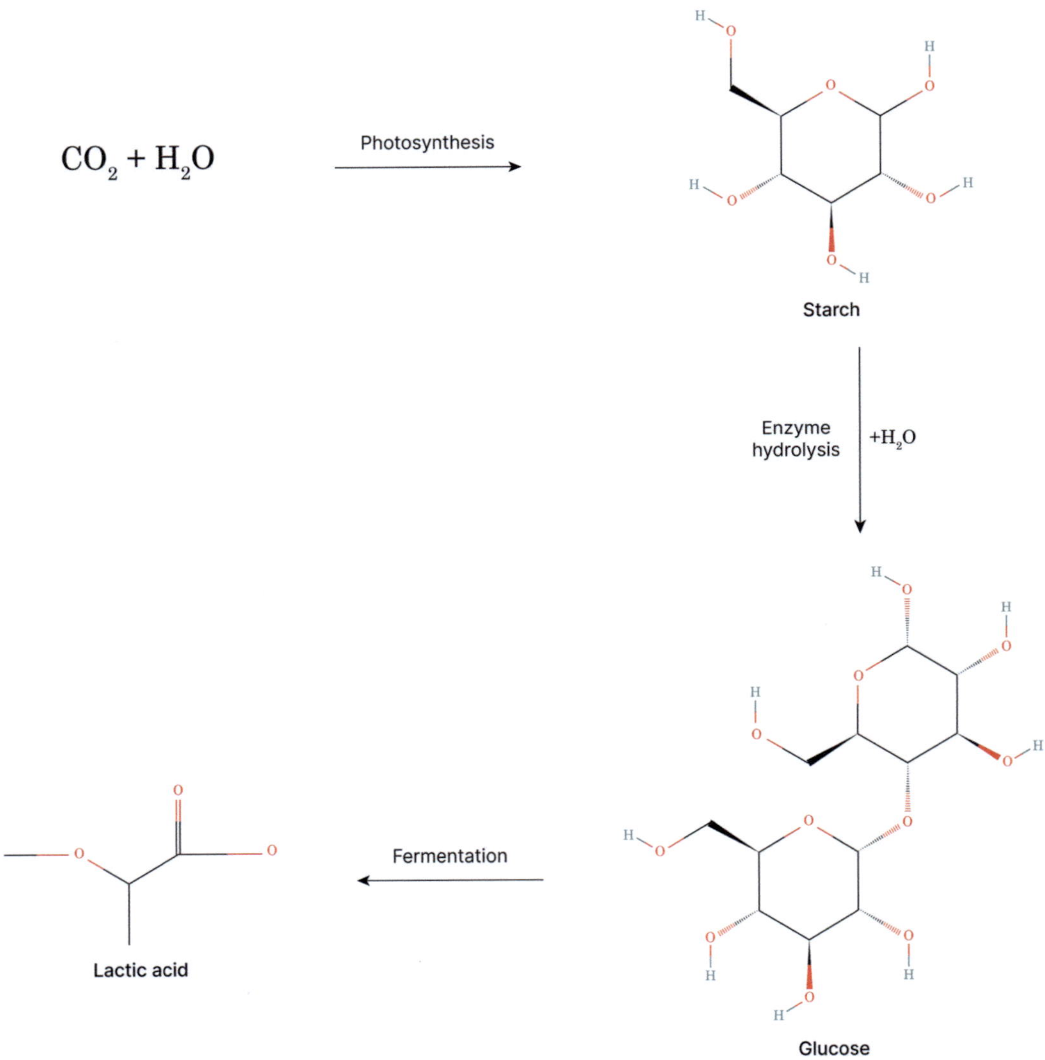

Fig. 4.3 Process of lactic acid production

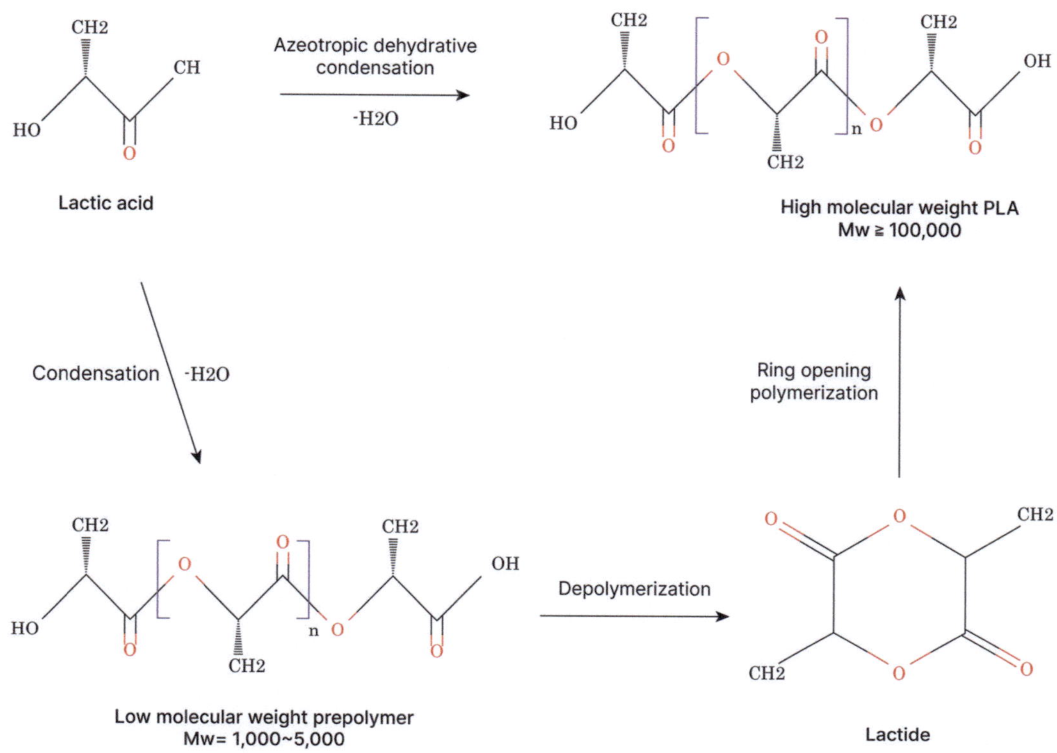

Fig. 4.4 Process of PLA production

Polycaprolactone (PCL) is a polymer compound primarily obtained through the ring-opening polymerization of ε-caprolactone (Fig. 4.5). Its degradation product, hydrohexanoic acid, is a substance that is fully absorbed by the body during metabolic processes, resulting in lower toxicity and good biocompatibility. PCL is semicrystalline and elastic, which contributes to its flexibility, leading to lower discomfort during in vivo use. Additionally, its hydrophobic properties result in a slower degradation rate, allowing it to be maintained for over 24 months (Table 4.2). However, due to its relatively low melting temperature (60 °C) and glass transition temperature (−60 °C), manufacturing can be challenging, and it is prone to deformation, making it difficult to handle. Furthermore, its flexibility limits its lifting effect. Therefore, it is often used in combination with other materials as a modifier. A representative example is PCLA (PLA + PCL), which exhibits different properties depending on the ratio of PLA to PCL. PCLA is known to combine the advantages of both PLA and PCL, maintaining the rigidity of PLA while incorporating the elasticity of PCL (Fig. 4.6).

Polypropylene (PP) is a material characterized by a very high melting temperature (300–500 °C) and does not fall under the conditions for degradation within the human body, making it nonabsorbable. Some literature claims that sutures made from PP can maintain lifting effects for the longest duration due to their non-absorbable nature. However, over time, the support provided by the cog may diminish, leaving only the suture in place. In fact, the author has encountered cases in patients who underwent facelift surgery where sutures inserted years ago were found to be ineffective. Analysis using 1H nuclear magnetic resonance (NMR) confirmed that these sutures were made of PP (Fig. 4.7).

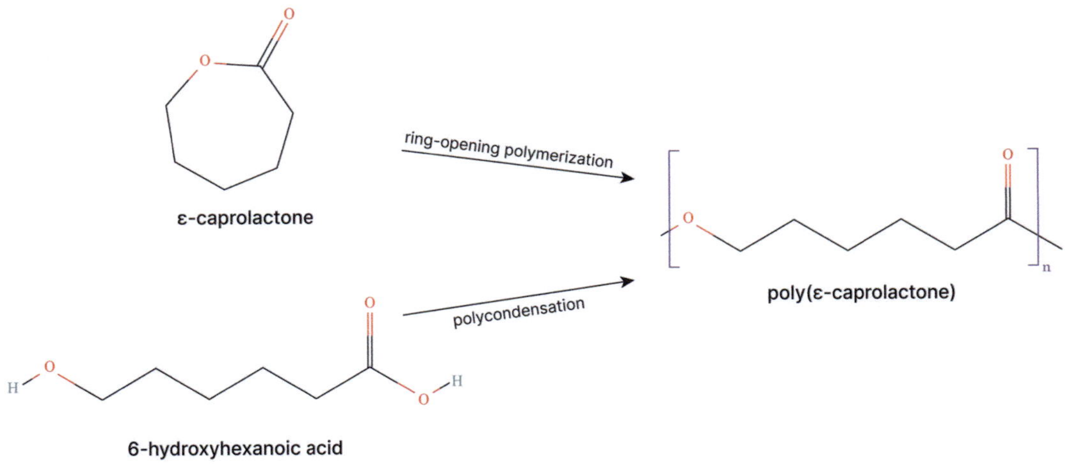

Fig. 4.5 PCL manufacturing process

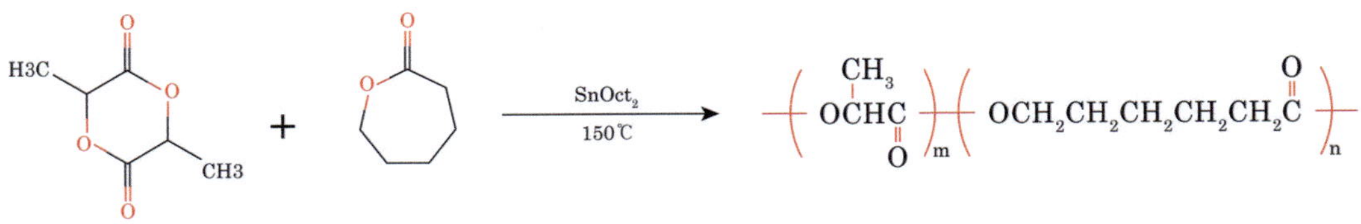

Fig. 4.6 PLCL manufacturing process

Fig. 4.7 1H NMR results of PP sutures

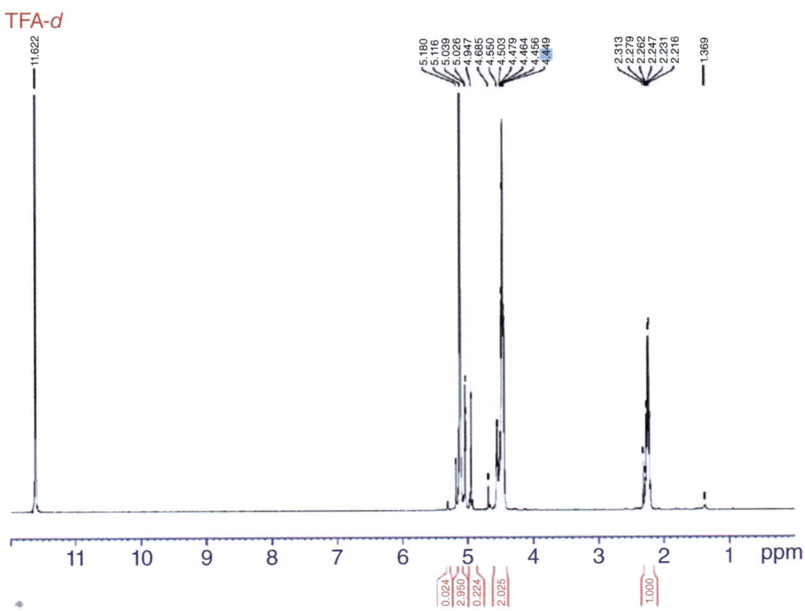

4.2.2 Spinning and Annealing

The high-molecular-weight polymer sutures obtained through the polymerization process are produced into thin and long suture materials via spinning and subsequent annealing processes. A representative method for producing suture material is melt spinning (Fig. 4.8). During this process, crystallization occurs through molecular orientation. The quality of the thread is determined by the high crystallinity and the uniform distribution of amorphous and crystalline regions (Fig. 4.9) [1]. The resulting thin and elongated threads are packaged in spool form according to length (e.g., 300 m, 500 m).

4.2.3 Manufacturing: Cogged Thread

There are three main methods for producing cogged threads using raw thread: cutting, molding, and pressing methods. Each method has its own advantages and disadvantages, and the differences in these processes can also affect the characteristics of the threads, making it more appropriate to use them selectively.

4.2.3.1 Cutting Method

The cutting method is the earliest technique used to create cogged threads by using a sharp blade to create notches in the thread, forming a cog shape (Fig. 4.10). Since the cog is carved from the core, this method results in a thinner core, making the cog weaker and thinner compared to threads produced by other methods (Fig. 4.11). This method was not widely used due to issues with precision when using automated machines, but recently, a new and more precise cutting method has been developed to address the aforementioned disadvantages (Fig. 4.12).

4.2.3.2 Molding Method

The molding method was developed to address the limitations of the cutting method, particularly the thinning of the core and to create larger and sturdier cogs. Initially, a cylindrical thread (T1) is flattened into an oval shape (T2), and then a mold designed in the shape of a cog is used to stamp the thread in a cookie-cutter fashion (T3)

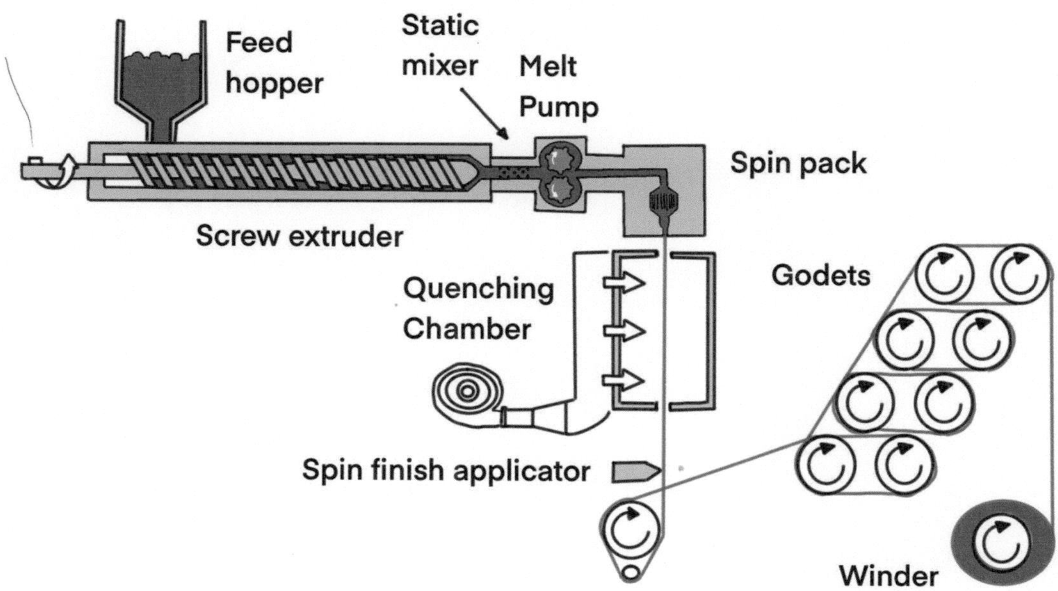

Fig. 4.8 Spinning and annealing process. The purple area indicates the process of the thread being drawn out [2]

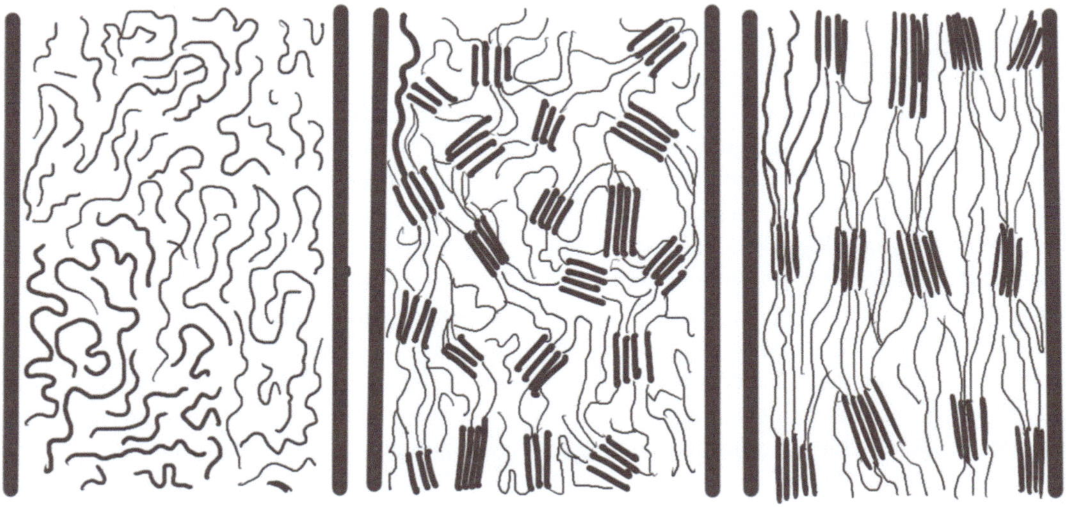

Fig. 4.9 In this process, as the amorphous arrangement within the polymer increases in crystallinity, a stable arrangement is achieved, ensuring the tensile strength and retention of the thread

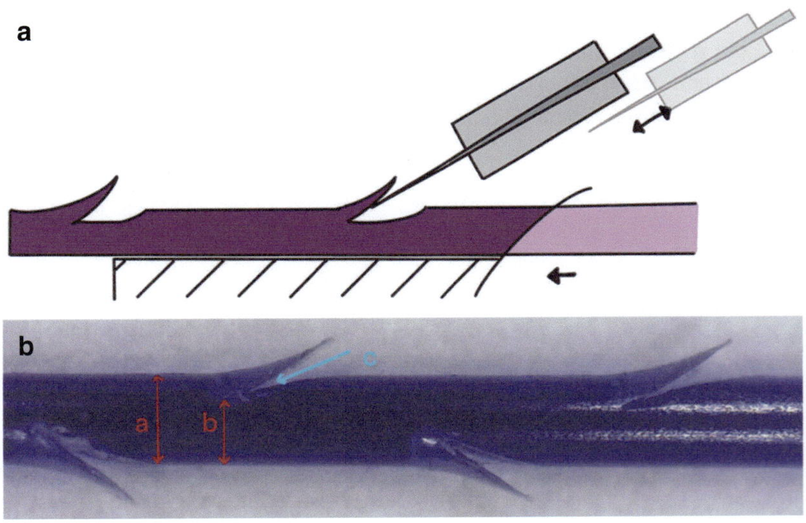

Fig. 4.10 Early cutting method. The cutting is performed by a simple diagonal movement of the blade. Over time, as the blade dulls, there is a possibility of cog defects and mechanical errors leading to excessive notching, which weakens the core. (**a**) Schematic diagram of the cutting method. (**b**) Magnified view of the thread produced by the cutting technique

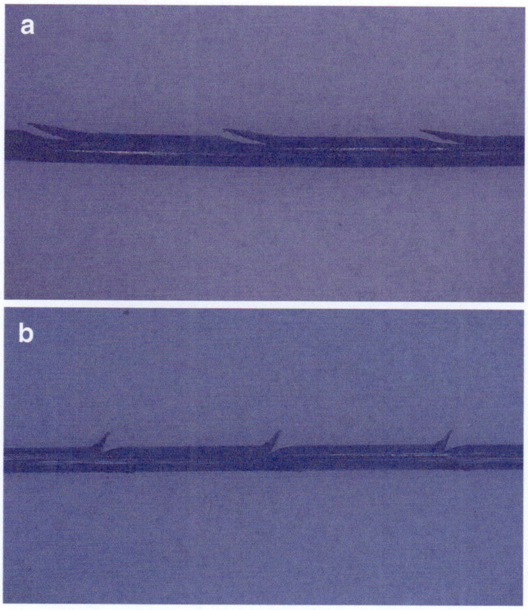

Fig. 4.11 Various threads produced by the early cutting method. (**a**) Product A. (**b**) Product B

(Fig. 4.13). By creating molds according to the shape of the thread and overlapping the cuts, the cogs can be produced thicker and sturdier compared to the cutting method. However, excessive flattening into an oval shape can thin the core (center thickness), potentially weakening its strength, and there are limitations in the height of the cogs that can be achieved (Fig. 4.14).

4.2.3.3 Press Molding Method

The press molding method involves applying strong pressure to the thread against a designed mold to form the cog, eliminating the need for the initial flattening process used in the molding method. This technique requires high pressure, which necessitates the use of large press equipment, leading to spatial constraints. However, it offers the advantage of being able to produce cogs with greater height compared to the molding method. A disadvantage of this method is that

Fig. 4.12 Recent cutting method. To overcome the limitation of the previous method, which resulted in a thin core to create larger cogs, the direction of the machine blade's joint was modified to allow for secondary processing in one operation. (**a**) Schematic diagram of the cutting method. (**b**) Microscopic view of the actual product. (**c**) Microscopic view of another product

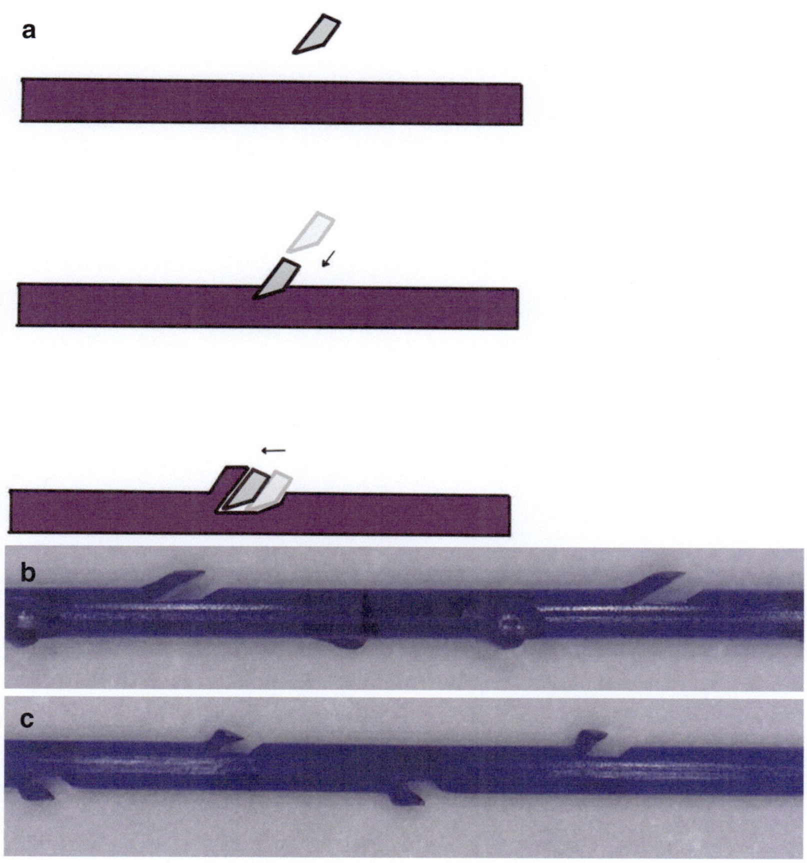

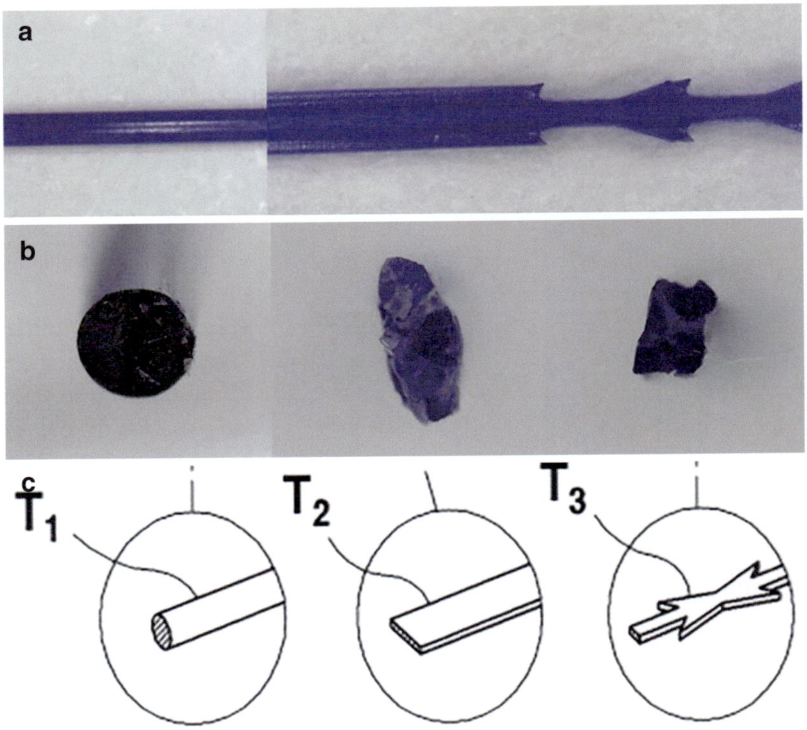

Fig. 4.13 Three-step cross-sectional view of the molding method. T1: Cross-section of the cylindrical thread. T2: Flattened to an oval shape. T3: Cross-section after being stamped with a cookie-cutter designed in the shape of a cog. (**a**) Shape of the thread. (**b**) Cross-section of the thread. (**c**) Schematic diagram

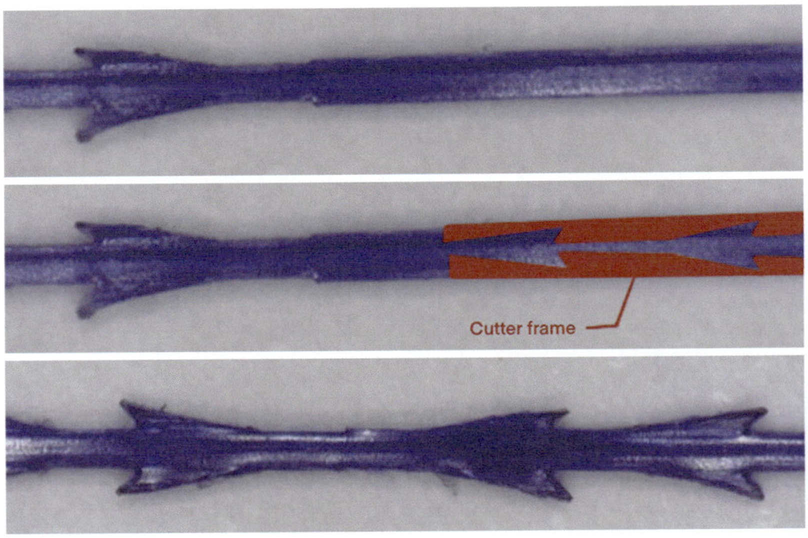

Fig. 4.14 State after pressing into shape T3 using a cutter frame from the T2 state

the strong pressure alone can lead to the formation of fine burrs on the thread. Recently, advancements have been made to reduce mold processing errors, resulting in products with minimal burrs (Figs. 4.15 and 4.16).

4.2.3.4 Other Methods

In addition, an ultrasonic molding method that applies the principles of the molding method has been developed. In this method, the thread is first flattened into an oval shape, and then a sudden

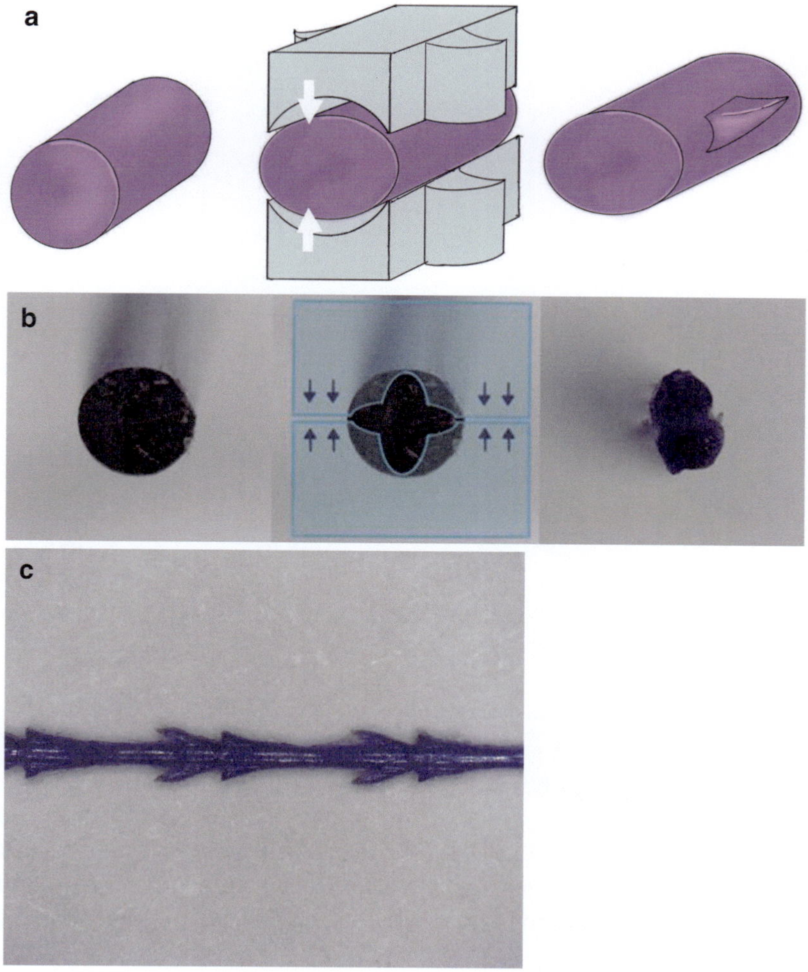

Fig. 4.15 Press molding method. (**a**) Schematic diagram. (**b**) Cross-section of the thread. (**c**) Thread produced by the press molding method

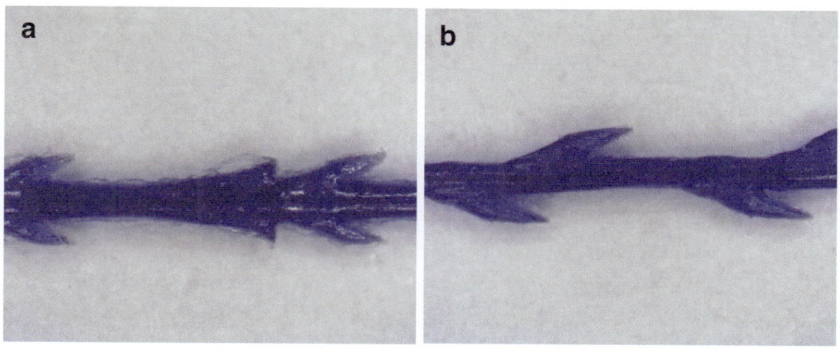

Fig. 4.16 Press molding thread. (**a**) Burrs that occurred around the thread during the initial press molding method. (**b**) Recent improvements in products that have addressed this issue

pressure and ultrasonic vibrations are generated at the interface between the horn (the part that shapes the thread) and the zig (the flat base) to create the cog shape (Fig. 4.17). Another method involves using an insert injection molding technique to manufacture products with a thin thread core.

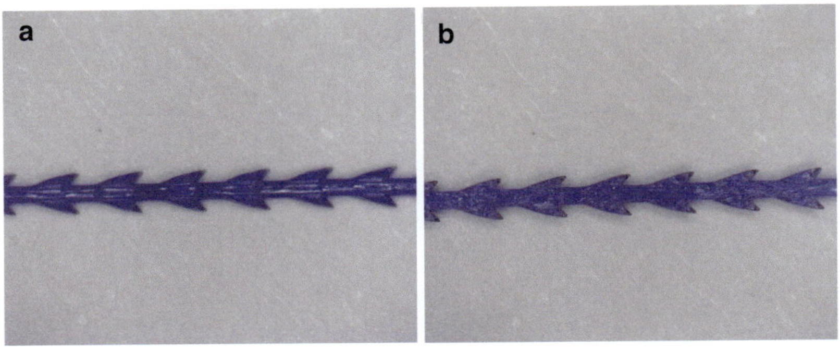

Fig. 4.17 Photos of ultrasonic molding products. (**a**) Upper part in contact with the horn. (**b**) Lower part in contact with the zig

Table 4.3 Cannula sizes. Needle gauge chart ISO 9626

Needle size		OD range			
Metric	Gauge	OD min	OD max	Minimum ID	
1.10	19	1.030	1.100	RW	0.648
				TW	0.750
				ETW	0.850
				UTW	0.891
1.20	18	1.200	1.300	RW	0.790
				TW	0.910
				ETW	1.041

OD outer diameter, *ID* internal diameter, *RW* regular wall, *TW* thin wall, *ETW* extra thin wall, *UTW* ultrathin wall

4.2.4 Packaging and Sterilization

Once the manufacturing of the cogged thread is complete, it is cut to the appropriate length and inserted into a cannula for packaging. The cannula typically uses an outer diameter (OD) of 18 gauge or 19 gauge. Since the cannula is manufactured according to specified standards (ISO 9626), the inner diameter (ID) is predetermined (Table 4.3). The core of the thread (the thickness of the thread) is closely related to the strength of the product, while the height of the cog is closely associated with lifting and fixation capabilities. This is why the core thickness and cog height cannot be adjusted indefinitely; the thread must fit within the limited inner diameter of the cannula.

Various sizes of cannulas are used depending on the type of thread inserted into the cannula. Sometimes, when a thick, grooved thread is used, it is necessary to use a larger cannula, which can be a disadvantage (Fig. 4.18).

A representative component of cogged threads, PDO, undergoes hydrolysis due to exposure to moisture from the moment it is exposed to air. To minimize this effect and maintain its efficacy over time, it is essential to include a desiccant (silica gel) in the packaging or to use vacuum packaging or nitrogen packaging (Fig. 4.19). Typically, each pack contains 2 to 10 threads.

After the packaging is completed, sterilization is performed, which is the time when the thread is exposed to the most extreme conditions since its manufacture. Threads made from biodegradable polymers, which are sensitive to external environments, cannot undergo sterilization methods such as autoclaving (moist heat) under high temperature and humidity or radiation sterilization using X-rays, gamma rays, or electron beams, as these methods significantly weaken their physical properties. Therefore, EO gas sterilization is employed. This method involves introducing ethylene oxide (EO gas), a toxic gas, into a vacuum-sealed environment while maintaining specific

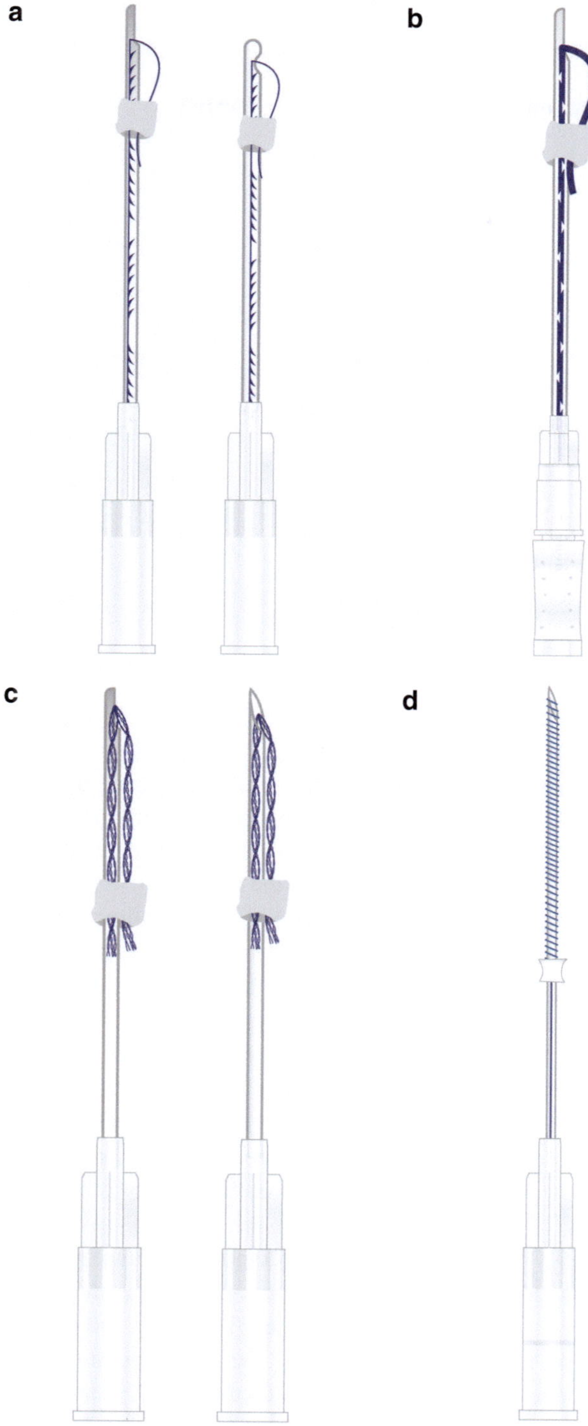

Fig. 4.18 Sizes of needles or cannulas according to the shape of the threads. (**a**) Multidirectional cogged thread (N Cogged Multi). (**b**) Micropunching thread (NFix). (**c**) Multifilament thread (N scaffold). (**d**) Spring type (N derma spring)

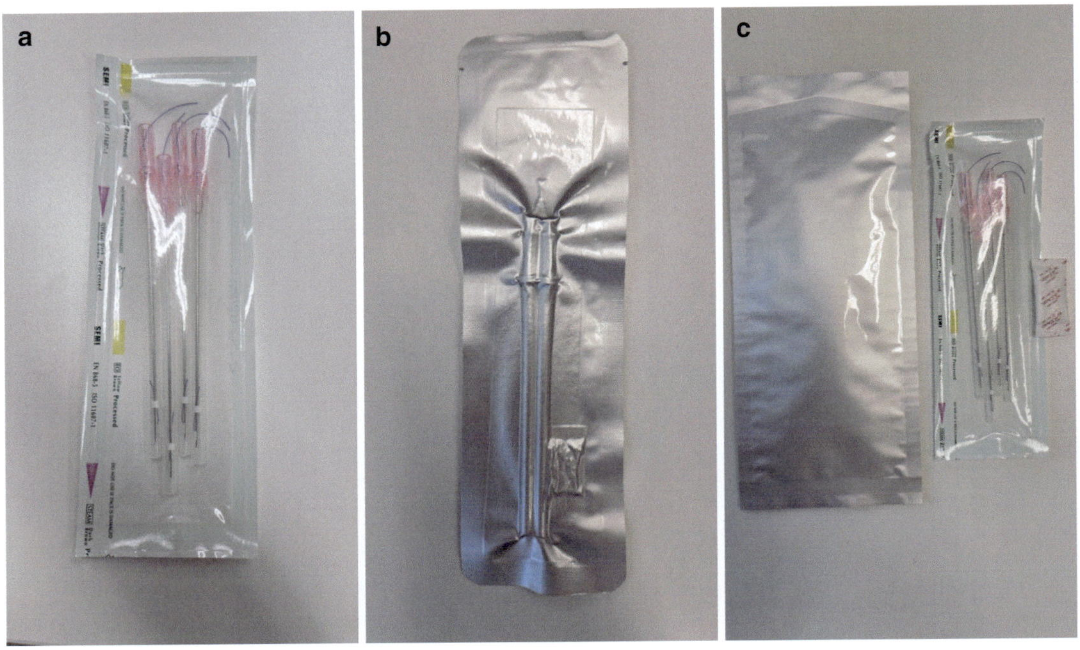

Fig. 4.19 Packaging. (**a**) Primary packaging (EO gas packing pouch). (**b**) Vacuum packaging. (**c**) Secondary packaging (aluminum pouch + silica gel)

conditions of temperature and humidity to eliminate surface bacteria. Afterward, sufficient aeration is performed to remove and purify the EO gas (Fig. 4.20).

EO gas sterilization is conducted under specific conditions of temperature and humidity, typically at a temperature of about 38–60 °C and a relative humidity of 40–80%. The sterilization time ranges from 1 to 6 hours. After sterilization is complete, a repeated process of vacuum and air infusion is carried out to ensure aeration for at least 3 hours, which is essential for the complete removal of the toxic EO gas.

4.2.5 Labelling and Storage

Most thread manufacturers set the expiration date based on the time when the product is exposed to the most extreme conditions, typically labeling only the date related to sterilization with a lot number (Fig. 4.21). However, some companies occasionally engrave a serial number that includes both the production date and the sterilization date to inform about the management status of the product.

The typical duration from the start to the end of production is between 5 and 7 days, and the shorter this period, the better it minimizes the thread's exposure to moisture in the air. Additionally, since the manufacturing process does not complete in a single day, the method of labeling and storing finished products, semifinished products, packaged products, etc., at the end of each workday is also very important. The longer the thread is exposed in a cleanroom where temperature and humidity are maintained, the more gradual the degradation of the thread becomes. Therefore, the method and duration of storing the thread in an environment with well-maintained humidity are critical factors that determine the quality of the thread used during procedures (Fig. 4.22).

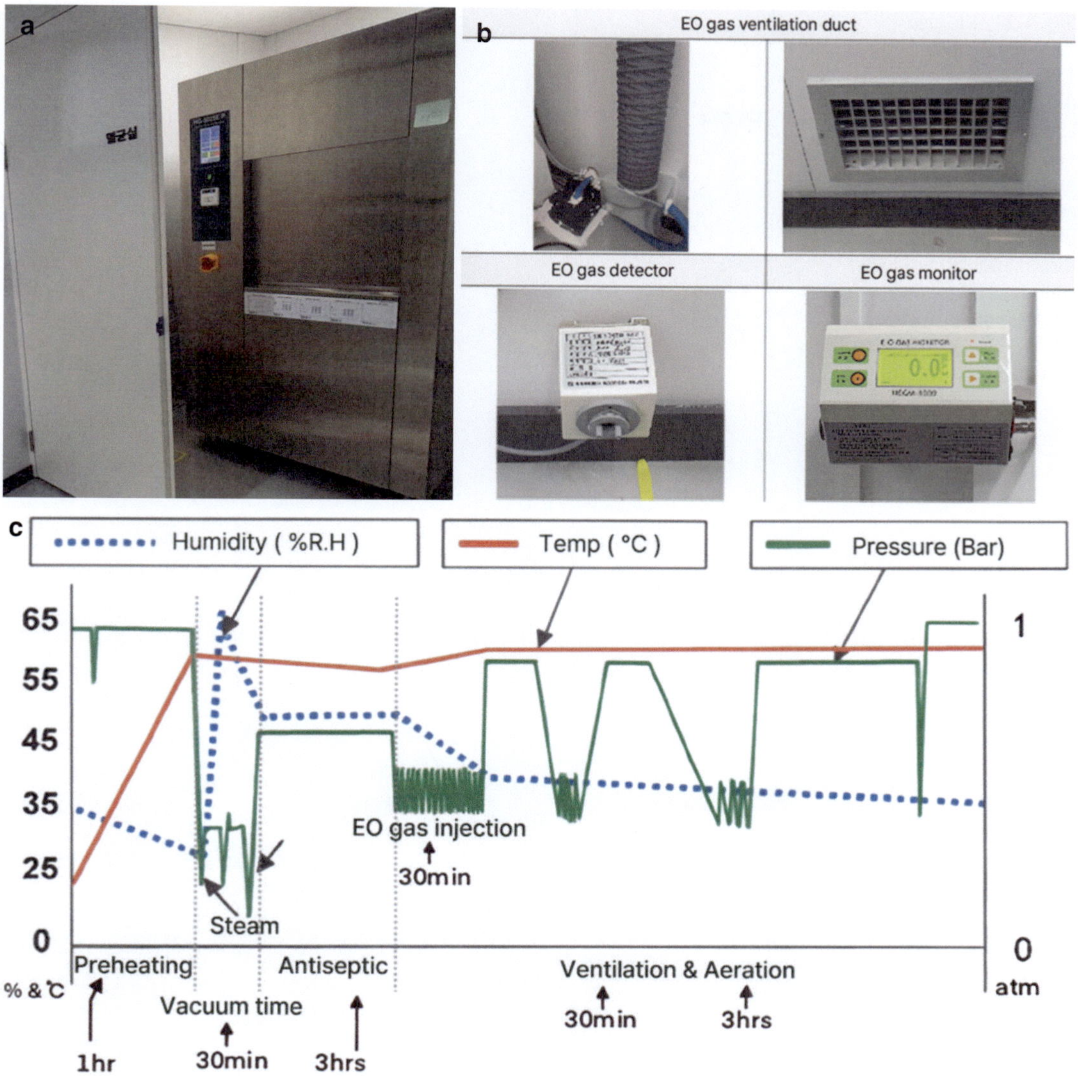

Fig. 4.20 Temperature and humidity exposure of the thread during the sterilization process. The sterilization process occurs under conditions where the thread is most susceptible to degradation. (**a**) Sterilization machine. (**b**) EO gas sterilization system. (**c**) Appropriate humidity and temperature (RH relative humidity)

Fig. 4.21 Labeling. N Fix (NFinders Co., South Korea)

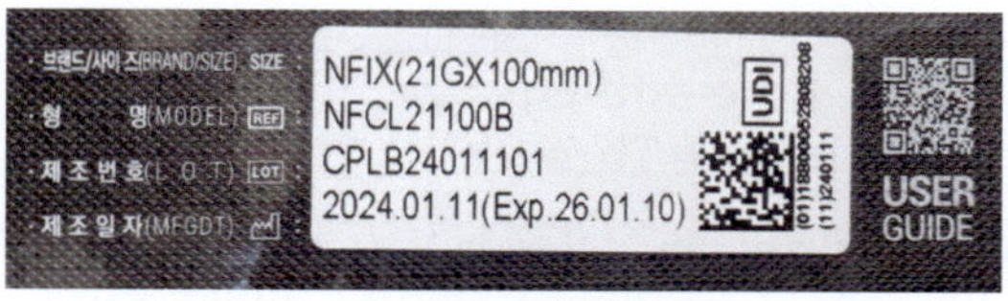

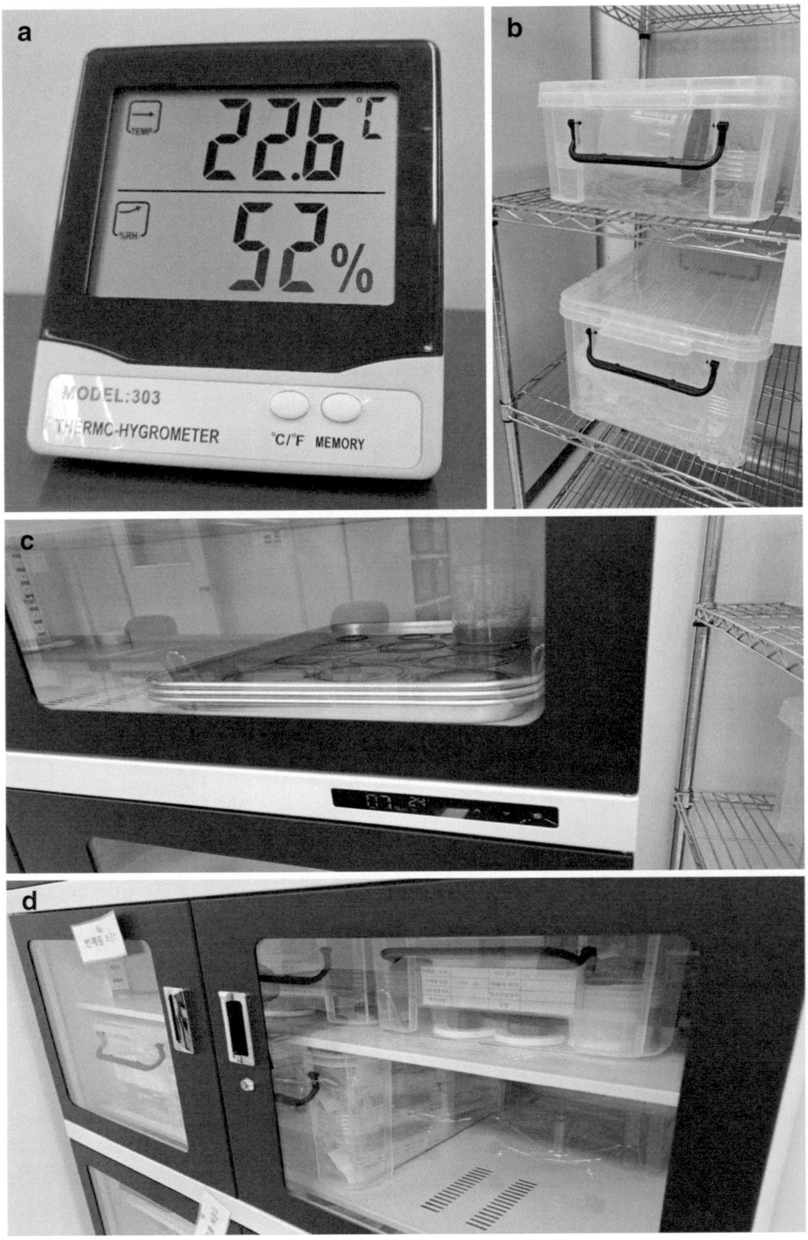

Fig. 4.22 Storage conditions. (**a**) Thermohygrometer in the cleanroom. (**b**) Living boxes are vulnerable to cleanroom humidity. (**c**) Storage conditions after the end of the workday. (**d**) Raw thread, molded products, semifinished products, storage conditions: 24 °C, 7% RH (relative humidity)

4.3 Role and Effects of the Thread

The role of the thread used for lifting can be broadly divided into two main functions. One is the physical role of the thread's structure and shape, which supports sagging tissue and holds it in place to prevent it from descending. The other is the chemical effect as a foreign body that stimulates collagen formation (fibrosis) in the surrounding tissue.

The mechanical effect depends on whether the cog or cone is designed to effectively engage the tissue, whether it is strong enough to maintain the tissue in place, and whether the core is robust enough to withstand the forces exerted by the facial muscles and gravity while the tissue is elevated. Additionally, since lifting involves pulling down tissue upward and maintaining that position, the ability to keep the elevated tissue from descending is also crucial. If the thread slips from the fixation point, the entire thread that is engaged with the tissue may migrate downward, negating the lifting effect. Consequently, the mechanical effect is determined by the size and design of the cog, the method of production, and the USP size of the thread.

The chemical effect primarily involves the well-known foreign body reaction (Figs. 4.23 and 4.24). This includes an inflammatory response, collagen stimulation, material degradation, and simultaneous collagen accumulation [3]. Protein absorption begins with neutrophil and macrophage infiltration upon insertion. The second aspect is the ability to act as a scaffold through cell-to-cell reactions, mediation, and attachment. A fibrosis process forms around the PDO thread, which is associated with myofibroblasts and giant cell macrophages. Generally, many studies describe the formation of a collagen column following the mechanical effect, with a duration of over one year reported in the literature. However, in patients who have undergone thread lifting, there are cases where strong fibrosis remains after a facelift and cases where it does not (Fig. 4.24). Therefore, the thickness of such capsules can vary due to multiple factors, indicating that further research is needed.

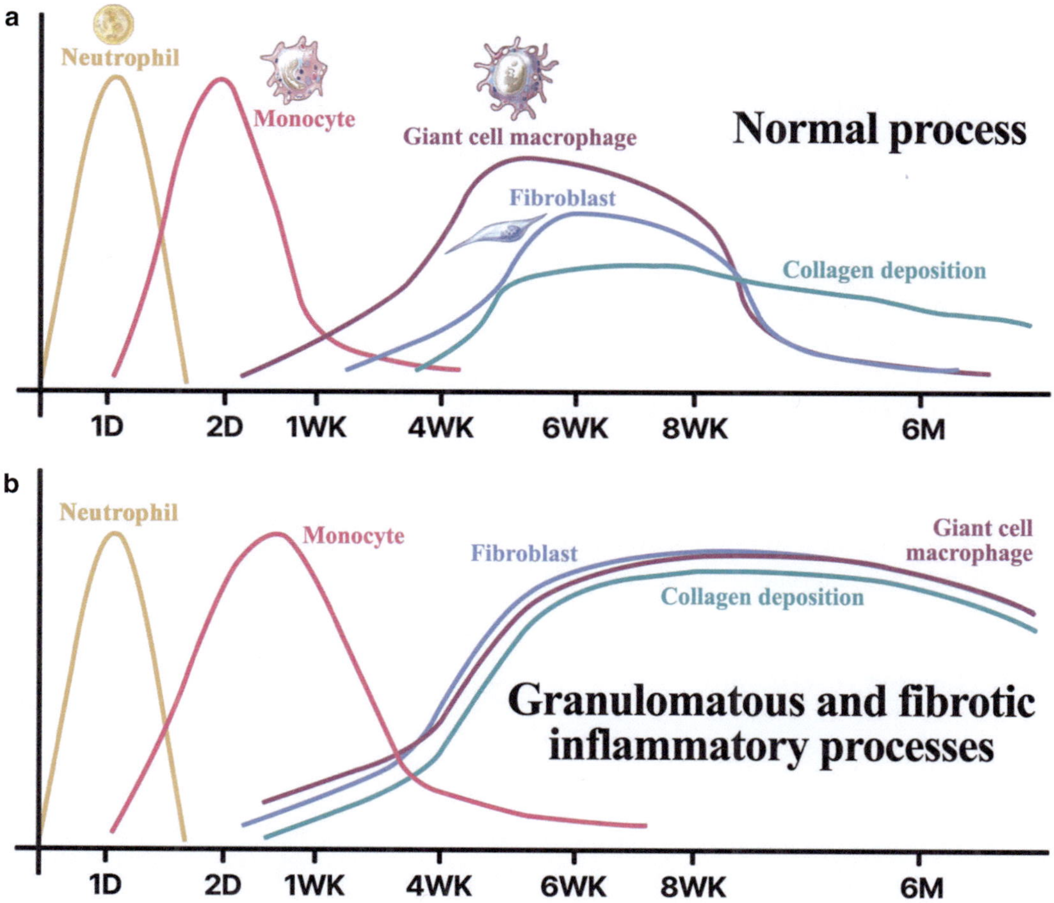

Fig. 4.23 Normal wound healing process (**a**) and foreign body reaction (**b**)

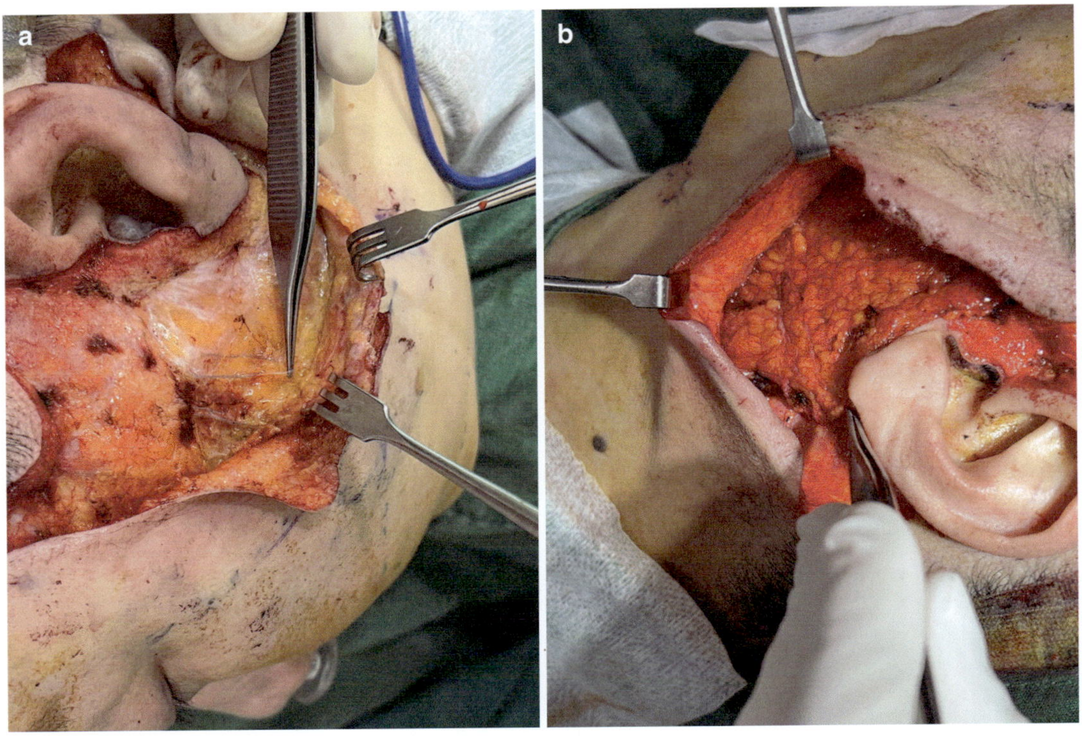

Fig. 4.24 Previously inserted thread discovered during rhytidectomy surgery. The collagen column (fibrosis) surrounding the thread generated by the chemical effect. (**a**) Thread found in the midface and the surrounding collagen column. (**b**) Thread found in the lower face and the surrounding collagen column

4.4 Differences in Properties Based on Types and Shapes of Threads

Threads can be classified based on various criteria. First, by shape, there are cogged threads, mesh types, screw types, cog-mesh, and mono threads. Mono threads are available in several forms, including simple mono threads, double-mono threads, and multi-mono thread types.

4.4.1 Cogged Thread Form

Cogged threads are generally categorized into three types: bidirectional cog, which have cogs oriented in opposite directions on either side of a non-cog area; monodirectional cogs, which lack a non-cog area; and multidirectional cogged threads, which have cogs distributed in various directions within a certain range. These threads are designed to lift tissue and may also include bidirectional cogs paired to prevent already lifted tissue from sagging again (Fig. 4.25). However,

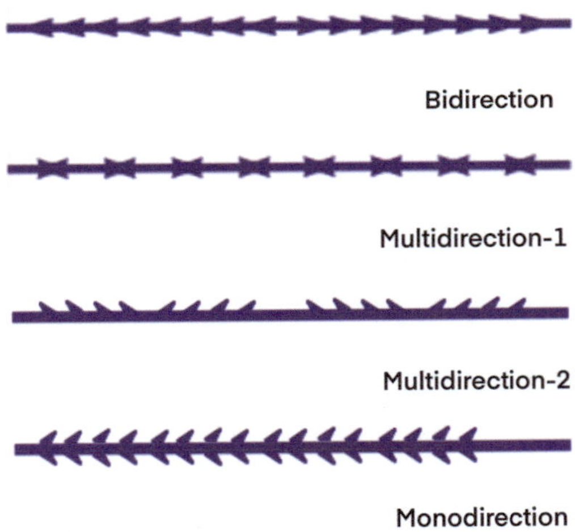

Fig. 4.25 Various types of threads based on cog direction

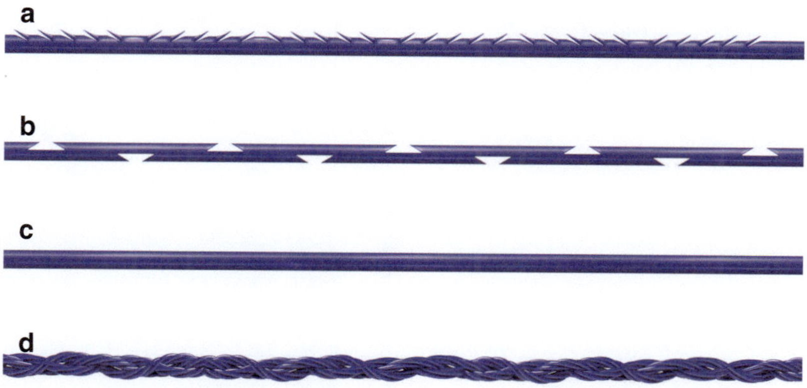

Fig. 4.26 Types of threads from Nfinders company. (**a**) Multidirectional cogged thread (N Cogged Multi). (**b**) Micropuncture thread (NFix). (**c**) Plain thread. (**d**) Scaffold volumizing thread

since each company may have different designs that are subject to approval or patent, the shapes can vary (Fig. 4.26).

Cogged threads can be divided into two main parts: the cog and the core. The thickness of the core is related to the degree of mass degradation of the thread, which affects how long the mechanical effect can be maintained. The cog determines how well it attaches to the tissue (attachment) and whether it detaches easily (detachment).

Factors influencing the capability of the cog include its shape (height, base area, total length, angle, etc.), surface differences due to manufacturing methods, and elasticity. The shape of the cog is primarily related to its ability to engage tissue, while the total length and angle determine the potential area for tissue engagement; a larger area allows for a more stable tissue hold (Fig. 4.27, Table 4.4). The base area and total length of the cog affect its strength, which is beneficial for heavier patients, but can complicate matters if dimpling occurs. Surface roughness impacts the surrounding tissue response; higher roughness enhances cell adhesion, strength, and proliferation, promoting a foreign body reaction. Molding-type threads typically exhibit relatively high roughness, and in contrast to other biomaterials, PDO threads, which are absorbed in a short time, may benefit from slight roughness in terms of chemical effects.

4.4.2 Volumizing Thread

Mesh type and screw type threads are products designed for volumizing. The mesh type aims to generate a significant amount of new collagen through the foreign body reaction that occurs around multiple threads. While a uniformly shaped mesh thread has the advantage of covering a relatively wide area, it may deform into a planar structure under vertical pressure once inserted into the body. Mesh threads made by twisting several mono threads together are used to achieve volumizing effects in a relatively narrow area and are often inserted just beneath the dermis for rejuvenation purposes (Fig. 4.28). The screw type serves the same role and purpose but is thought to have a greater structural integrity while causing less foreign body reaction compared to mesh. However, improper insertion can lead to nodules due to capsulization.

Cog-mesh threads are designed to combine the advantages of cog threads and mesh. Based on the premise that the foreign body reaction occurs at the interface between the thread and tis-

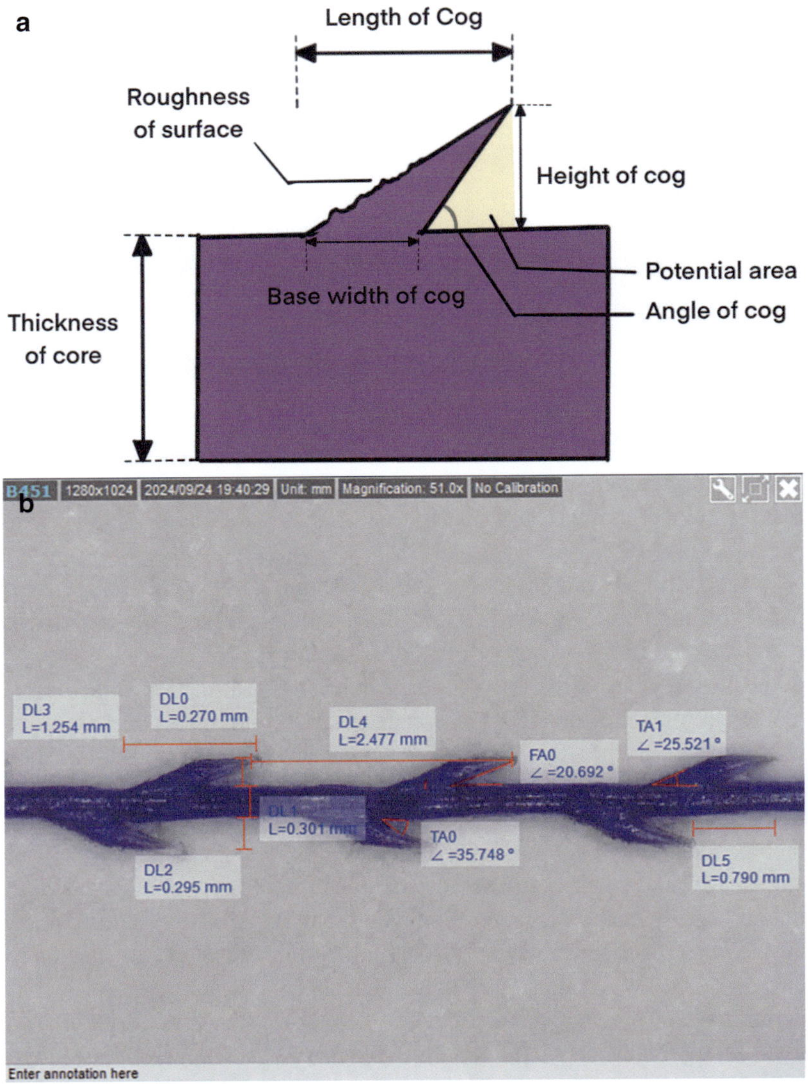

Fig. 4.27 Comparison of various cogged thread parameters. (**a**) Schematic diagram. (**b**) Actual thread measurement

sue, cog-mesh threads leverage the neocollagenesis capability of mesh while compensating for the difficulty in maintaining shape with cogged threads, allowing for a lifting effect as well (Fig. 4.29). However, since the cogs are stacked on the mesh, the height of the cogs that can actually engage the tissue is limited.

Mono threads are very thin products designed for direct insertion into the dermis, aiming to induce collagenesis in the dermal layer for skin rejuvenation effects. The sharp cannula containing the thread is designed to ensure that the entire thread is inserted into the dermis during the insertion and removal process, allowing for multiple

Table 4.4 Comparison of various cogged thread parameters

Product	Total length	Length for each section (mm)	Thickness of core	Ht of cog	Length of cog	Inter-cog distance	Number of cogs	Angle of cog
A product	185	20/30/6/58/71	0.30	0.28	1.2	2.5	12 + 24	35
B product	183	25/35/7/46/70	0.31	0.33	1.1	2.0	18 + 24	50
C product	183	20/38/7/49/69	0.30	0.23	2.0	3.0	13 + 17	30
D product	150	25/36/8/48/33	0.29	0.32	1.1	1.5	24 + 32	52
E product	182	27/89/66	0.38	0.25	1.6	2.1	28	40
F product	152	24/59/69	0.29	0.18	1.9	1.9	16	55
G product	175	25/41/5/49/55	0.33	0.19	0.6	1.5	27 + 32	33

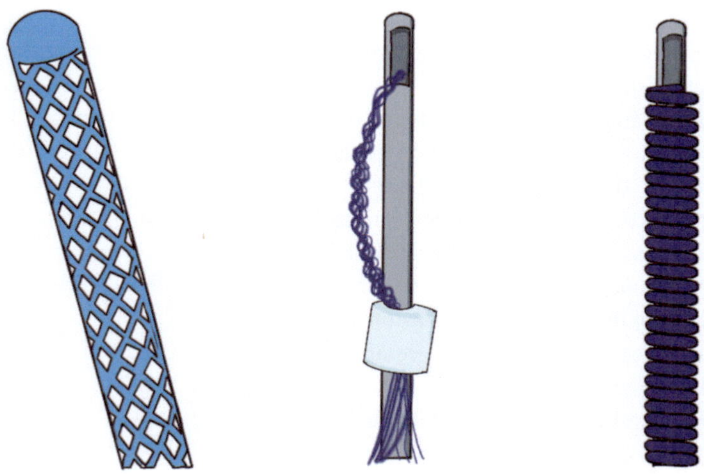

Fig. 4.28 Mesh type and screw type threads for volumizing effects

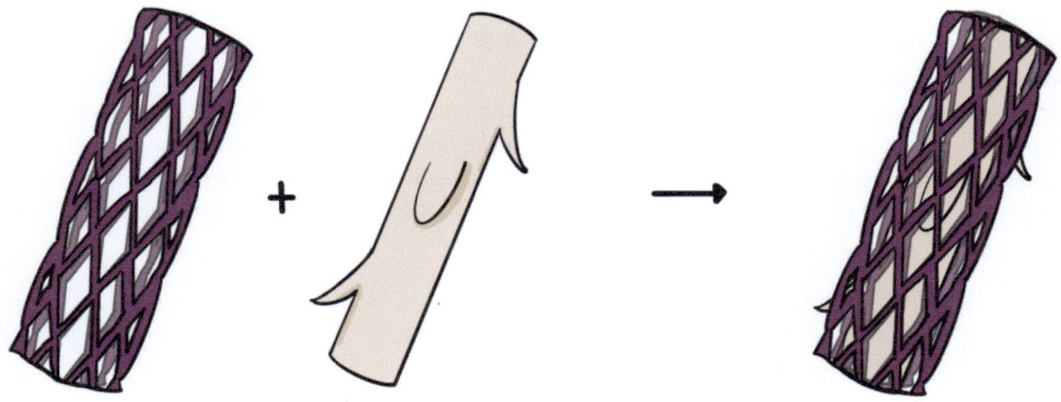

Fig. 4.29 Form of threads combining mesh and cogged threads

threads to be placed in a single motion, which is why they are often produced as double mono or multiple mono threads.

4.4.3 Thickness of the Thread

The thickness of the thread is a crucial factor that the practitioner must decide upon during the procedure, along with the length of the thread, the number of threads, the shape of the thread, the insertion method, and the insertion location. The thickness of the thread largely determines the size of the cannula used.

Thread thickness is a fundamental aspect that can predict physical strength. Factors to consider when selecting thickness include the patient's skin thickness, the degree of soft tissue sagging, the history of previous foreign body insertions, surgical history, and the desired movement of the soft tissue, including the amount and direction of movement, as well as the location on the face.

Thicker threads facilitate the movement of soft tissue using strong physical properties, but patients may experience a sensation of foreignness, and undesirable outcomes such as protrusion or skin transparency may occur. Conversely, thinner threads may result in a relatively diminished physical lifting effect.

The insertion location should be deeper for thicker threads and shallower for thinner threads, and the dual-layer technique based on thickness will be described in Chap. 5. All threads are labeled with USP, which is defined according to the United States Pharmacopeia. The standards for synthetic absorbable surgical sutures and nonabsorbable surgical sutures differ slightly in the pharmacopeia. The USP and EP (European Pharmacopeia) present slightly different specifications, and this section will describe the USP (Fig. 4.30).

USP	METRIC	Sutures Diamater in mm
3	6	0.600-0.699
2	5	0.500-0.599
1	4	0.400-0.499
0	3.5	0.350-0.399
2/0	3	0.200-0.249
3/0	2	0.150-0.199
4/0	1.5	0.100-0.149
5/0	1	0.070-0.099
6/0	0.7	0.050-0.069
7/0	0.5	0.040-0.049
8/0	0.4	0.030-0.039
9/0	0.3	0.030-0.039
10/0	0.2	0.020-0.029

Fig. 4.30 Thickness of threads

4.5 Conclusion

Thread lifting is a widely used procedure worldwide, but various results can occur depending on the practitioner and the patient, leading to ongoing skepticism regarding its effectiveness and durability. However, better outcomes are observed in patients with more favorable indications, especially when performed using techniques that effectively utilize vectors. Additionally, understanding the technique, the materials of the threads, the shapes of the cogs, and the manufacturing processes is crucial for achieving better results. It is particularly important to recognize that PDO threads exhibit weaknesses in the amorphous region and that differences in packaging methods exist among manufacturers. Furthermore, understanding polymers and the advantages and disadvantages of currently marketed polymers such as PDO, PLLA, PCL, and PP is essential.

References

1. Márquez Y, et al. Influence of pH on morphology and structure during hydrolytic degradation of the segmented GL-b-[GL-co-TMC-co-CL]-b-GL copolymer. Fibers. 2015;3(3):348–72.
2. Hufenus R, Yan Y, Dauner M, Kikutani T. Melt-spun fibers for textile applications. Materials (Basel). 2020;13(19):4298. https://doi.org/10.3390/ma13194298.
3. Yoon JH, Kim SS, Oh SM, Kim BC, Jung W. Tissue changes over time after polydioxanone thread insertion: an animal study with pigs. J Cosmet Dermatol. 2019;18(3):885–91. https://doi.org/10.1111/jocd.12718.

5 Thread Lifting Techniques

Contents

Thread lifting is considered one of the most invasive procedures among minimally invasive techniques. This indicates that patients desire more noticeable effects, which can be a burden for the physician. While many literatures report effective thread lifting techniques, it is often challenging to select a standard procedure. One of the main reasons for this difficulty is that most studies are based on clinical experiences, making it hard to exclude the subjective perceptions of the practitioners. There needs to be a more fundamental consideration and analysis in designing an effective thread lifting method. Additionally, understanding the limitations and finding the meaning and effects of thread lifting for each patient is essential for performing a more sophisticated thread lifting procedure. In other words, thread lifting is a procedure that inevitably yields varying results

W. Lee, K. H. Jung, *Lifting Techniques in Plastic Surgery*,
https://doi.org/10.1007/978-981-96-4820-7_5

depending on the physician's skills, the patient's condition, and the advantages and disadvantages of the threads used. This chapter will outline the general knowledge necessary for thread lifting procedures and emphasize that physicians should have their own methods tailored to individual patients among the various techniques described.

5.1 Indications for Thread Lifting

Generally, the suitable patient population for thread lifting includes those who (1) have mild skin laxity and (2) exhibit mild to moderate sagging of the skin and subcutaneous tissue, typically aged 30 to 49 years. In patients over 50, the effectiveness of thread lifting lasting more than 6 months is reported to be only 18%, with a significantly higher risk of dimpling or infection [1]. However, in practice, many patients outside these criteria seek thread lifting, and a considerable number of individuals in their 50s also pursue this procedure. Furthermore, many patients have been consistently receiving treatments such as fillers, fat grafting, or energy-based devices (EBD), making it difficult to judge solely based on age.

Based on the following conditions, if the degree of effectiveness and duration can be anticipated and sufficient explanations are provided to the patient, thread lifting can be considered a procedure applicable to all patients. First, if skin laxity is mild, patients can be included in the group eligible for thread lifting regardless of the degree of volume loss. Even if skin laxity is moderate, significant effects can still be achieved if the volume loss is not severe (Table 5.1). Here, volume loss does not refer to an absolute amount of fat. If volume restoration has been performed through fillers or fat grafting, it should be evaluated based on the degree of reduction. Similarly, if a patient has undergone a facelift to improve skin laxity, good results can be obtained with thread lifting alone. However, patients who exhibit decreased elasticity when pinching the cheek skin may not see significant effects.

Additionally, in patients with a high body mass index (BMI), excessive fat in the face can hinder the lifting effect due to weight, and even if the lower facial tissues are adequately lifted, there may be issues with maintenance or an overly wide midface appearance, necessitating caution.

Table 5.1 Indications for thread lifting. Both variables are variable

Skin laxity / Volume loss	Mild	Moderate	Severe
Mild	Thread lifting	Thread lifting	Mini-lifting Conventional facelift
Moderate	Thread lifting Mini-lifting	Thread lifting Mini-lifting	Conventional facelift
Severe	Thread lifting Mini-lifting	Conventional facelift Mini-lifting	Conventional facelift
Relative contraindication: severe skin ptosis and minimal soft tissue elasticity			

5.2 Principles of Thread Lifting

When patients are asked why they seek thread lifting, responses vary from improvement of wrinkles, changes in facial shape, to improve of deepening lines when making expressions. However, fundamentally, the reason patients seek thread lifting is the desire to "look younger." Therefore, rather than being led by the patients, practitioners must have their own criteria and principles for judgment.

The principles of thread lifting should follow the "principles of lifting" described in Chap. 2. As people age, volume deflation, bone absorption, and skin loosening cause tissues to sag, leading to a face that appears divided into multiple units due to retaining ligaments (Fig. 5.1). The horizontal axis can be broadly divided into the midface and lower face, while the vertical axis distinguishes between medial and lateral. Ultimately, the goal of lifting should be to elevate the tissues that have descended downward to the midface (lateral cheek fat compartment repositioning), move the tissues that have shifted medially back to the lateral side (jowl fat and malar fat pad repositioning), and connect the separated malar fat pad and nasolabial fat to restore a smooth face, making it appear as a single unit again.

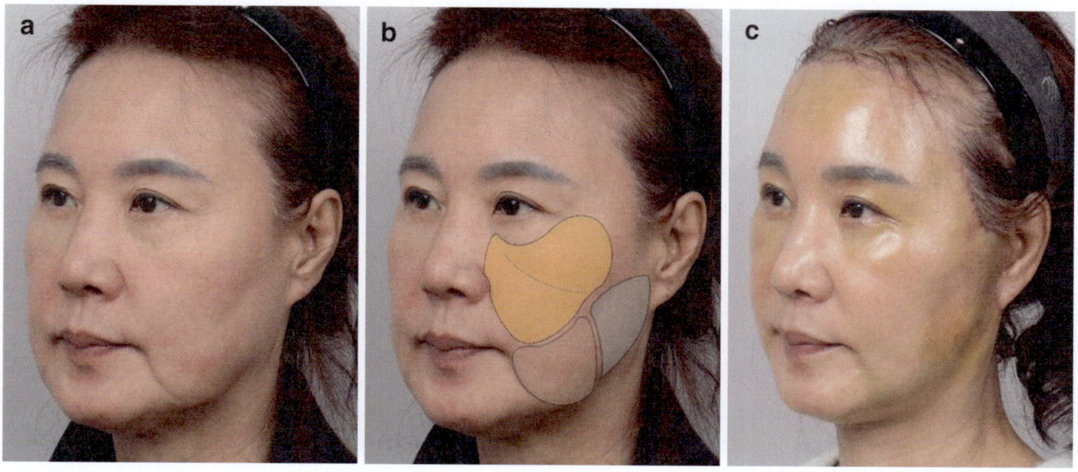

Fig. 5.1 Patients with a multi-unit appearance of the face due to aging. (**a**) Preoperative. (**b**) Schematic diagram. The boundary between the midface (orange) and lower face becomes distinct, with the lower face divided into medial (brown color) and lateral (gray color) areas by the masseteric ligament, and the midface appearing divided into two regions by the zygomatic cutaneous ligament. (**c**) Post-rhytidectomy, the boundaries disappear, restoring a single unit appearance

5.3 Vectors of Thread Lifting

The vector of thread lifting is traditionally described as "perpendicular to the wrinkle," with the direction being superolateral. This indicates that the tissues have descended in an inferomedial direction. There are two main reasons for this inferomedial descent of tissues: gravity (inferior) and the facial expression muscles (medial or lateral). While gravity applies uniformly to everyone, the facial expression muscles vary from person to person and by facial region, necessitating the consideration of these factors when determining the vector.

The facial muscles of the midface consist of four main muscles: the levator labii superioris (LLS), the levator labii superioris alae nasi (LLSAN), the zygomatic major (Zmj), and the zygomatic minor (Zmi). The LLS and LLSAN exhibit vertical movement, while the Zmj and Zmi have oblique movements (Fig. 5.2). Therefore, to lift tissues that are positioned laterally to the mid-pupil, a superolateral vector should be used, while a superior vector should be employed to lift tissues that have descended medially to the mid-pupil.

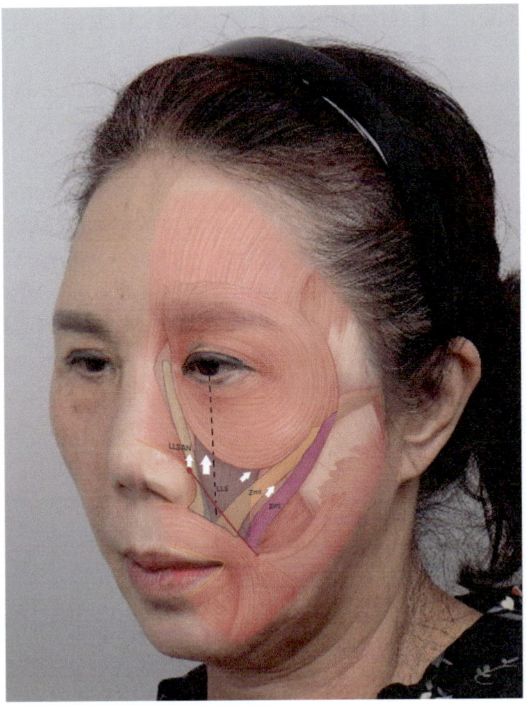

Fig. 5.2 Direction of movement of midface facial muscles. Medial is shown as a vertical direction, while lateral exhibits a superolateral vector based on the mid-pupil. LLSAN (levator labii superioris alae nasi), LLS (levator labii superioris), Zmi (zygomatic minor), Zmj (zygomatic major)

In the lower face, the medial area, based on the masseteric retaining ligament, is significantly influenced by the depressor anguli oris (DAO) and the platysma. Particularly, the hyperactivation of the DAO due to aging exerts a strong force that moves tissues inferomedially, especially in the medial direction, while the loosening of the platysma tends to pull tissues inferiorly (Fig. 5.3). Therefore, using both vertical and lateral vectors in this area can yield good results.

The masseter muscle, particularly its superficial part, occupies the largest area of the lower lateral face. Originating from the maxillary process of the zygomatic arch and inserting at the angle of the mandible, it moves the soft tissue and skin superomedially. Consequently, the sagging of tissues in this region tends to follow an inferolateral direction, necessitating the use of a superomedial vector (Fig. 5.4).

By utilizing different vectors for each region, the threads naturally criss-cross, which offers advantages in retention compared to the fan technique when inserting the threads (criss-cross technique).

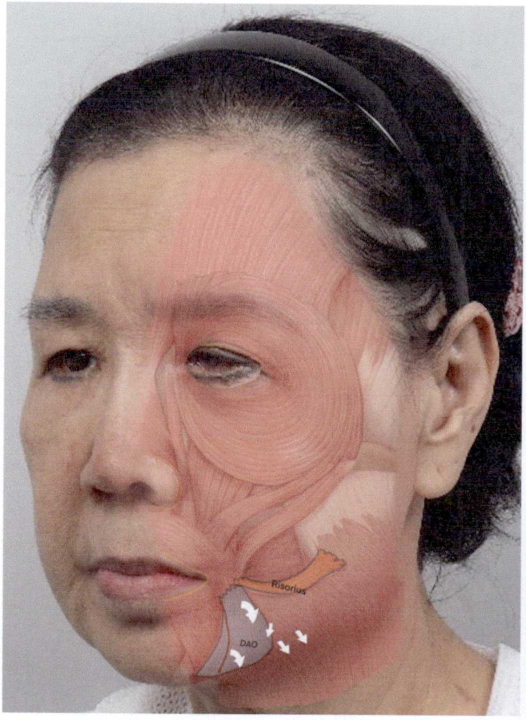

Fig. 5.3 Vector of the lower face. The lower-medial area is most affected by the DAO, contracting inferomedially around the modiolus, resembling the folding of a traditional fan

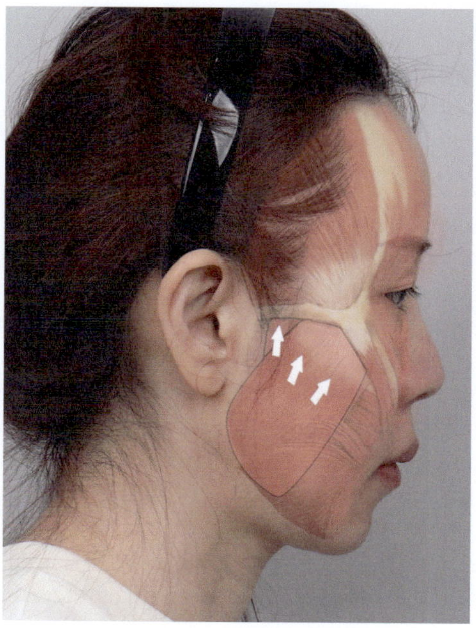

Fig. 5.4 Vector of the lower-lateral area. This area is most influenced by the masseter muscle, where the deep part exhibits a vertical vector while the superficial part shows a superomedial vector

5.4 Criss-Cross Technique

The criss-cross technique is a fundamental method of thread lifting that utilizes different vectors to maximize the lifting effect. Specifically, instead of using a fan technique with multiple threads emerging from a single entry point, this method involves inserting threads from 3 to 4 entry points in various directions to induce a more comprehensive lifting effect [2]. It is crucial to carefully assess the patient's sagging and understand the vectors before inserting the lifting threads (Figs. 5.5 and 5.6).

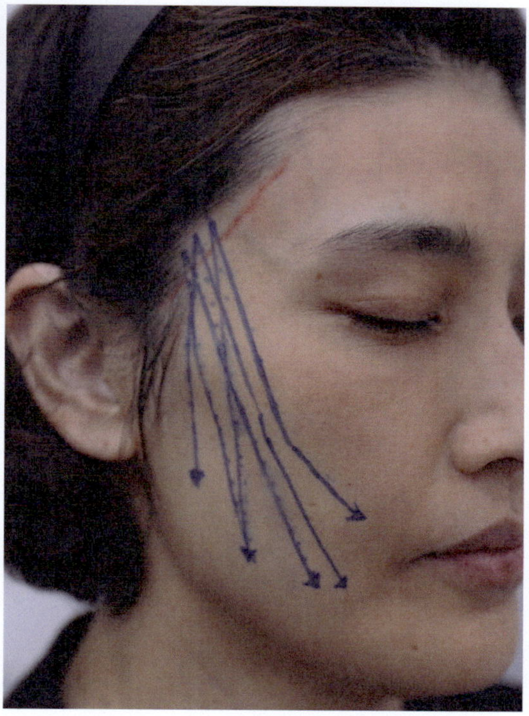

Fig. 5.5 Basic method of thread lifting. Insertion of threads using the criss-cross method based on the entry point

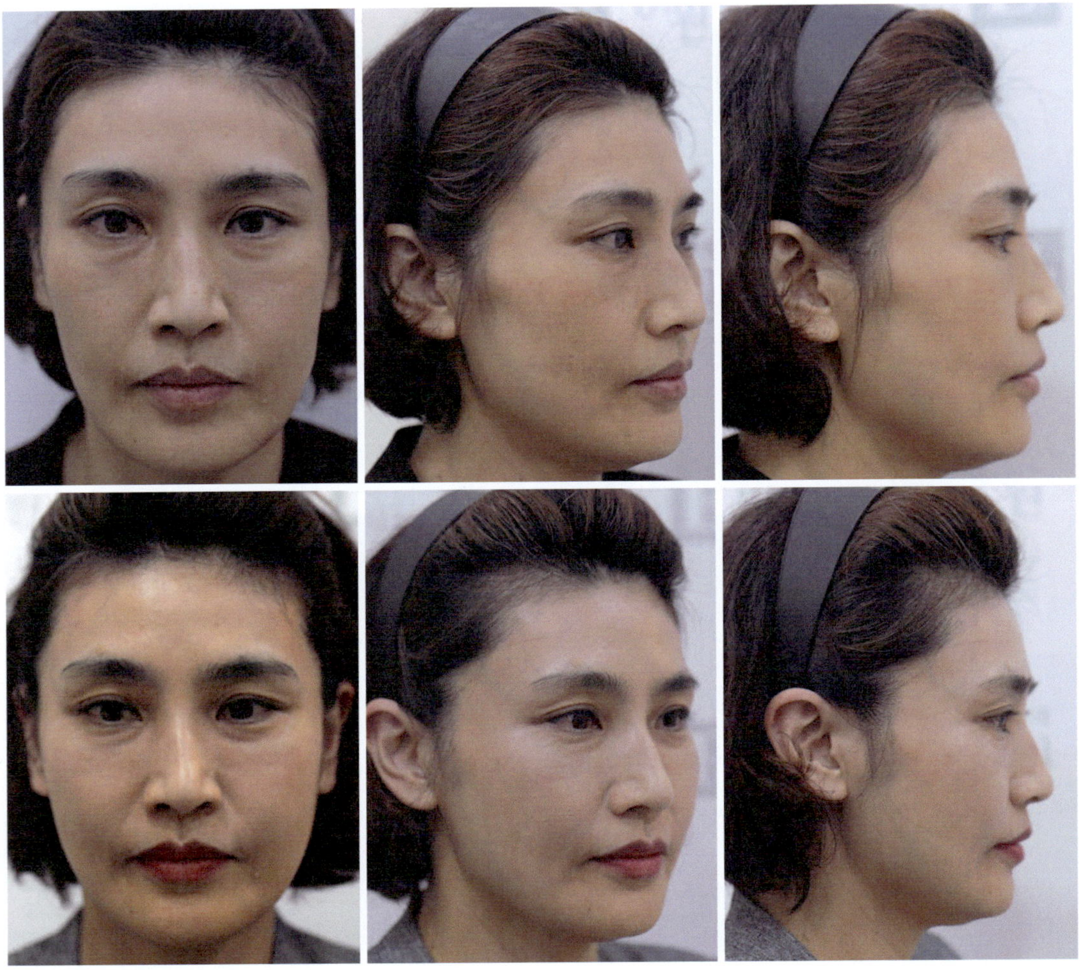

Fig. 5.6 Before and 3 months after thread lifting (criss-cross)

5.5 Reverse Technique

The typical direction for thread insertion is to anchor the upper part (anchoring fixed point) while treating the sagging lower part as the movable area. The reverse insertion technique involves inserting the thread in the opposite direction, starting from the movable area below and pulling the tissue upward. This method simplifies the procedure and allows for direct visualization of the area being lifted, potentially making it more effective. However, there is a risk of soft tissue depression or pigmentation at the entry point, necessitating proper post-procedure care. It is essential to inform patients that the insertion site may be noticeable immediately after the procedure and to take precautions to prevent complications such as protrusion of the threads over time.

For patients with a wide zygomatic arch, inserting the threads in the forward direction can lead to the cannula becoming shallow as it passes over the zygomatic arch, increasing the risk of dimpling. Therefore, the reverse insertion technique is particularly effective in these cases. However, most existing lifting threads are designed for forward insertion, which may limit their use in reverse insertion. It is advisable to select threads specifically designed for reverse insertion. Additionally, threads inserted in reverse tend to be positioned slightly lower than those inserted in the forward direction, so a combination of both methods can be beneficial.

5.6 Depth of Thread Insertion

Threads are inserted using a cannula, which typically navigates through loose planes between layers, regardless of the operator's attempts to manipulate them. There are two planes where the cannula can easily enter: the subcutaneous layer and the sub-SMAS layer. The commonly used entry points, such as the temporal area and parotid region, have a structure where subcutaneous fat lobules are stacked by fibrous septae, allowing for variable depth of insertion in the subcutaneous layer.

The optimal depth for thread placement is within the subcutaneous layer. Inserting threads at this depth allows for lifting based on the deep insertion pivot point of the retaining ligaments, resulting in more significant surface changes. Additionally, this method applies less load to the threads to achieve the same changes. However, if threads are inserted too superficially within the subcutaneous layer, the cogs may directly engage the dermis, leading to dimpling, or even if they do not directly contact the dermis, they may strongly pull on fibrous structures close to the dermis, causing wavelike deformations (Fig. 5.7). Therefore, using thinner threads for patients with thin skin can reduce this risk (double-layer technique).

Inserting threads into the surface layer of the SMAS is intended to tighten the SMAS rather than the skin. The SMAS has significantly lower stress-relaxation and creep properties compared to the skin, which may result in less visual lifting effect than inserting into the subcutaneous fat, but it can maintain the effect for a longer duration (Fig. 5.8).

The author does not recommend inserting threads into the sub-SMAS layer, as this plane

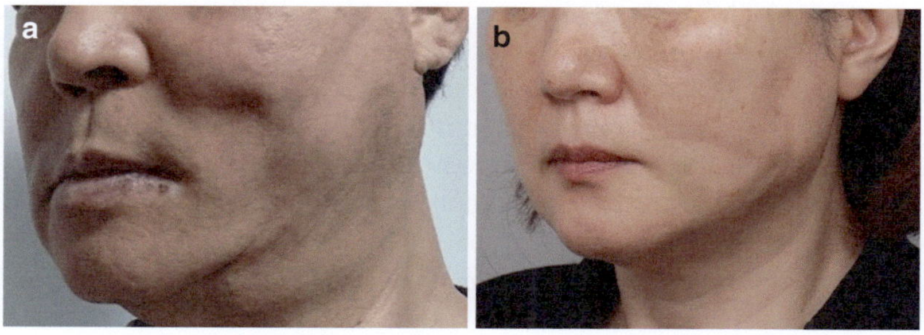

Fig. 5.7 Wavy appearance deformation. Inserting into the subcutaneous fat layer close to the dermis can lead to dimpling or wavelike deformations. (**a**) Strong dimple. (**b**) Wavy appearance

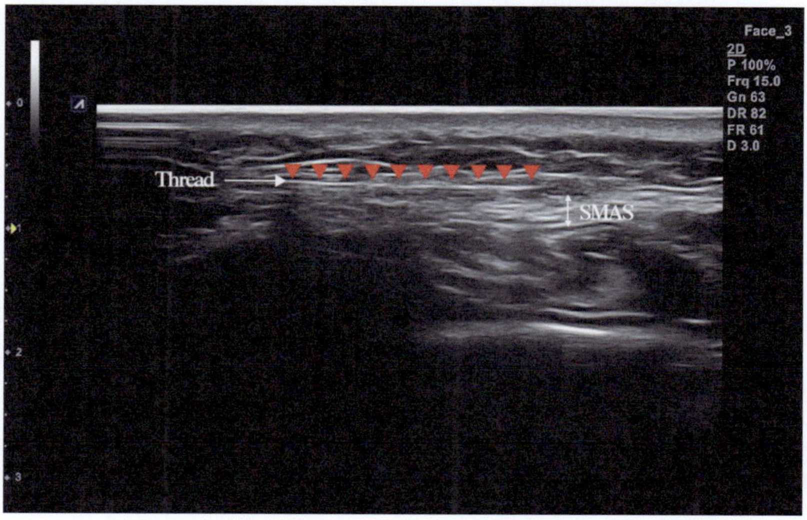

Fig. 5.8 Ultrasound image showing threads inserted just above the SMAS

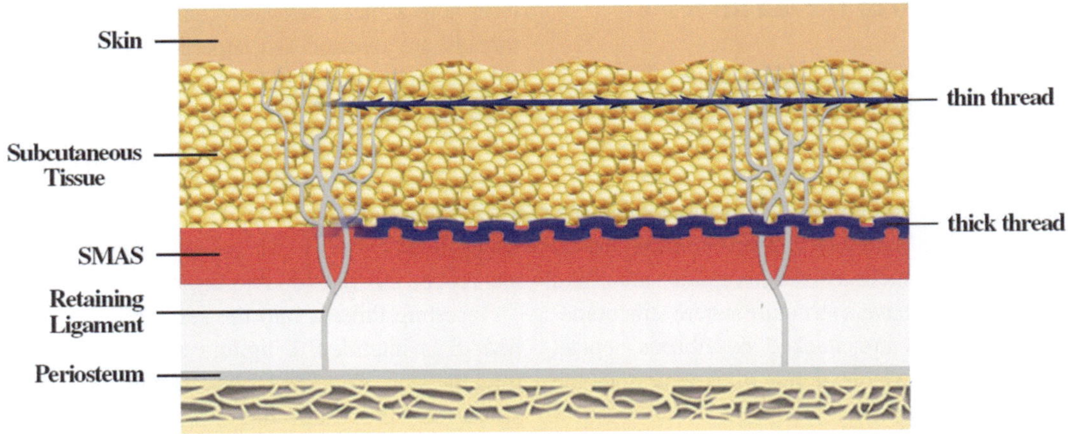

Fig. 5.9 Double-layer technique. Thinner threads are used in the subcutaneous fat layer, while thicker threads are used closer to the SMAS

contains numerous thick and firm deep parts of the retaining ligaments, making it difficult for the threads to function effectively and achieve a lifting effect. Additionally, if the cogs engage the masseteric muscle fascia, discomfort may occur with mastication, and there is a risk of damaging the transverse facial artery perforator. If this vessel is damaged, it can lead to severe hematoma throughout the cheek, including the oral mucosa, due to its connection to the buccal space.

Therefore, combining insertion methods into the not-too-superficial subcutaneous layer and the surface of the SMAS can yield better long-term results. When using the double-layer technique, it is safer to use thinner threads (N cog multi, 2-0, 21G, 150 mm, NFinders, South Korea) in the subcutaneous layer and relatively thicker threads (N Fix, No3, 19G 100mm, NFinders, South Korea) in the SMAS surface. In some cases, it may also be beneficial to use a pulling method that penetrates multiple layers to target the desired area (Fig. 5.9).

5.7 Double-Layer Technique

As mentioned above, the double-layer technique involves inserting thicker threads just above the SMAS and thinner threads into the subcutaneous fat. For threads like NFix, which have a strong cog design, the No. 3 thickness is quite substantial, increasing the risk of dimpling if inserted too close to the dermis, and they may also be palpable from the outside. Therefore, it is ideal to insert them closer to the deeper SMAS layer. However, to achieve a more pronounced lifting effect, the threads should be closer to the skin layer. In this case, using thinner threads to provide additional lifting in the subcutaneous fat layer is a very effective method (Figs. 5.10, 5.11, and 5.12).

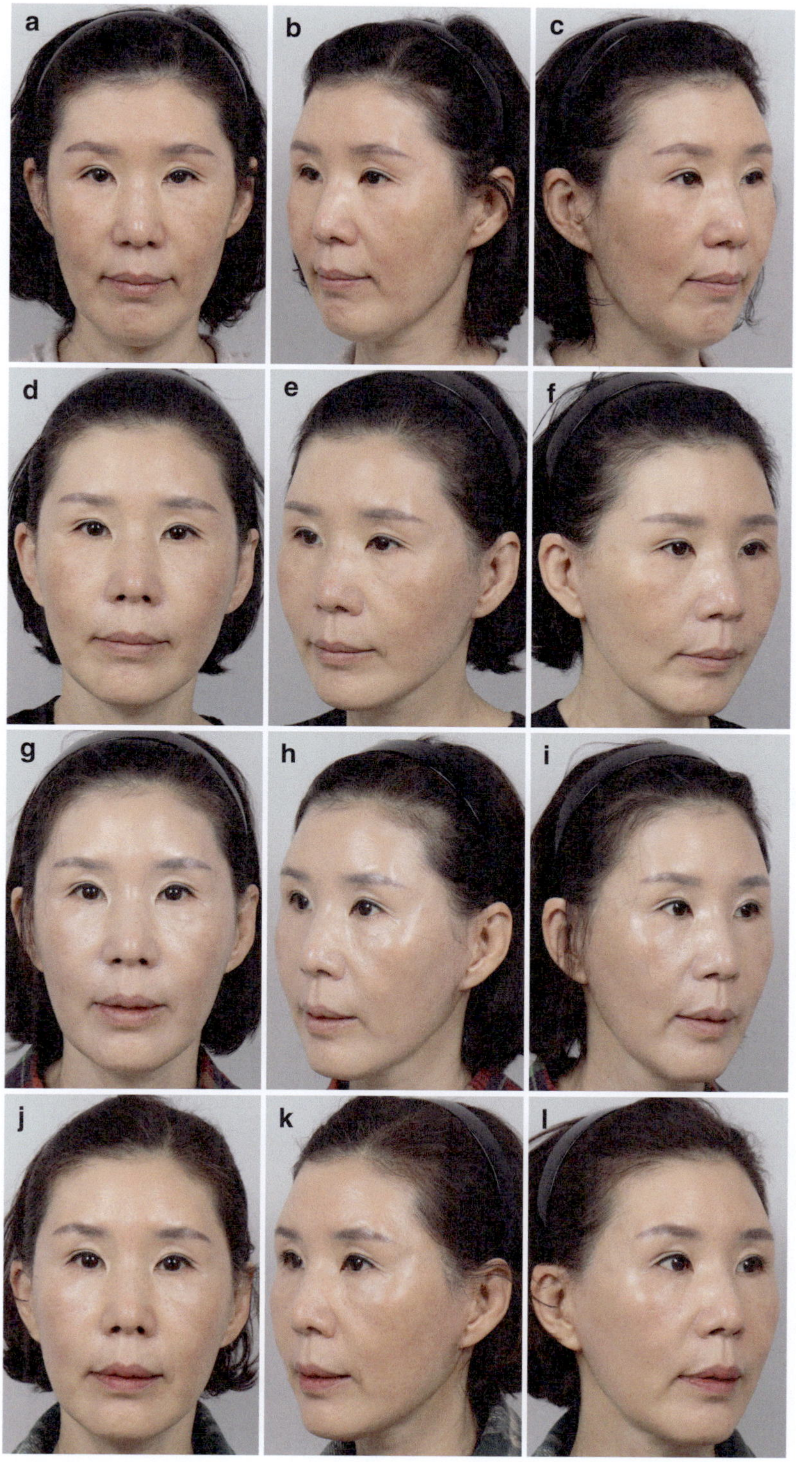

Fig. 5.10 Double lifting in a 60-year-old female patient. (**a–c**) Preoperative; (**d–f**) 1 month postoperative; (**g–i**) 3 months postoperative; (**j–l**) 6 months postoperative

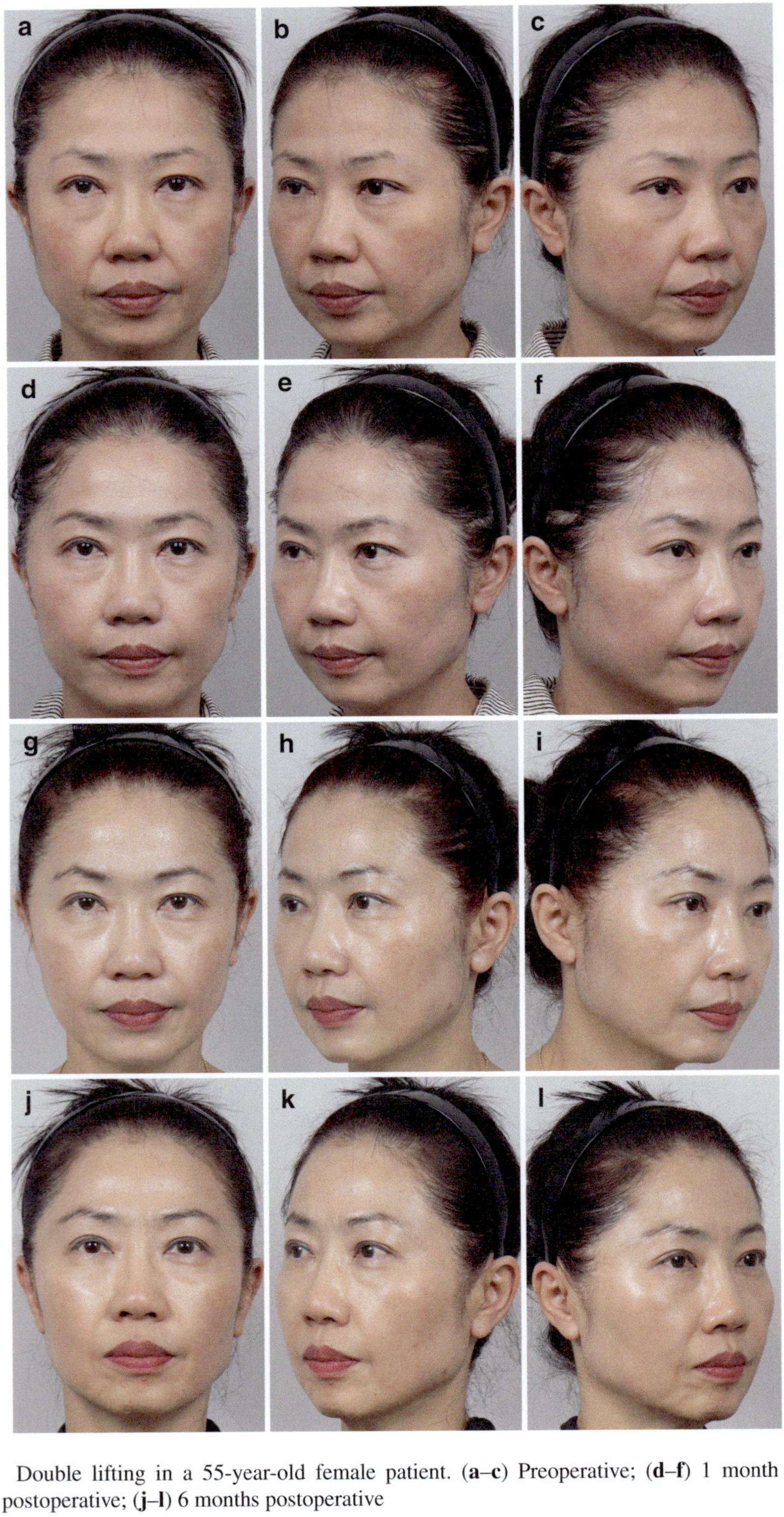

Fig. 5.11 Double lifting in a 55-year-old female patient. (**a–c**) Preoperative; (**d–f**) 1 month postoperative; (**g–i**) 3 months postoperative; (**j–l**) 6 months postoperative

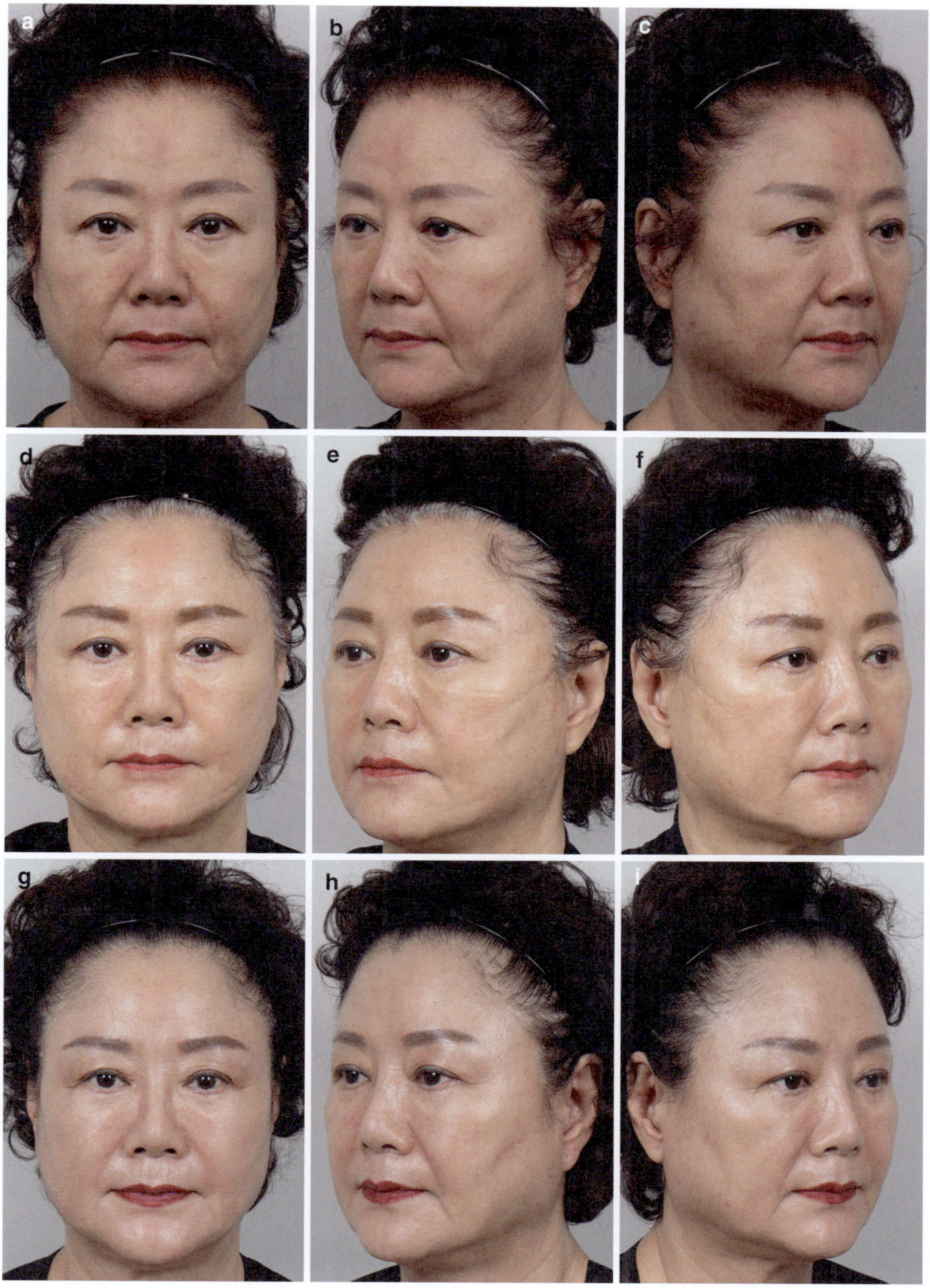

Fig. 5.12 Double lifting in a 55-year-old female patient. (**a–c**) Preoperative; (**d–f**) 3 months postoperative; (**g–i**) 6 months postoperative

5.8 Thread Lifting Method

To utilize the advantages of the criss-cross technique and prevent excessive widening of the zygomatic area, it is advisable to use multiple entry points. Typically, entry points are established along the temporal hairline, with the height determined between the lateral canthus and the eyebrow. The reasons for this are as follows: (1) using this area as an entry point allows the non-cog section of the commonly used floating type bidirectional thread to be positioned in the submalar hollowness beneath the zygomatic arch; (2) it tightens the zygomatic cutaneous ligament, enhancing its anchoring ability; and (3) it utilizes the zygomatic cutaneous ligament as a safety structure to prevent thread migration.

However, the entry points should be adjusted slightly for each patient based on their facial shape (length and size). The entry point is determined for anchoring purposes, but since the thread will settle approximately 0.5–1 cm lower than the insertion point, it is recommended to set the entry point slightly higher than the desired anchoring location. Therefore, placing the entry point inside the hairline increases the likelihood that the thread will be positioned where expected (Fig. 5.13).

5.8.1 Basic Method of Thread Lifting 1: Improvement of the Midface and Lower Face

While the thread lifting method may vary for each patient, a basic approach applicable to all patients is as follows: the midface is restored to fullness using short threads, while the tissue that has descended in the lower face is lifted and gathered from below the zygomatic arch (Fig. 5.14). In this process, the tissue in the lower medial area is lifted, indirectly supporting the midface tissue and achieving a natural improvement effect.

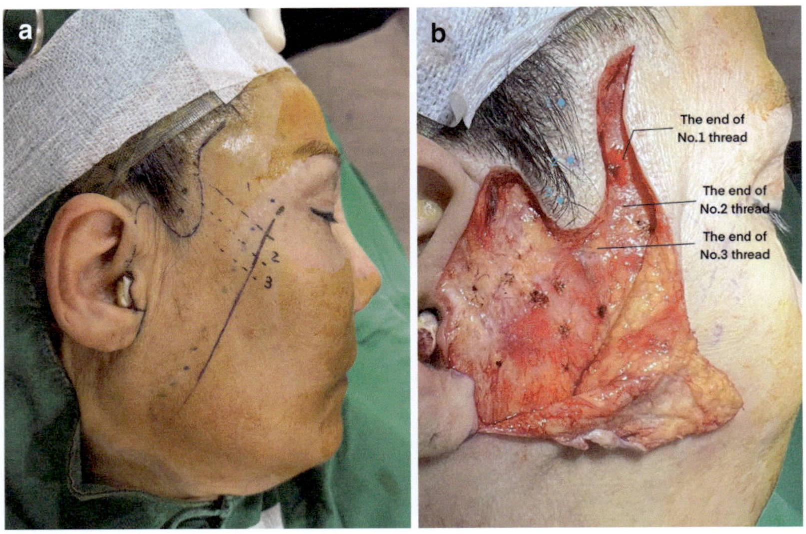

Fig. 5.13 Relationship between entry point and thread anchoring point. In a patient dissatisfied with the results of thread lifting who underwent facelift surgery, the anchoring point of the thread moved approximately 0.5–1 cm lower than the entry point. In case No. 1, where a single thread was inserted, it also settled lower, and in cases No. 2 and No. 3, where the threads were sutured together to form a loop, the anchoring point also settled lower. (**a**) preoperative design, (**b**) operative finding

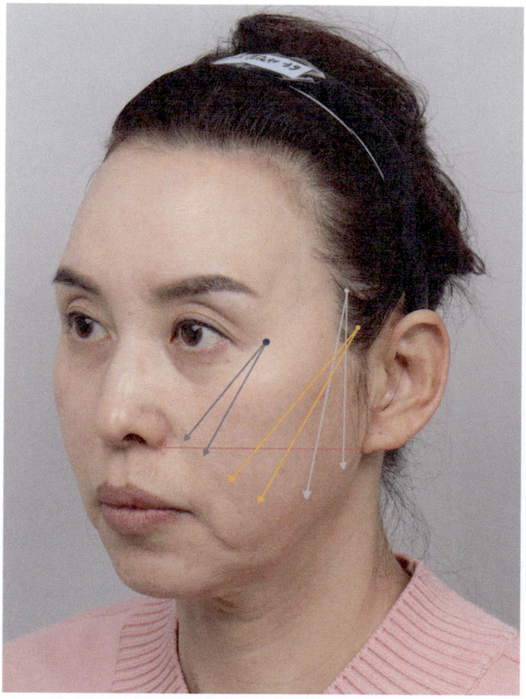

Fig. 5.14 Basic thread lifting method 1. Two threads are inserted from two entry points at the temple area, crossing at the zygomatic arch, with the midface being gathered from the lateral orbital rim to the malar fat pad and nasolabial fat pad. Pink horizontal line: the line connecting the nasal ala to the otobasion, serving as a baseline to separate the midface and lower face

5.8.2 Basic Method of Thread Lifting 2: Midface Reinforcement Method

For patients desiring more significant improvement in the midface, inserting threads targeting the nasolabial fold at the mid-pupil height along the lateral line of the hairline can minimize widening of the zygomatic area while improving bulging nasolabial fat (Fig. 5.15). If an excessively high entry point is used to lift the midface, the malar fat pad may shift to the malar eminence, leading to the zygomatic medial cutaneous ligament being pulled, which can create or deepen a mid-cheek groove.

5.8.3 Basic Method of Thread Lifting 3: Strengthening the Lower-Medial Area

For cases requiring more improvement in the lower-medial area, in addition to inserting threads in the superolateral direction of the jowl fat, if the marionette line is vertical due to medial descent, inserting threads from an entry point behind the ear targeting the marionette line can yield

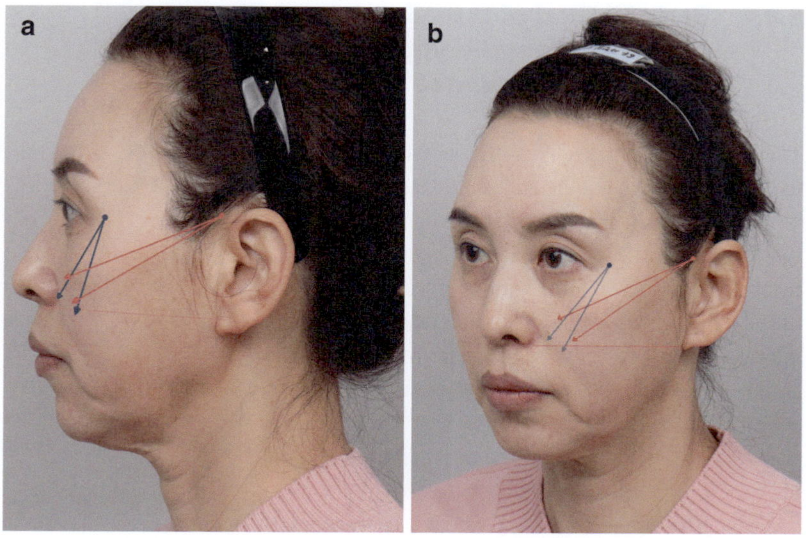

Fig. 5.15 Basic method of thread lifting 2 for midface reinforcement. Inserting threads targeting the nasolabial fold at the mid-pupil height along the lateral line of the hairline improves the nasolabial fat while pushing it back in lateral view, thereby reducing the nasolabial fold. (**a**) Lateral view. (**b**) Three quarter view

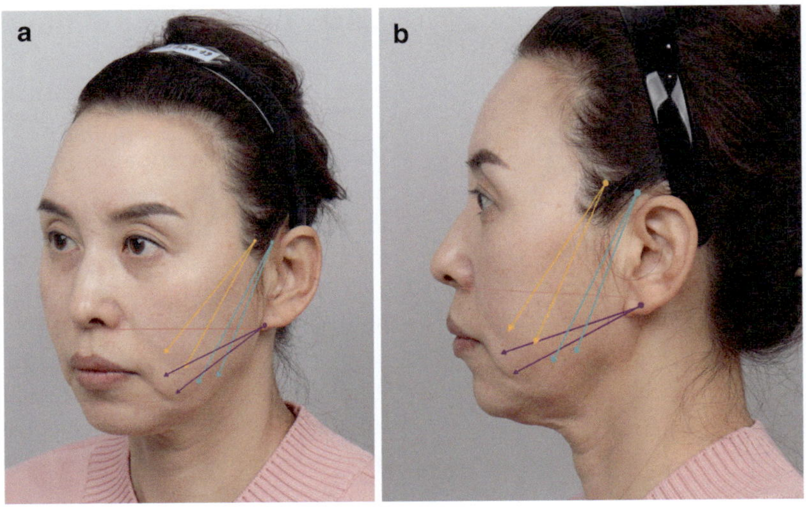

Fig. 5.16 Basic method of thread lifting 3 for strengthening the lower face. In addition to inserting threads in the superolateral direction of the jowl fat, inserting threads from an entry point behind the ear targeting the marionette line or setting the entry point at the mid-pupil height along the lateral line of the temporal hairline to target the lower bulging area can achieve better results. (**a**) Three quarter view. (**b**) Lateral view

additional effects. For patients with significant lower bulging lateral to the marionette line, setting the entry point at the mid-pupil height along the lateral line of the temporal hairline and inserting threads can provide even greater benefits (Fig. 5.16).

5.8.4 Basic Method of Thread Lifting 4: Strengthening the Lower-Lateral Area

The lower-lateral area is a region where pulling tissue with a nearly vertical vector can yield significant effects (Fig. 5.17). However, for patients with less volume in the face, it is necessary to insert threads in a superomedial direction to gather tissue that has descended inferolaterally due to the masseter muscle vector back to the midface. It is generally recommended to set the entry point at eyebrow height; this is because if a lower entry point is chosen, the distance to the mandible angle is short, which may prevent the effective use of the thread. If the thread engages tissue below the mandible border, it can lead to tissue gathering downward, reducing the lifting effect.

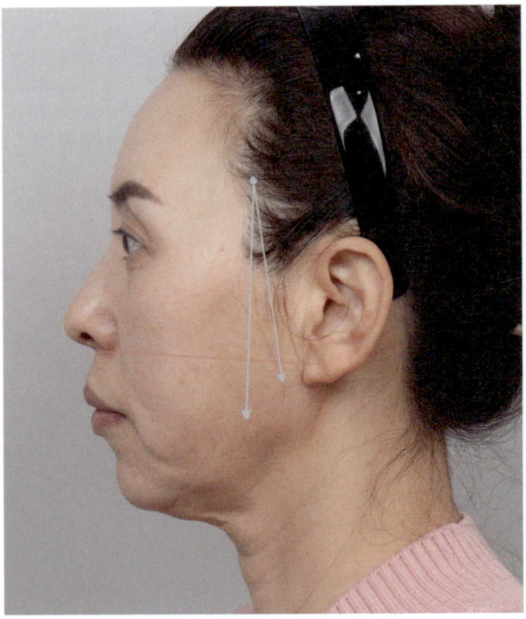

Fig. 5.17 Basic method of thread lifting 4. Strengthening the lower-lateral area tissue in the lower-lateral area requires complete vertical vector tissue movement, and adding a superomedial vector enhances tissue repositioning effects. The entry point is set at a relatively high eyebrow height compared to other areas

5.8.5 Basic Method of Thread Lifting 5: Improving the Neckline

By inserting threads to secure the fascia of both sternocleidomastoid muscles (SCM) at the virtual cervicofacial angle position along the midline, improvement in the neckline can be observed (Fig. 5.18). Additionally, inserting long cog threads with long needles into the neck can help restore the cervicofacial angle and enhance the clarity of the jawline. Typically, threads are inserted with the entry point at the center of the cervicofacial angle, securing them to the fascia of both SCMs. The dermis at the entry point should be made free using Metzenbaum scissors to minimize the appearance of pinching after the procedure. Furthermore, if the threads are inserted too superficially, dimpling or translucency may occur, while inserting them too deeply can damage some platysma muscle fibers due to the cog when the patient moves their neck, potentially leading to delayed hematoma and bruising.

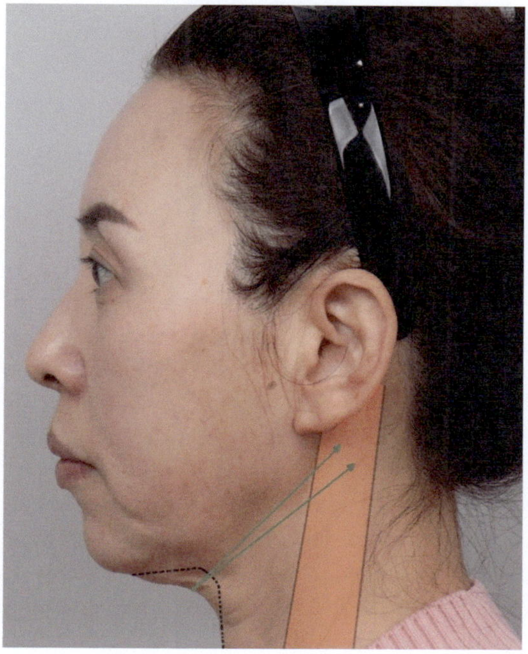

Fig. 5.18 Basic method of thread lifting 5 for improving the neckline. Threads are inserted to secure the fascia of both sternocleidomastoid muscles (SCM) at the virtual cervicofacial angle position along the midline

5.9 Longevity of Thread Lifting

When discussing the duration of effects, it is important to consider the perspective from which the evaluation is made. The duration of immediate effects can be maintained without change for up to 2 months, but after that, they gradually diminish, with a slow loss occurring between 6 months and 1 year. However, while the physical effects may fade, the benefits of neocollagenesis in preventing tissue loosening can last up to 1.5 years. If nonabsorbable threads are used, the physical effects may last longer, but they are also expected to diminish between 1.5 and 2 years.

Therefore, when performing thread lifting with the goal of achieving more long-term effects, it is reasonable to explain and conduct the procedure with consideration for the chemical effects of neocollagenesis rather than just the immediate effects. Repeated thread lifting procedures can accumulate tightening and lifting effects, leading to longer-lasting results (Fig. 5.19).

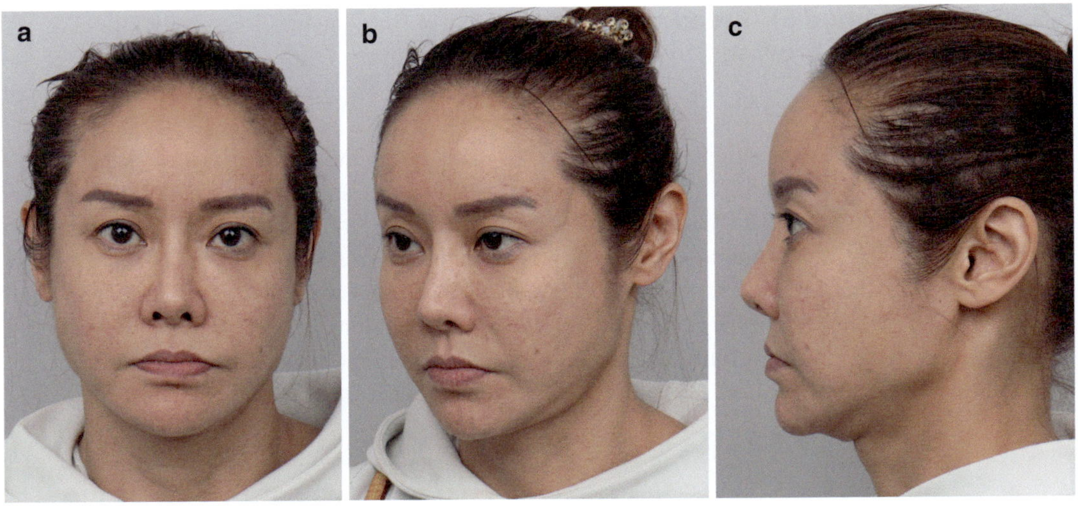

Fig. 5.19 A 45-year-old female patient who received facial thread lifting consistently over six sessions at 2–3-month intervals, showing less sagging in the face compared to the neck skin. (**a**) Frontal view. (**b**) Three quarter view. (**c**) Lateral view

5.10 Effective Accompanying Procedures

Since thread lifting alone cannot solve all problems, combining it with procedures that create a synergistic effect can yield better results. The most accessible option is fillers. When used in conjunction with thread lifting in areas such as the anterior cheek and lateral cheek where volume deflation begins, fillers can more effectively improve facial fullness and irregularities (Fig. 5.20). However, there is still controversy regarding the scientific understanding of the interactions that occur when threads and fillers meet in the same space (for instance, whether hyaluronic acid fillers gather water from the surrounding area, accelerating the hydrolysis of the threads, or whether the interaction between foreign substances (fillers and threads) promotes fibrosis or granuloma formation). Therefore, when using fillers together with threads, it is necessary to either place the filler in areas where the threads are not inserted or to inject it into deeper layers to avoid unexpected complications.

The buccal fat pad is a fat tissue located in a deeper layer than the sub-SMAS, serving as a gliding pad and cushion. As one ages, the ligaments and capsule supporting the buccal fat weaken, causing the buccal extension, which is part of the posterior lobe of the buccal fat pad, to sag and push the jowl downward, resulting in bulging. The challenge is that to target this tissue directly with threads, they must be inserted at a very deep layer, which is not easy. Even if access is successful, the weakened capsule may tear, leading to a "cheese wiring" effect and causing the tissue to sag again. Therefore, in patients with significant buccal fat extension, simply removing the buccal fat can paradoxically lead to a loss of fullness and an increase in skin fine lines. In obese patients (as there is a high correlation between visceral fat and buccal fat [3]), improvement is limited with thread lifting alone; thus, performing deep fat removal in conjunction with thread lifting can achieve greater improvement.

Botulinum toxin can also create a synergistic effect when used together. Specifically, injecting botulinum toxin into the hyperactivated depressor anguli oris or platysma, which are responsible for downward movement of the tissue, can provide additional lifting effects and reduce the load on the threads, thereby prolonging their effectiveness. Injecting botulinum toxin into the mentalis muscle, which is not effectively lifted by the threads, is another method to maximize improvement in the perioral area when performed alongside thread lifting (Fig. 5.21).

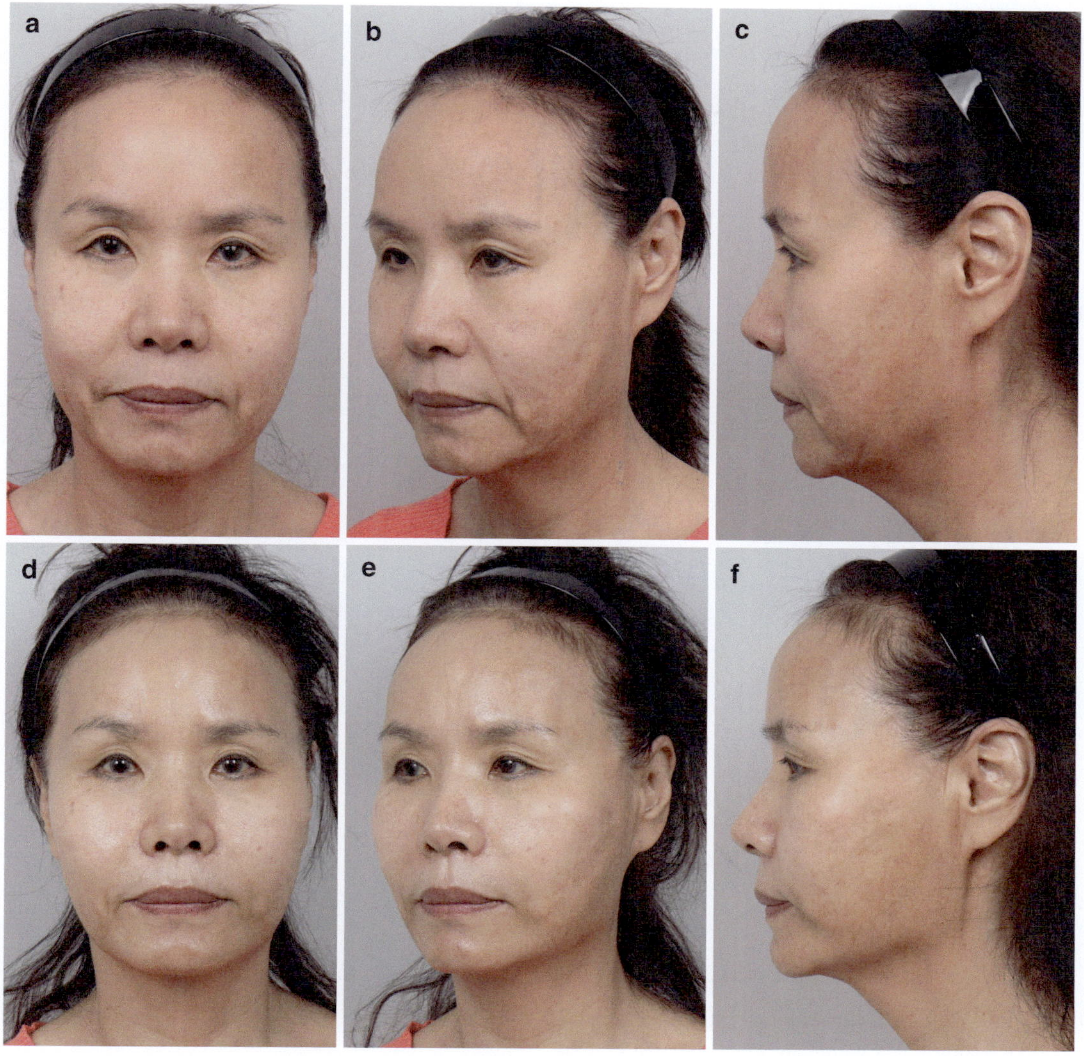

Fig. 5.20 A 65-year-old female patient. A total of 1.2 cc of filler injected in conjunction with thread lifting in the anterior cheek and mid-cheek groove. (**a**–**c**) Preoperative; (**d**–**f**) postoperative 45 days

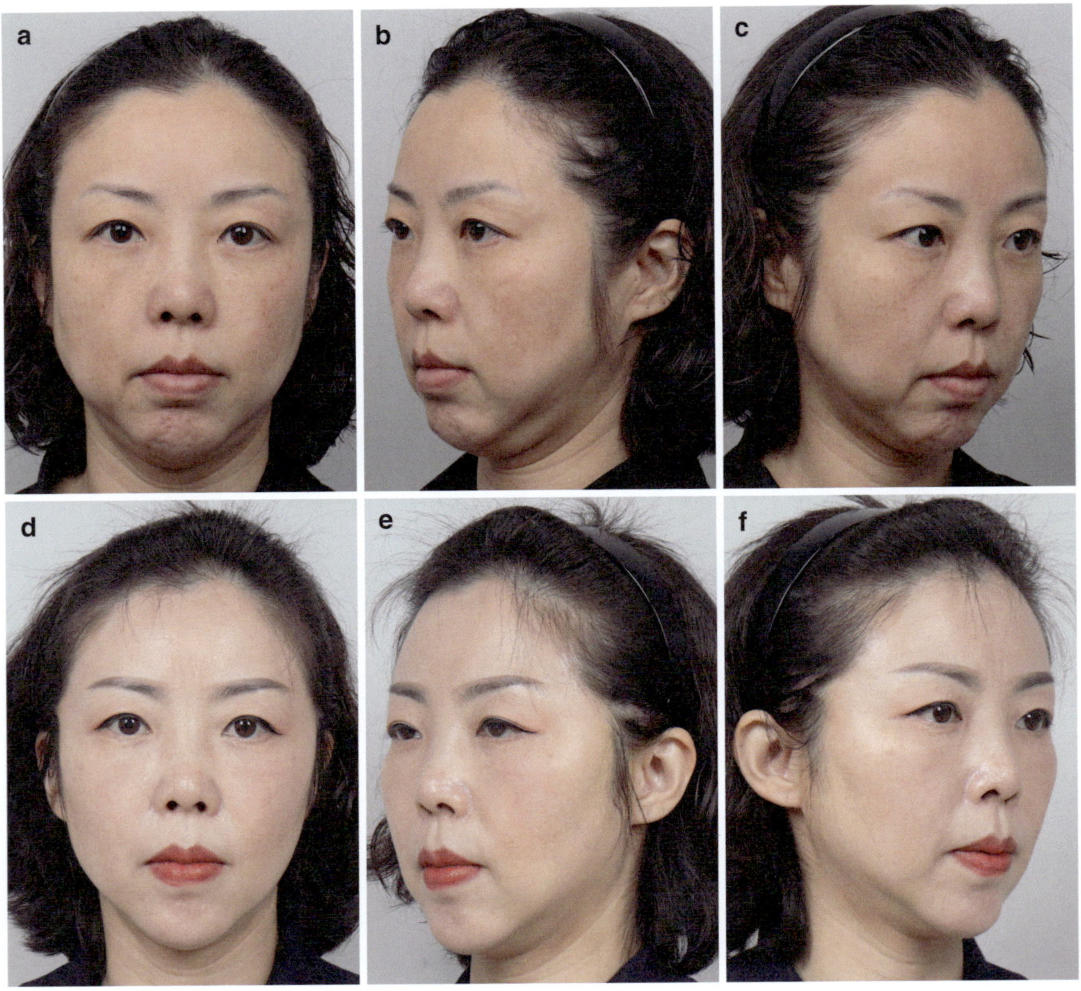

Fig. 5.21 A 48-year-old female patient. Thread lifting, deep fat removal, and botulinum toxin injection into the mentalis muscle were performed together. (**a–c**) Preoperative. (**d–f**) Postoperative 2 weeks. Significant improvement in the jawline

References

1. Niu Z, Zhang K, Yao W, et al. A meta-analysis and systemic review of the incidences of complications following facial thread-lifting. Aesth Plast Surg. 2021;45(5):2148–58.
2. Song JK, Chang J, Cho KW, Choi CY. Favorable crisscrossing pattern with polydioxanone: barbed thread lifting in constructing fibrous architecture. Aesthet Surg J. 2021;41(7):NP875–86. https://doi.org/10.1093/asj/sjab153.
3. Levine JA, Ray A, Jensen MD. Relation between chubby cheeks and visceral fat. N Engl J Med. 1998;339(26):1946–7. https://doi.org/10.1056/NEJM199812243392619.

Complications of Thread Lifting

6

Contents

Upon reviewing the literature related to thread lifting, most papers either introduce company products claiming good efficacy or discuss complications associated with the procedure. Thread lifting is a minimally invasive surgical technique performed similarly to filler injections, using a blind technique that does not allow direct visualization of the internal structures. Occasionally, during the procedure, when the surgeon uses their fingers to estimate the thickness of the tissue in the patient's mouth and face, they may realize that the facial tissue is thinner than expected. There are various layers within this thin tissue, and accurately inserting threads into these layers can be quite challenging, leading to unexpected complications (Fig. 6.1).

W. Lee, K. H. Jung, *Lifting Techniques in Plastic Surgery*,
https://doi.org/10.1007/978-981-96-4820-7_6

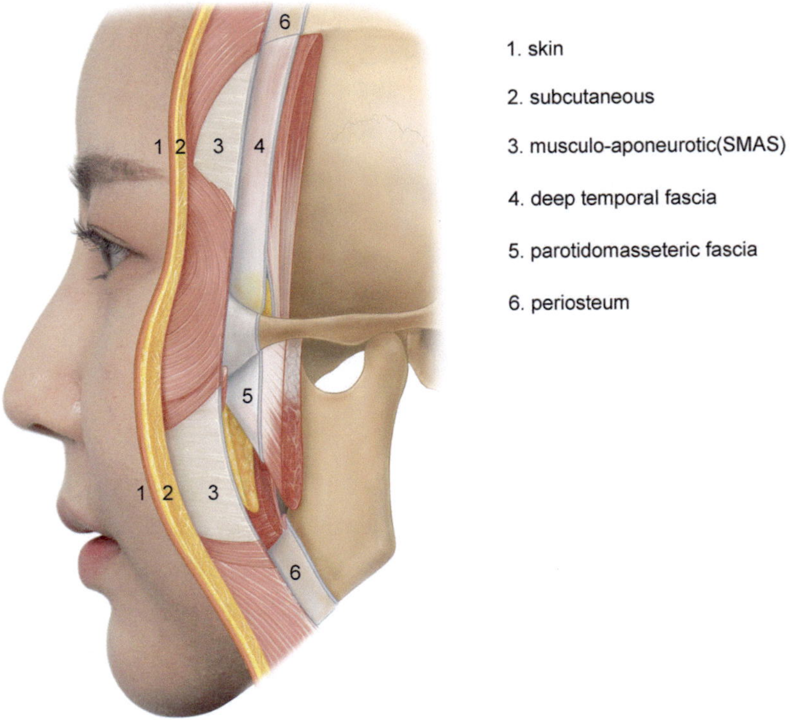

Fig. 6.1 Layers of the face

Nevertheless, the practitioner must insert the appropriate threads in the correct locations based on the patient's condition to achieve good results. Preoperative assessment of factors such as how much the skin has sagged, the thickness of the subcutaneous fat layer, and the prominence of the cheekbones is crucial. Additionally, understanding the precise causes of even minor complications and addressing them is of utmost importance.

6.1 Parotid Gland Injury

Injuries to the parotid gland due to thread lifting are very rare. However, some patients may exhibit parotid gland hypertrophy. Many patients frequently receive botulinum toxin injections in outpatient settings. In these cases, performing thread lifting, which has been routinely done, may lead to parotid gland injury (Fig. 6.2). Furthermore, as observed in Chap. 5, if the practitioner is not

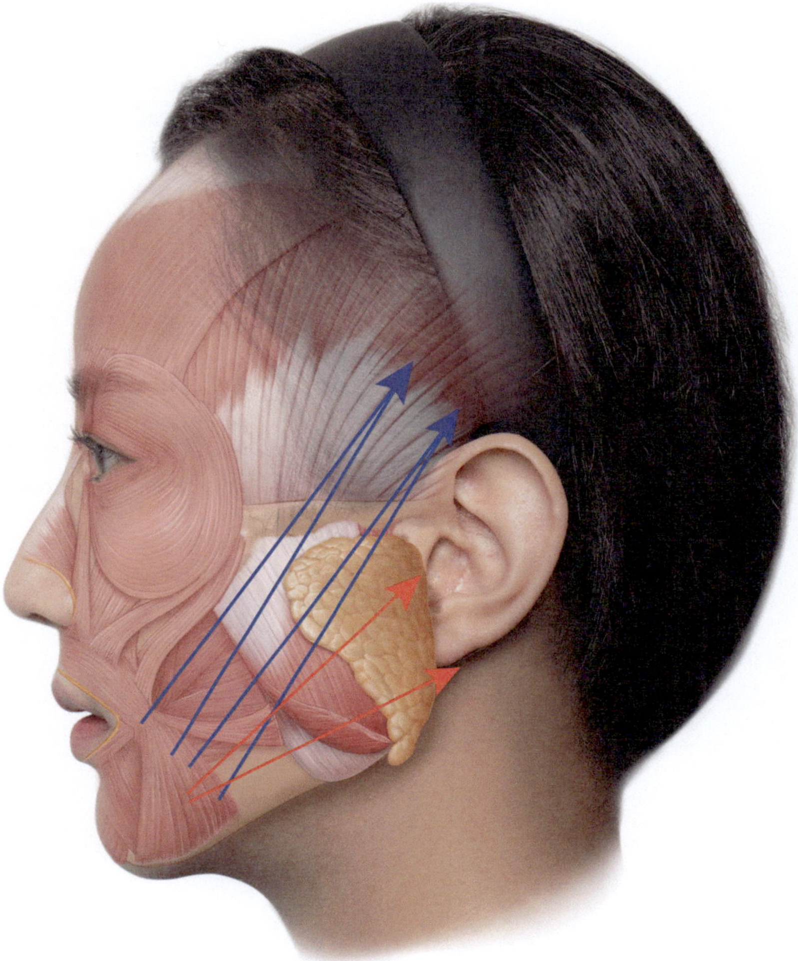

Fig. 6.2 Mechanism of parotid gland injury. Deep thread lifting that invades the gland or occurs in patients with benign parotid gland hypertrophy

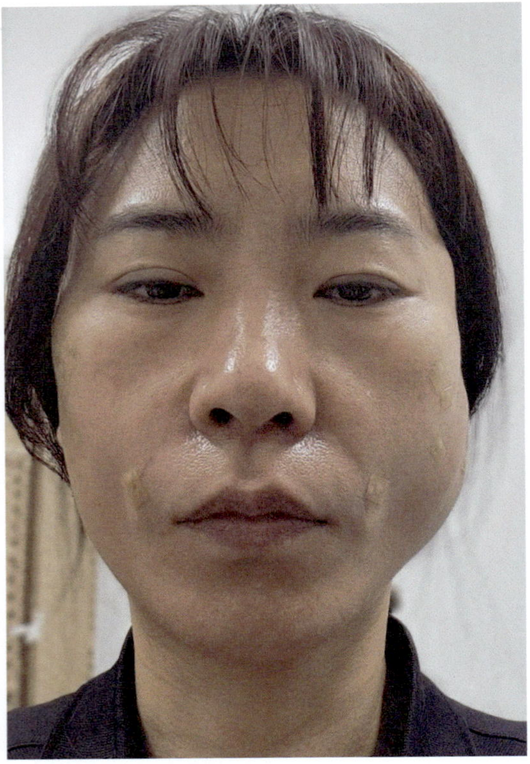

Fig. 6.3 Left parotid gland injury. Two days post-thread lifting

always aware of the parotid gland area during the procedure, even a slight increase in depth can result in damage to this structure.

Typically, patients will report swelling without bruising starting the day after the procedure, which worsens during meals. This symptom is usually subsided with anti-inflammatory drugs, but inflammation may persist, and if the parotid duct is damaged, symptoms can last for up to a month [1] (Fig. 6.3).

In cases of parotid gland injury following thread lifting, ultrasound can reveal the presence of threads within the gland. The position of the threads is usually confirmed above the masseter muscle within the parotid gland (Fig. 6.4).

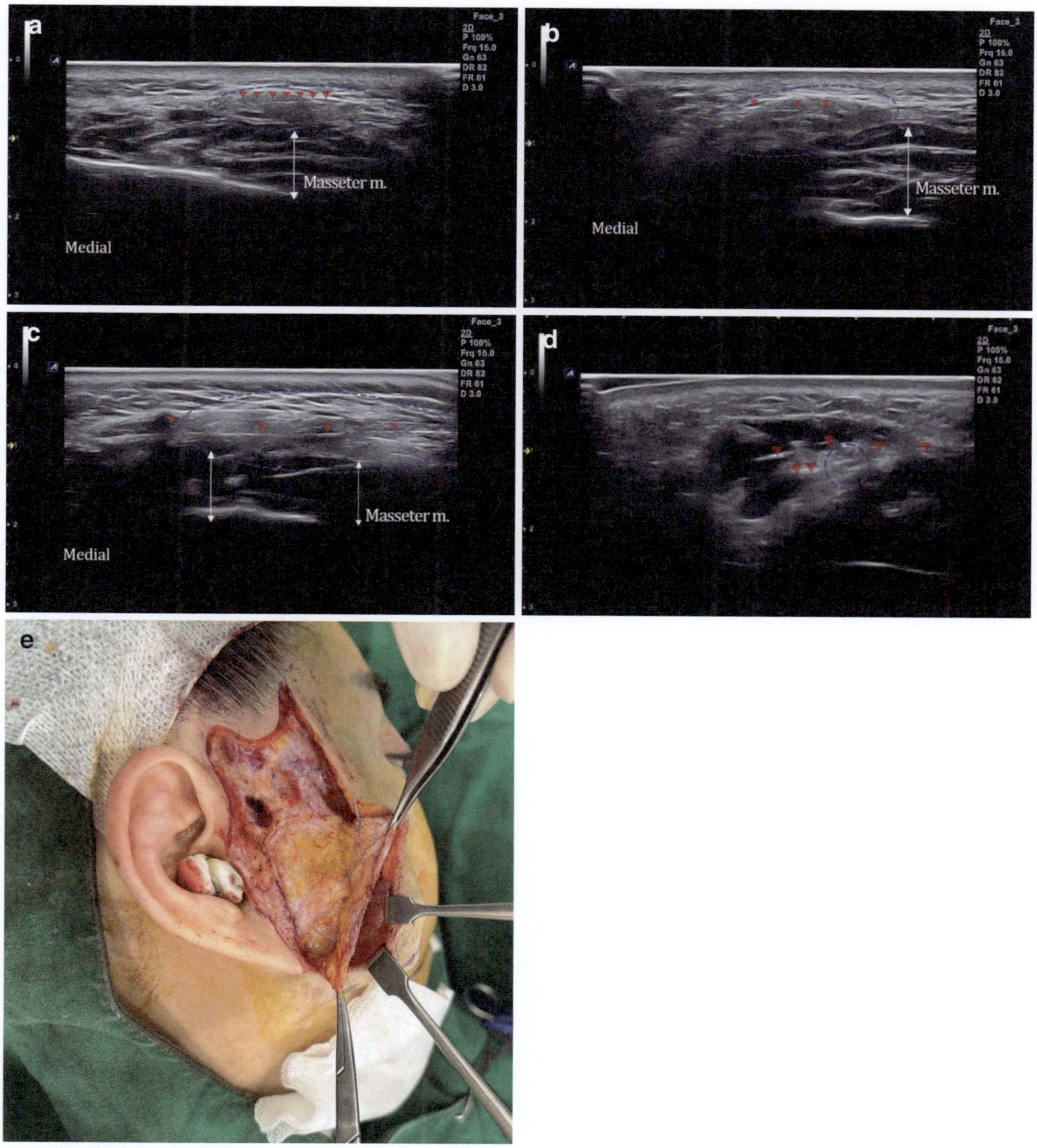

Fig. 6.4 Threads located within the parotid gland. (**a**, **b**, **c**) Ultrasound findings showing threads within the parotid gland. (**d**) Ultrasound findings showing fluid collection due to parotid duct damage. (**e**) Threads penetrating the salivary gland observed during facelift surgery

6.2 Worsening of the Mid-Cheek Groove

The mid-cheek groove, often referred to as the "Indian crease," is caused by the zygomatico-cutaneous ligament. However, this groove may become more pronounced after lifting. This groove is accentuated by the ligament and becomes more distinct due to fat deflation and bone absorption [2]. While the skin may sag slightly, resulting in a mild line, lifting can cause the surrounding tissue to tent, making the groove

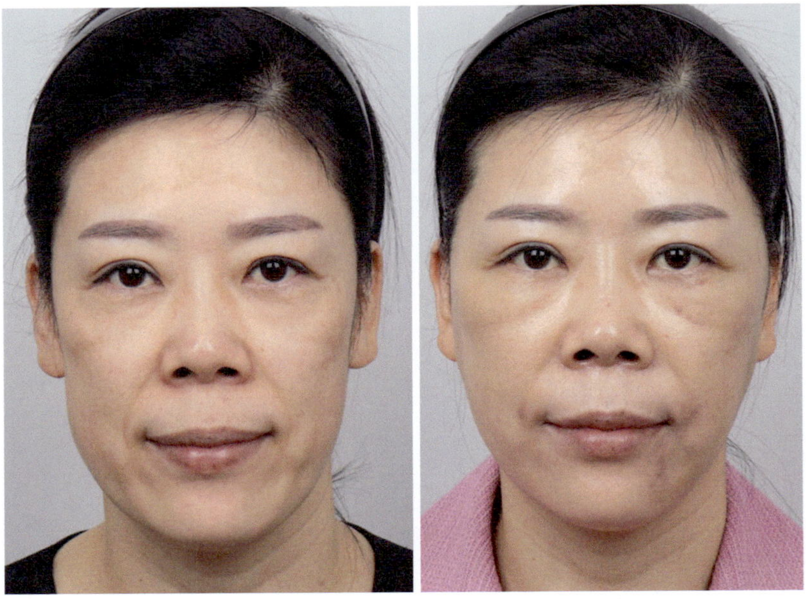

Fig. 6.5 Worsening of the mid-cheek groove after lifting procedure. Left: preoperative; Right: postoperative 1 week

more prominent (Fig. 6.5). Therefore, it is essential to recognize and explain the mid-cheek groove preoperatively, and if it becomes more pronounced postoperatively, it may be necessary to use hyaluronic acid fillers to alleviate the appearance.

6.3 Thread Migration and/or Protrusion

PDO threads, commonly used, gradually degrade within the body, leading to a decrease in strength over time. Occasionally, during periods of prolonged humidity, the storage conditions (packaging) of the threads may result in their use in a partially degraded state. Consequently, when such threads are inserted, it is rare but possible for them to break in the middle and migrate inward toward the face after 1–2 months. Protrusion can also occur, which is aesthetically unpleasing and may cause discomfort for the patient, making removal advisable (Fig. 6.6). Most importantly, it is crucial to understand the manufacturing process of the threads and to verify whether there are any issues with the manufacturer's packaging.

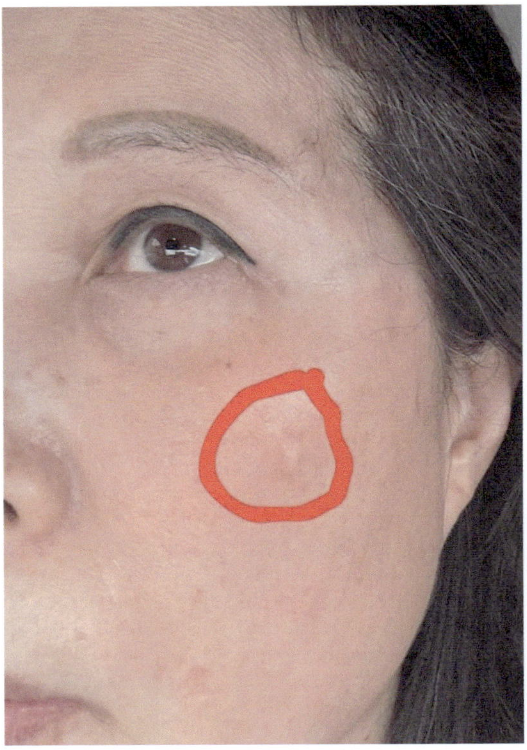

Fig. 6.6 Thread protrusion after 2 months post-thread lifting. A sound of the thread breaking was heard, followed by the protrusion of the thread through the skin. The thread is removed after skin puncture

6.4 Skin Dimpling and Irregularity

The primary cause of dimpling is the insertion of threads too close to the dermal layer. When threads are inserted from the temple towards the mouth, they are likely to pass through the zygomatic arch and be placed in the superficial layer, increasing the risk of dimpling (Figs. 6.7 and 6.8). Therefore, the most common locations for dimpling are at the ends of the inserted threads or just below the zygomatic arch. In cases where a reverse technique is used to insert threads toward the temple after puncturing the face, the risk of dimpling is relatively low. However, caution is necessary for patients with very thin dermal and subcutaneous fat layers, as well as for those who have undergone significant energy-based procedures, which may lead to atypical collagen fiber formation and a higher likelihood of dimpling.

Additionally, many patients may report skin irregularity even in the absence of visible dimpling. It is important to assess this after the swelling has resolved, as irregularities are more likely to occur when thicker threads are inserted close to the dermal layer.

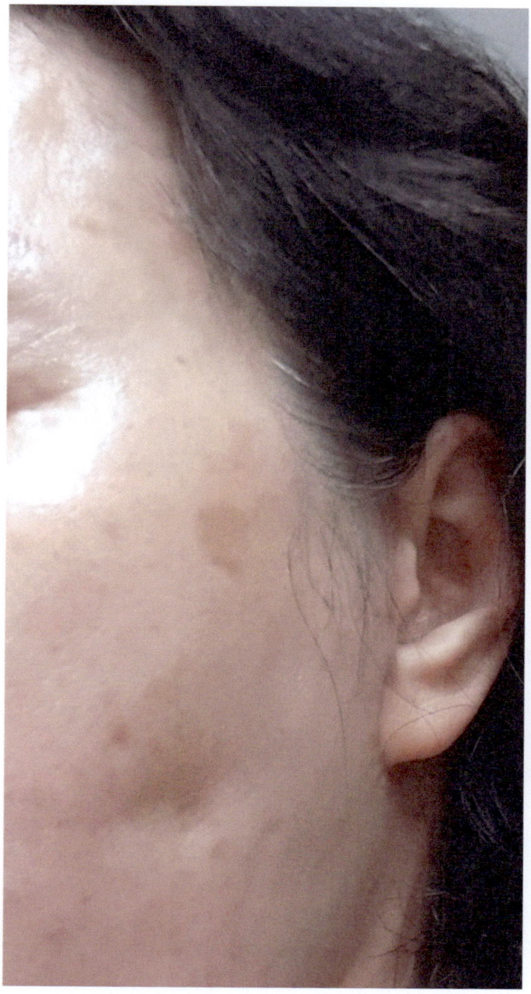

Fig. 6.7 64-year-old female patient. Dimpling under the zygomatic arch after thread lifting

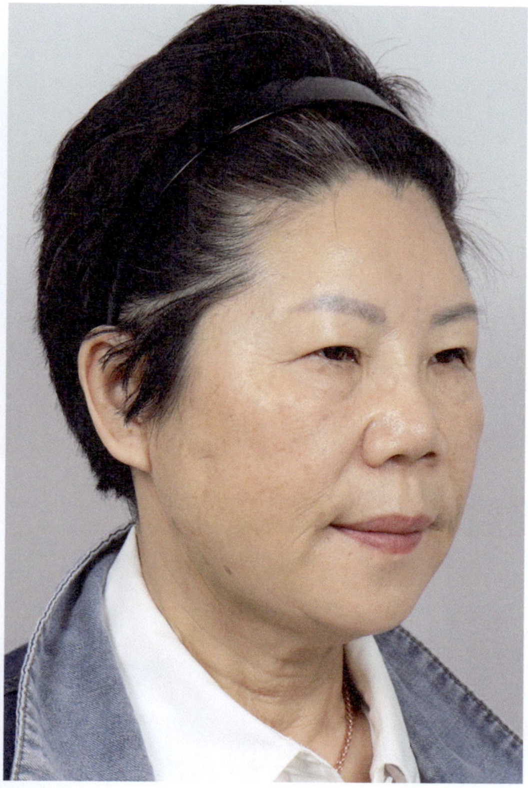

Fig. 6.8 61-year-old female patient. Dimpling under the zygomatic arch

6.5 Hematoma and Bruising

Bruising is the most common complication associated with thread lifting. The face contains numerous blood vessels, and bruising can occur due to capillary or venous bleeding. However, most bruises resolve within 2–3 weeks. The real concern arises when larger blood vessels are punctured. For larger veins or arteries, understanding their anatomical pathways is essential for minimizing the risk of hematoma. As mentioned in Chap. 1, the veins in the temple area can be detected using near-infrared techniques. For arteries, it is crucial to recognize their basic pathways and to feel for pulsation manually; more importantly, using ultrasound for pre-procedural assessment can enhance safety. The frontal branch of the superficial temporal artery is one of the most critical vessels in the temple area (Fig. 6.9). Additionally, when performing procedures that elevate the jawline or extend beyond the nasolabial folds, it is important to understand the course of the facial artery, as damage can lead to hematoma formation in the oral cavity (Fig. 6.10). Hematomas can also occur in the mouth if the transverse facial artery perforator is damaged. Therefore, recognizing the vessels that may be encountered during thread insertion is vital, and performing the procedure gently and slowly is essential (Fig. 6.11).

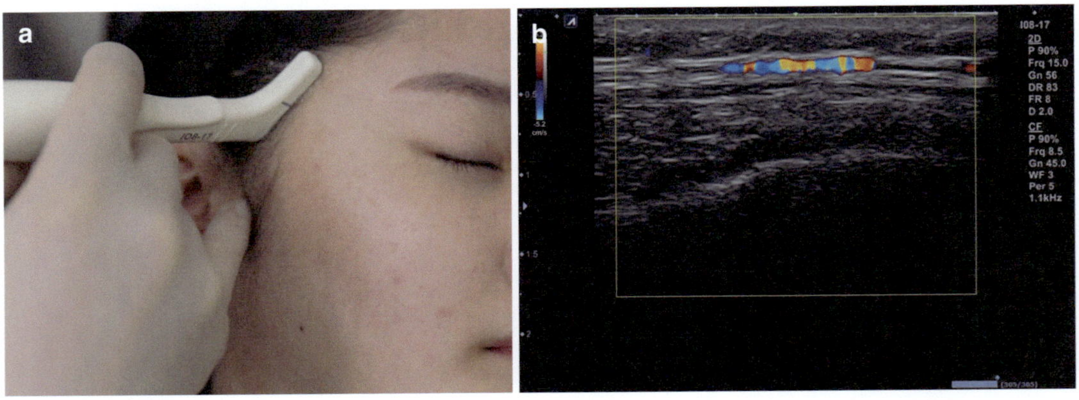

Fig. 6.9 Ultrasound findings of the temple area. (**a**) Hairline position detection probe. (**b**) Frontal branch of the superficial temporal artery at the superficial temporal fascia

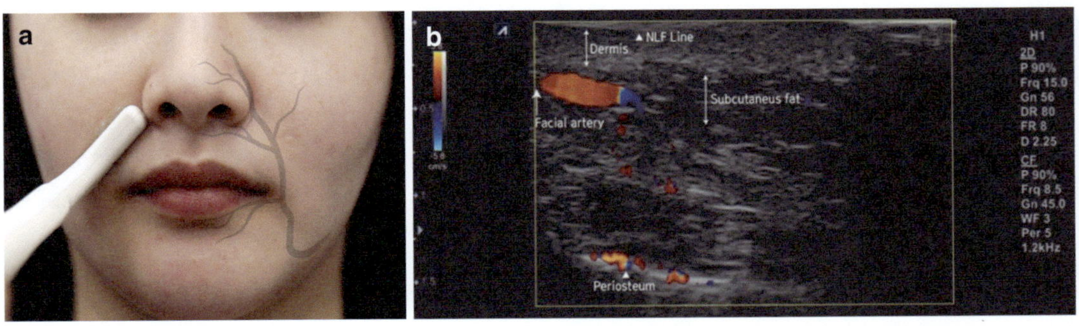

Fig. 6.10 Ultrasound findings at the nasolabial fold area. (**a**) Nasolabial fold detection probe. (**b**) Facial artery

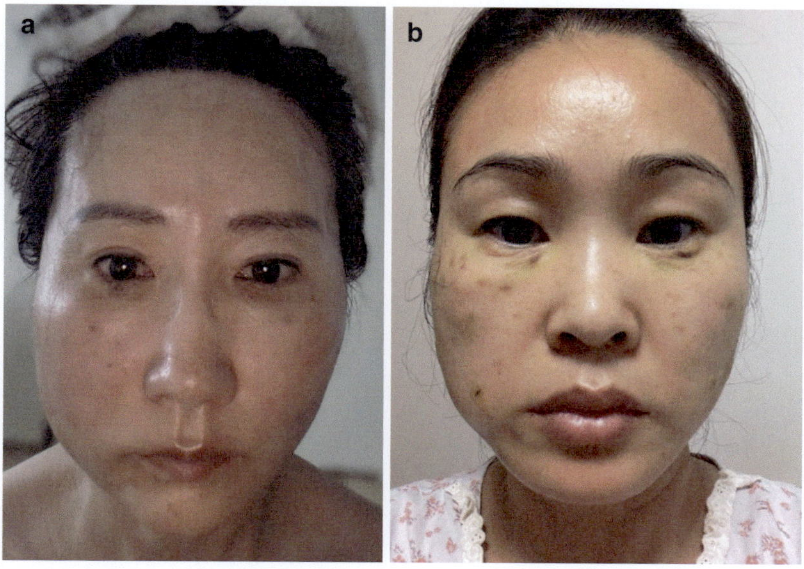

Fig. 6.11 Hematoma after thread lifting. (**a**) 54-year-old female patient. Post-thread lifting day 1. Hematoma in the right cheek area. (**b**) 45-year-old female patient. Post-thread lifting day 2. Hematoma in the right cheek

6.6 Pain

Pain that may occur after thread lifting is primarily due to the barbs on the threads. This pain typically manifests around the mouth and neck and can persist from 1 day to 2 weeks post-procedure. Therefore, it is important to be aware of the sensory nerves that may be affected and to perform the procedure cautiously (Fig. 6.12). Additionally, when lifting the neck, care should be taken regarding the course of the great auricular nerve at the entry point.

Patients who experience no significant pain or discomfort immediately after surgery may later present with sudden sharp pain weeks or months later. The areas most commonly reported are around the zygomatic arch or temple, likely due to stimulation of the zygomaticofacial nerve, zygomaticotemporal nerve, or auriculotemporal nerve. Initially, this may not be due to direct stimulation but rather from ongoing facial expressions that irritate the area due to the threads' barbs. When taking anti-inflammatory pain relievers and avoiding wide mouth opening can help reduce irritation. As time passes, the threads adapt to the tissue and degrade, making it important to explain the symptoms and their causes to the patient.

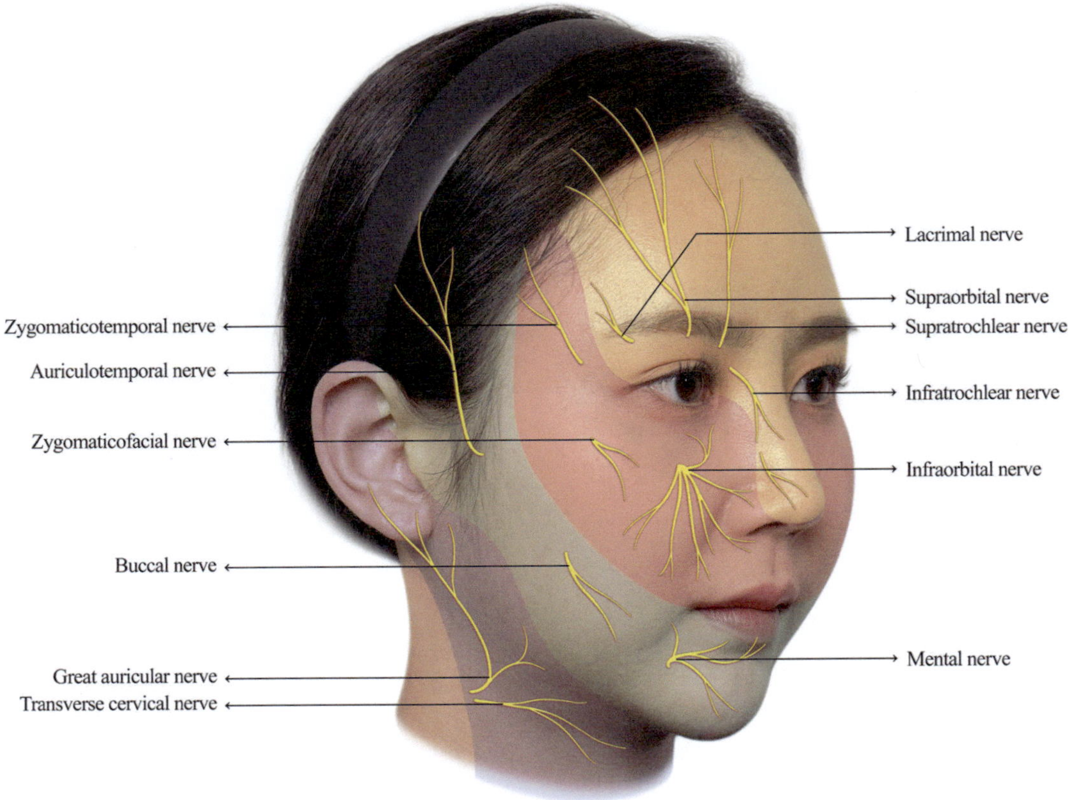

Fig. 6.12 Distribution of sensory nerves in the face

6.7 Asymmetry

Some patients request correction of asymmetry before the procedure, while others express dissatisfaction with asymmetry afterward. It is crucial to assess the degree of asymmetry preoperatively and to make the patient aware of it. Approximately 45% of Koreans already have asymmetry in their 20s [3], and for some, asymmetry that was previously masked becomes more apparent in their 40s. Therefore, many patients seeking lifting procedures often already have asymmetry (Fig. 6.13). In cases of bony frame asymmetry, the vectors of the facial muscles differ, resulting in varying angles of wrinkle lines. Differences in fat volume on both sides can also become more pronounced when aligning the lower face, and the ratio differences due to age-related fat deflation tend to worsen. Thus, it is essential to explain to patients that complete correction of asymmetry is challenging.

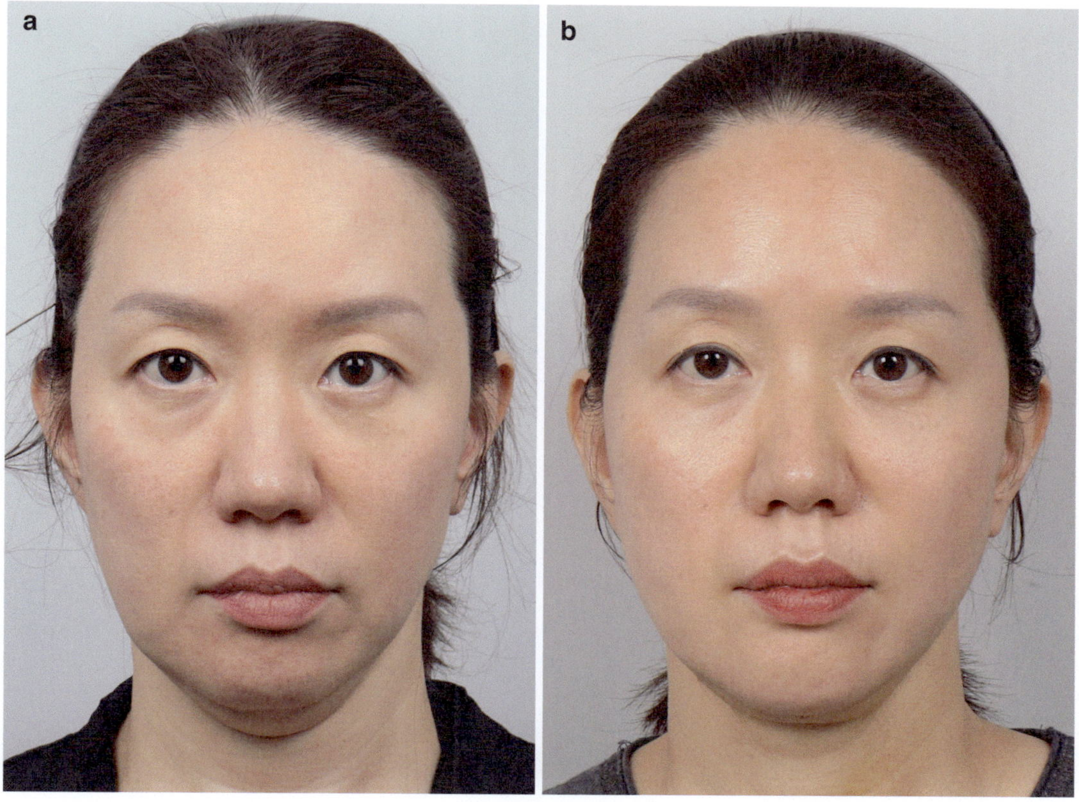

Fig. 6.13 A patient with significant asymmetry before surgery. (**a**) Preoperative findings show differences in the width of the zygomatic arch, eye height and depth, and tissue volume in the cheeks. (**b**) One-week post-thread lifting. Asymmetry remains uncorrected after the procedure

Many patients complain of asymmetry immediately after surgery. However, asymmetry within 3 days post-thread lifting is likely due to swelling (Figs. 6.14 and 6.15). Occasionally, noticeable differences in wrinkle lines may result from insufficient treatment, and in such cases, additional procedures may be necessary for partial correction. After completing the thread lifting, comparing both sides in an upright position to check for asymmetry before finishing the procedure can minimize the occurrence of immediate post-procedural asymmetry (Fig. 6.16). Additional treatments can be performed about 1 month later, with 1–2 threads being inserted.

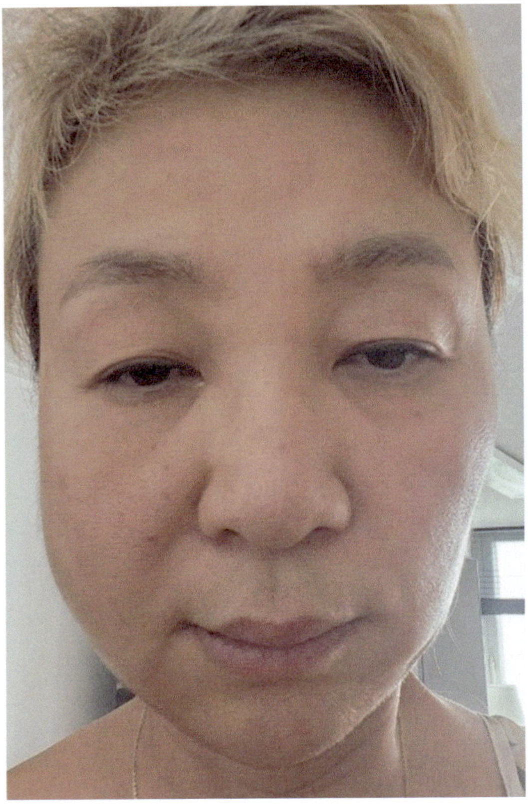

Fig. 6.14 A 56-year-old female patient complaining of asymmetry on postoperative 3 days after thread lifting. Notably due to swelling on the right side, highlighting differences in the NLF and mid-cheek groove

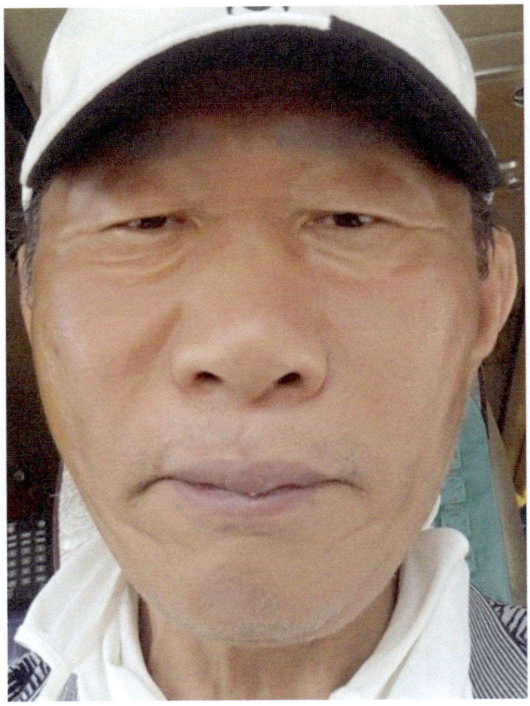

Fig. 6.15 A 76-year-old male patient complaining of asymmetry in the nasolabial fold 2 days post-thread lifting

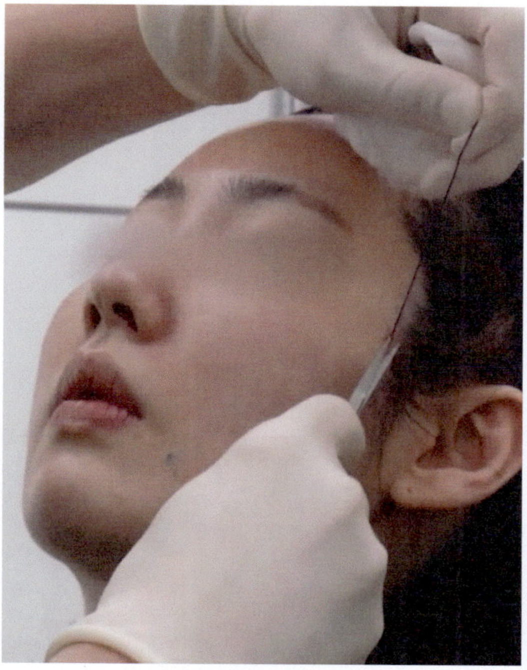

Fig. 6.16 Method to prevent asymmetry. Confirming asymmetry after assuming an upright position and cutting the threads to complete the procedure

6.8 Nodule and Granuloma

Threads can elicit a foreign body reaction in the body, and using an excessive amount indiscriminately, clustering them to achieve a volumetric effect in specific areas, or using them in spaces similar to fillers can lead to unwanted hyperactive immune responses, resulting in persistent inflammation or the formation of nodules. In severe cases, this can cause continuous granuloma formation beneath the skin, which can be distressing for the patient. In such cases, using ultrasound or CT to confirm the presence of threads can be helpful. If threads are still present, injecting non-cross-linked hyaluronic acid can promote hydrolysis, and physical massage can create cracks to facilitate rapid absorption. If more than 6 months have passed since the procedure or if the remaining threads are not visible, treatment with triamcinolone injection may be necessary to alleviate the nodule, and if this method is ineffective, surgical removal may be required (Fig. 6.17).

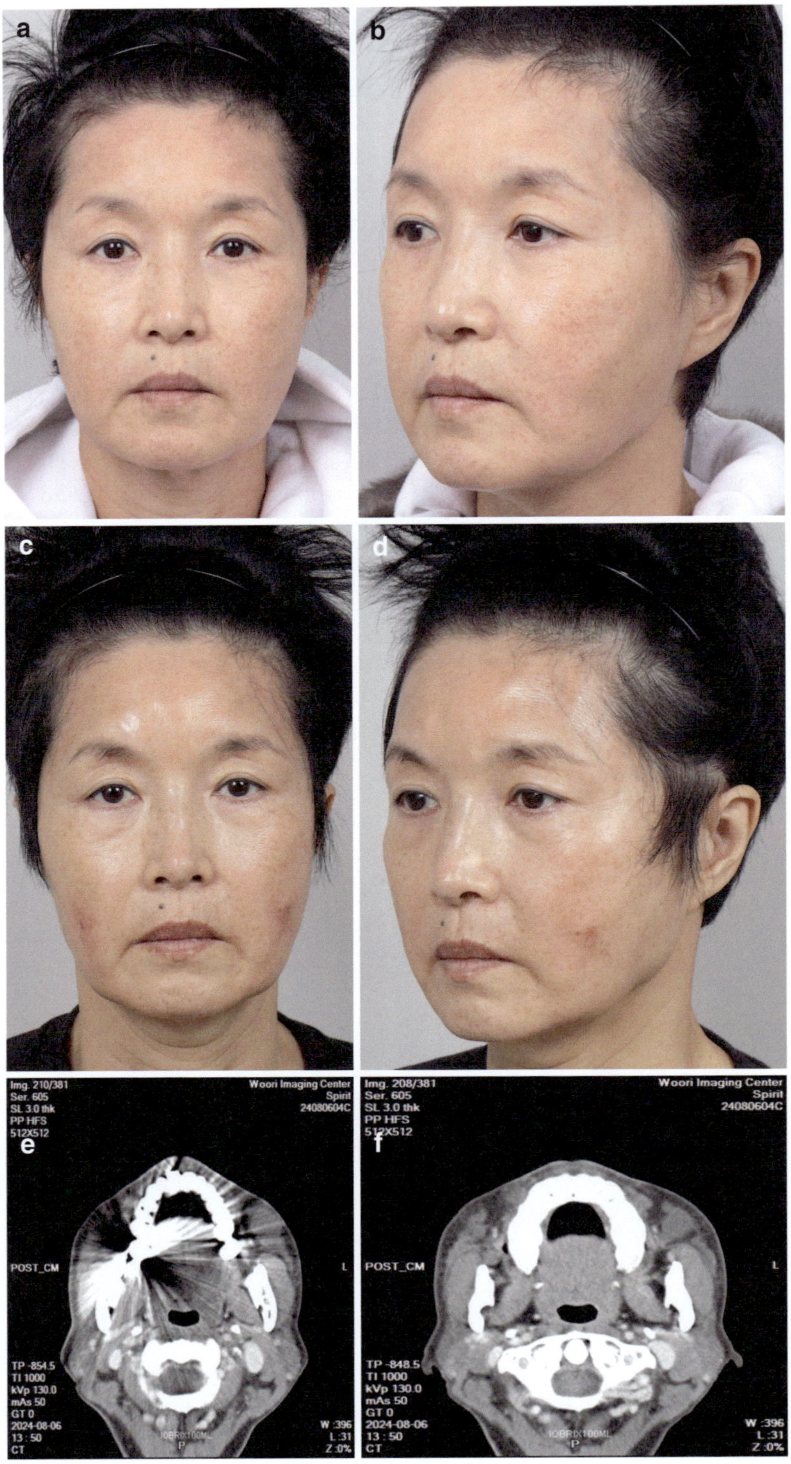

Fig. 6.17 A 58-year-old female patient with 30 threads from thread lifting and hyaluronic acid filler injected into the nasolabial folds. (**a**) Preoperative frontal view. (**b**) Preoperative lateral view. (**c**) Postoperative 3 years frontal view, showing granuloma formation in both cheeks. (**d**) Postoperative 3 years lateral view, showing cheek granuloma. (**e**, **f**) CT Findings—multiple/scattered soft tissue nodules/oval regions of bilateral buccal fat space—particularly about 20 mm on the long axis at the left buccal fat space, probably indicating the presence of foreign body and granuloma, mild mucosal thickening at both maxillary sinuses

6.9 Recurrence and Lack of Effectiveness

The primary drawback of thread lifting is its duration of effect. For PDO threads, the initial strength is maintained for about 2 months, after which the effects gradually diminish. In patients in their 20s and early 30s, the effects may last around 1 year, while patients in their mid-40s often experience a significant reduction in perceived effects by around 6 months. Consequently, it is common to encounter patients who visit for complaints about the effectiveness of the procedure. Although the temporary effects of thread lifting may fade, the benefits of collagenesis in preventing sagging tend to last longer. Therefore, explaining and making patients aware of this effect prior to the procedure can help avoid unnecessary disputes.

However, some patients may not notice significant effects from the beginning, or they may not recognize the changes even if they occur. This tendency is particularly evident in patients over 40 with moderate to severe skin laxity, where improvements may not be visible to the patient, indicating that they fall outside the indications for thread lifting. In such cases, it is important to explain that more invasive surgical options may be necessary for better results. In younger patients, those with a higher volume of fat often report limited changes, leading to complaints of insufficient effectiveness. For these patients, it should be emphasized during pre-procedural consultations that additional procedures to reduce fat may be necessary for effective outcomes (Fig. 6.18).

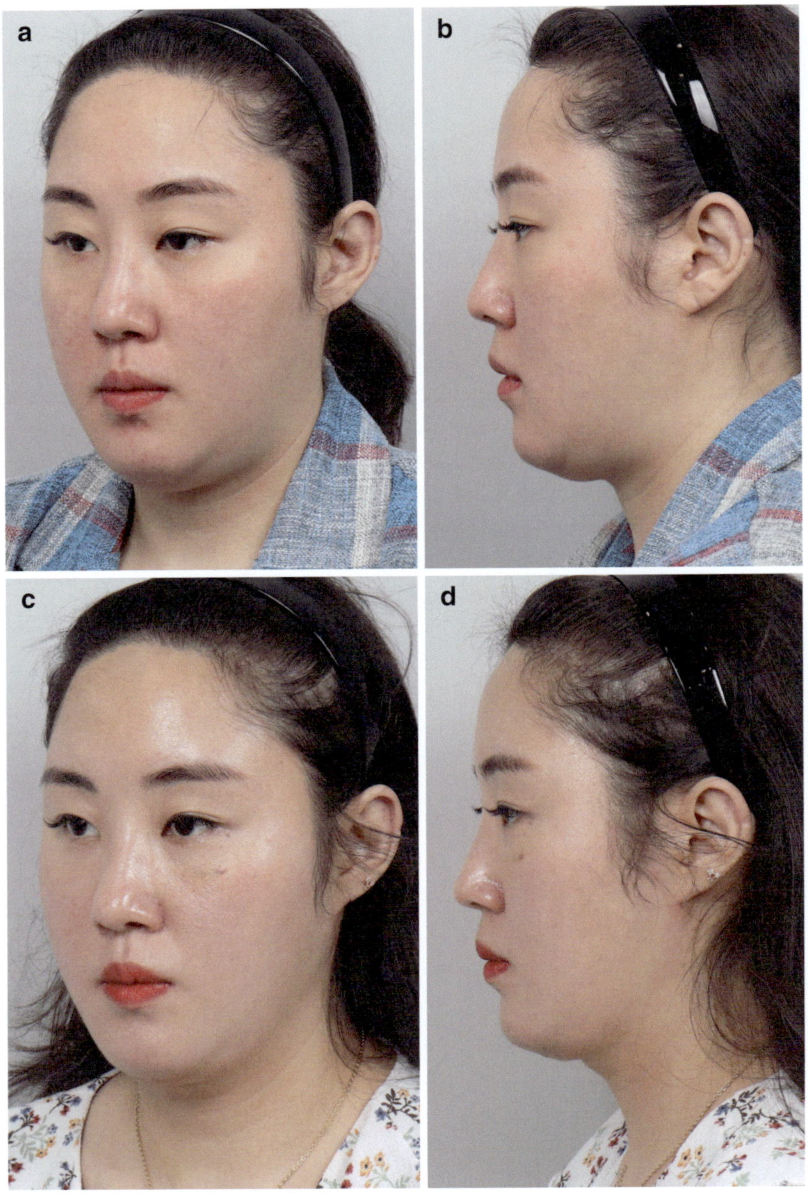

Fig. 6.18 A 21-year-old female patient who experienced improvement in the contours of the lower face and some enhancement of the cervicofacial angle after thread lifting, yet complained of insufficient effectiveness. (**a**) Preoperative three quarter view. (**b**) Preoperative lateral view. (**c**) Postoperative three quarter view. (**d**) Postoperative lateral view

6.10 Conclusion

Thread lifting results can vary significantly based on the surgeon's skill, the patient's condition, the type and thickness of the threads used, among other factors. Therefore, it is very challenging to generate objective data on this topic. While many studies have been conducted, most focus on the lifting results of actual cases or complications related to the procedure. A review of the literature indicates that using absorbable sutures tends to result in fewer complications compared to non-absorbable sutures. However, as discussed in this chapter, various complications can still arise. Preventive measures are crucial for many complications, and a deeper understanding of anatomy, skin thickness, and the threads themselves, along with appropriate patient selection, is of utmost importance.

References

1. Kim JS, Yang EJ, Kim WR, Lee W, Kim HJ, Yi KH. Ultrasound-guided thread lifting for the prevention of parotid gland and diagnosing parotid duct complications. Skin Res Technol. 2023;29(12):e13535. https://doi.org/10.1111/srt.13535.
2. Wong CH, Mendelson B. Facial soft-tissue spaces and retaining ligaments of the midcheek: defining the premaxillary space. Plast Reconstr Surg. 2013;132(1):49–56. https://doi.org/10.1097/PRS.0b013e3182910a57.
3. Song WC, Koh KS, Kim SH, Hu KS, Kim HJ, Park JC, Choi BY. Horizontal angular asymmetry of the face in korean young adults with reference to the eye and mouth. J Oral Maxillofac Surg. 2007;65(11):2164–8. https://doi.org/10.1016/j.joms.2006.11.018.

Mini-Lifting

7

Contents

The desire to maintain a youthful appearance has long been a reality, and the demand for cosmeceutical products has dramatically increased. For centuries, the aspiration for human beauty has existed, as evidenced by the story of Cleopatra bathing in fresh milk to keep her skin looking young [1]. Recently, with advancements in science, more evidence-based antiaging methods have been introduced. Surgical techniques for facelifts have also evolved, beginning with the removal of loose skin through subcutaneous tissue lifting [2]. Knowledge of facial anatomy has improved, leading to a better understanding of the superficial musculoaponeurotic system (SMAS) [3]. Various studies on facial retaining ligaments have shown that releasing these ligaments can yield greater lifting effects [4]. While more invasive techniques have been proposed to achieve larger lifting effects, increased invasiveness often leads to greater patient anxiety [5]. Consequently, less invasive methods have been developed in recent years. Ultimately, achieving minimal invasiveness with maximum effect has become a crucial factor. Although several studies have been conducted on short scar rhytidectomy to reduce scarring and complication risks, these surgical techniques are still perceived as invasive lifting procedures from the patient's perspective [6].

Noninvasive thread lifting was introduced in the early 1990s [7]. Since then, various thread

W. Lee, K. H. Jung, *Lifting Techniques in Plastic Surgery*,
https://doi.org/10.1007/978-981-96-4820-7_7

lifting methods have been developed, and numerous techniques have been introduced [8, 9]. Noninvasive thread lifting techniques have significantly increased their presence in the cosmetic market; however, the effectiveness of thread lifting is often questioned, suggesting that the threads may temporarily shift, leading to a loss of lifting effect [10]. Therefore, another solution combining minimal invasiveness with maximum lifting effect has been developed, resulting in the creation of mini-lifting, aimed at reducing invasiveness and improving patient satisfaction [11, 12].

7.1 Definition

"Mini-lifting" is described as a procedure that removes wrinkles in specific areas through relatively small incisions [13]. However, due to a lack of understanding of the SMAS, initial procedures only involved skin excision. After further research, lifting that includes the SMAS has been shown to improve facial contours and enhance skin elasticity through skin excision [14, 15]. Short scar rhytidectomy, which includes minimal incisions and facial contour improvement, has also been introduced, but all these techniques share a similar preauricular incision [16]. Therefore, the "mini-lifting" technique can be defined as a surgical method distinct from traditional short scar rhytidectomy, which aims to improve facial contours through skin excision within or along the hairline and surface fat repositioning for skin elasticity.

7.2 Indication

Selecting appropriate indications for mini-lifting is one of the most important factors for patient satisfaction. Sasaki et al. described the ideal candidate as a patient aged between 35 and 45, primarily suitable for those with early midfacial sagging due to the descent of the buccal fat pads [17]. Pontius et al. suggested candidates aged between 40 and 50, while also proposing brow lift procedures [18]. In conclusion, mini-lifting is suitable for patients with mild midfacial sagging, slightly sagging lower faces, and without severe skin laxity or volume loss. Mini-lifting can also be applied to male patients or those undergoing secondary lifting procedures [19].

7.3 Surgical Method

7.3.1 Incision

The surgical incision is typically made 1–2 cm behind the hairline, measuring 3–4 cm in length, corresponding to the upper part of the temporalis muscle and positioned between the superior and inferior temporal lines. Both anterior and posterior incisions relative to the hairline are possible, but most patients prefer incisions placed behind the hairline to avoid visible scarring (Fig. 7.1).

7.3.2 Insertion Points

After making the incision, the thread is inserted from the incision on the inside of the hairline towards the zygomatic area. The thread is then lifted through the skin layers, including the deep

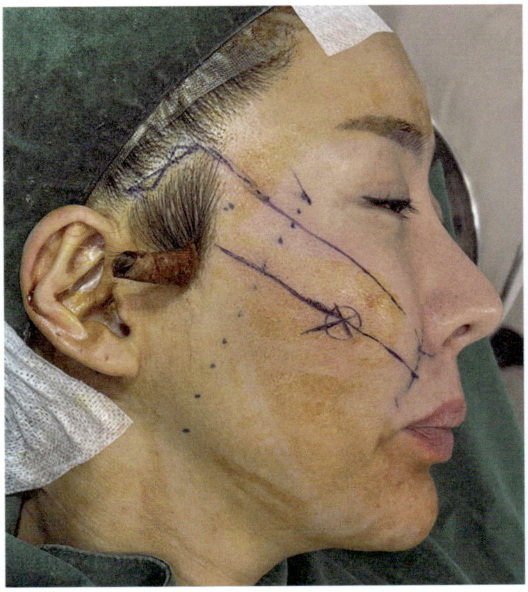

Fig. 7.1 Mini-lifting incision design

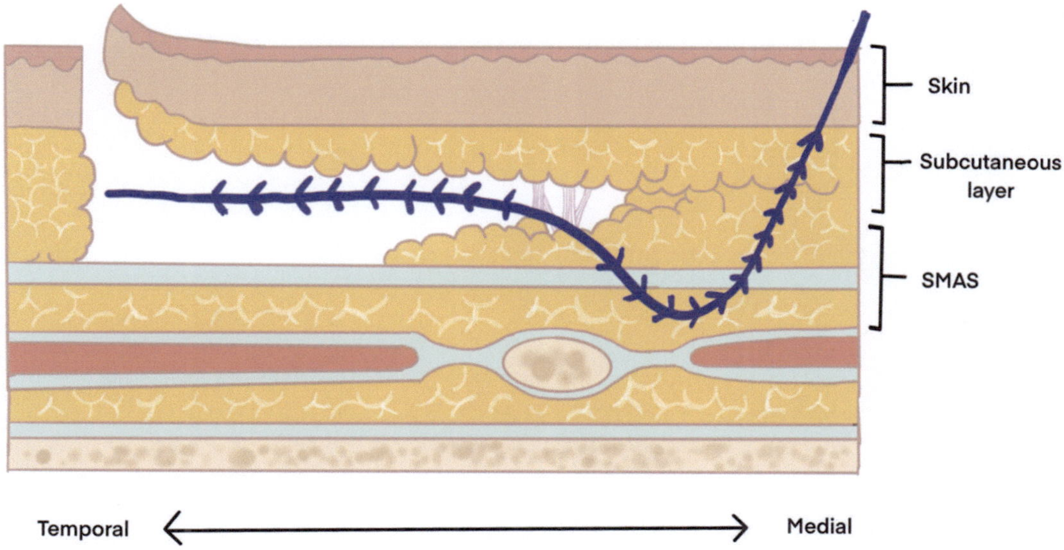

Fig. 7.2 Schematic diagram of thread insertion layer (SQ Subcutaneous layer, SMAS Superficial musculoaponeurotic system)

SMAS layer, and secured tightly at the incision within the hairline (Fig. 7.2).

Sasaki et al. described creating insertion points at the nasolabial fold area, with the second point positioned 1 cm laterally and inferiorly from the first point [17]. Laferriere et al. also described similar insertion points [20]. Since the movement of the malar fat pad is one of the primary objectives of this surgery, the insertion points are carefully considered. It is advisable to pinch the area between the arcus marginalis and the zygomatic ligament before creating the insertion points. After pinching, the most prominent two points are marked, and four additional points are marked along a horizontal imaginary line based on the alar base (Fig. 7.3).

7.3.3 Anesthesia

The procedure can generally be performed under intravenous sedation or local anesthesia. A 1% xylocaine solution containing 1:400,000 epinephrine may be used, or 2% lidocaine mixed with 1:100,000 epinephrine can be injected at a volume of 10–20 mL per side before surgery. An infraorbital nerve block may also be performed. However, large volumes of lidocaine or tumescent solutions are not recommended, as polydioxanone threads, commonly used, can degrade quickly upon exposure to moisture [21].

7.3.4 Procedure

After making the temporal incision, dissection is performed. A zigzag-shaped skin incision is primarily made within the hairline. In cases where a significant amount of remnant skin is expected, a backcut can be extended in the direction of the helix root. Dissection can be performed between the superficial temporal fascia (STF) and deep temporal fascia, but it is mainly conducted in the subcutaneous fat layer above the STF. Dissection is carried out using a Metzenbaum scissors or fingers, reaching medially to the vicinity of the Pitanguy line and inferiorly to the upper zygomatic arch, partially dissecting the zygomaticocutaneous ligament (Fig. 7.4).

After dissection is complete, six insertion points are created using an 18G needle, followed by the reverse technique with PDO threads (multidirectional cogged 21G 150 mm 2-0 N cog multi thread, N Finders Co., Seoul, South Korea).

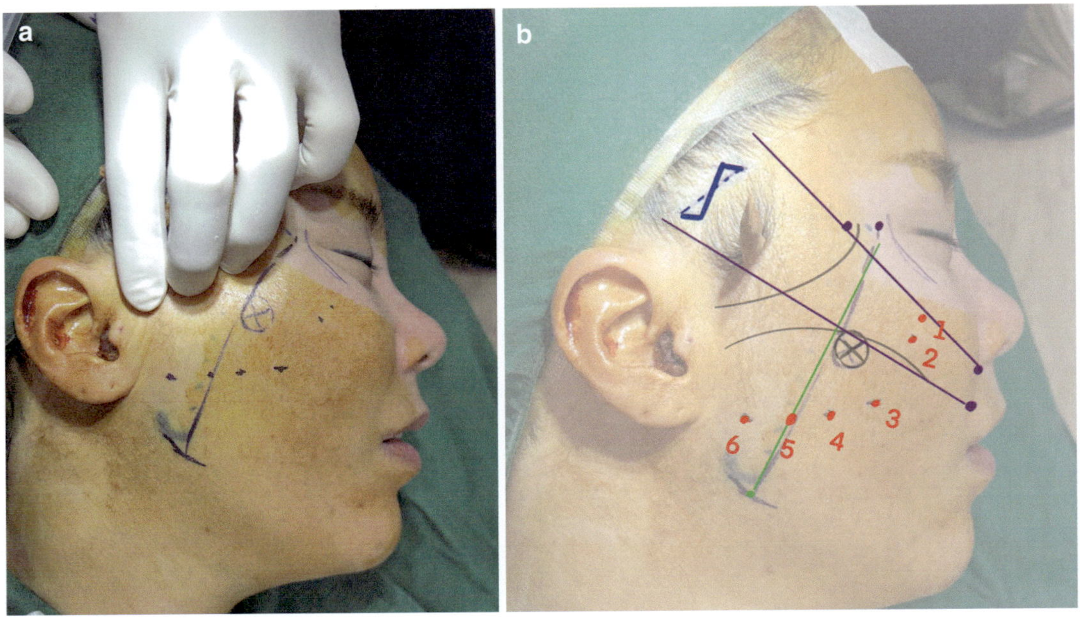

Fig. 7.3 Insertion points. (**a**) Marking four points by pulling the skin from the otobasion inferius to the subnasale. (**b**) Marking the two most prominent areas as points 1 and 2 after pinching the area between the arcus marginalis and the zygomatic ligament, with points 3 and 4 marked for lifting the jowl fat compartment and points 5 and 6 for lifting the lateral cheek fat compartment

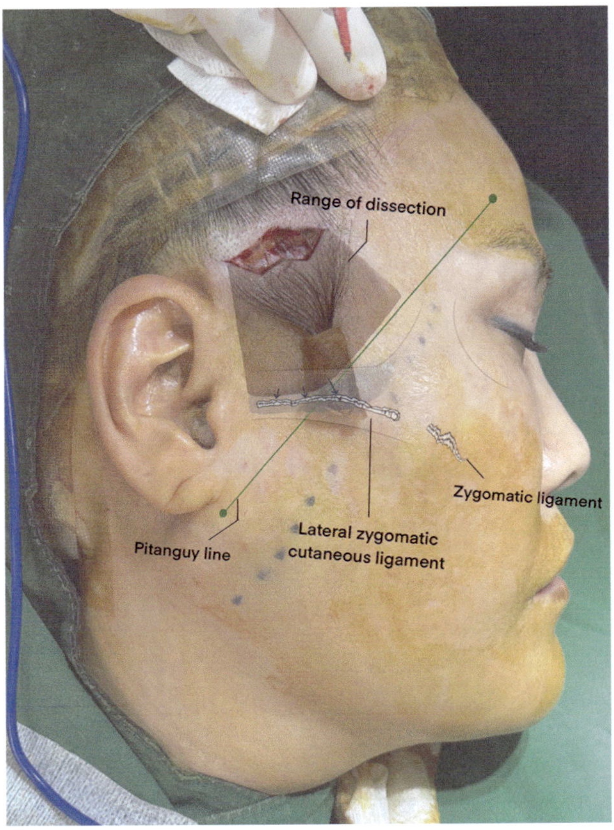

Fig. 7.4 Dissection range. Dissection (red line) performed using Metzenbaum scissors or fingers. Medially to the Pitanguy line (green line) and inferiorly to the zygomatic arch (blue line)

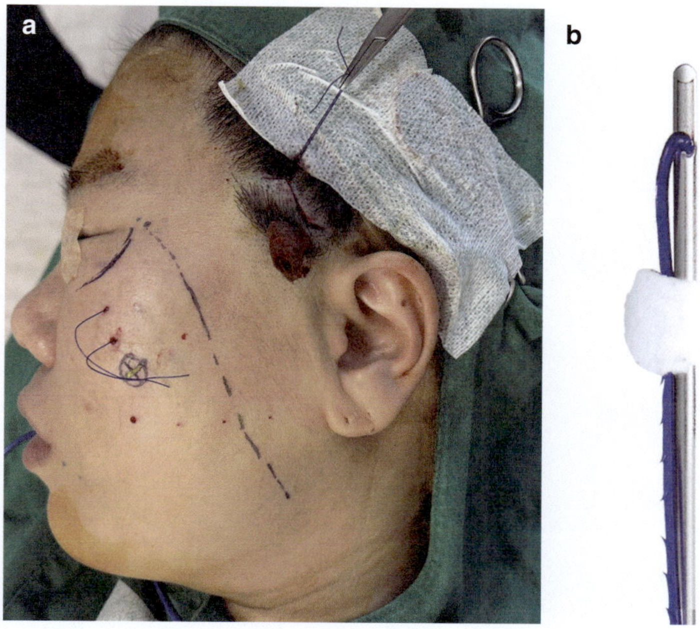

Fig. 7.5 Loop formation after thread insertion. (**a**) The two strands of thread are intertwined to form a loop, and the tension is checked after pulling. The loop is then sutured to the deep temporal fascia (DTF). (**b**) N Cog multi 21G 2-0 150 mm

The two threads that emerge from the scalp incision are tied together to form a loop. The repositioned tissue is then checked for tension by pulling on the threads to ensure it is not excessive (Fig. 7.5). If the tension is too high, there is a risk of scarring, so this must be confirmed before proceeding to the next step. The threads are then sutured to the deep temporal fascia with 2-0 PDO. The subcutaneous fat is sutured with 4-0 PDO, and the skin is closed with 5-0 nylon.

7.4 Longevity

Hamra reported that patients who underwent deep plane facelifts experienced midfacial repositioning effects lasting from 1 to 2 years [22]. Sasaki et al. reported that patient satisfaction after mini-lifting reached 85% over a 2-year period [17]. Keller et al. noted that the effects lasted for 1 year [19], while Laferriere reported in a 28-month follow-up study that lifting effects were maintained for 1 to 2 years [20]. Gualdi et al. also reported that using nonabsorbable sutures resulted in lifting effects lasting for 1 year [21]. According to the authors' experience, the duration of mini-lifting effects is approximately 1 year (Figs. 7.6, 7.7, 7.8, 7.9, 7.10, 7.11, and 7.12). However, the tensile strength of PDO decreases by up to 60% within 3 months post-insertion, indicating that the lifting effect observed immediately after surgery may last less than 1 year. Nevertheless, it is evident that performing mini-lifting 2–3 times results in less tissue sagging. PDO threads are expected to provide not only mechanical lifting effects but also chemical effects such as collagen production.

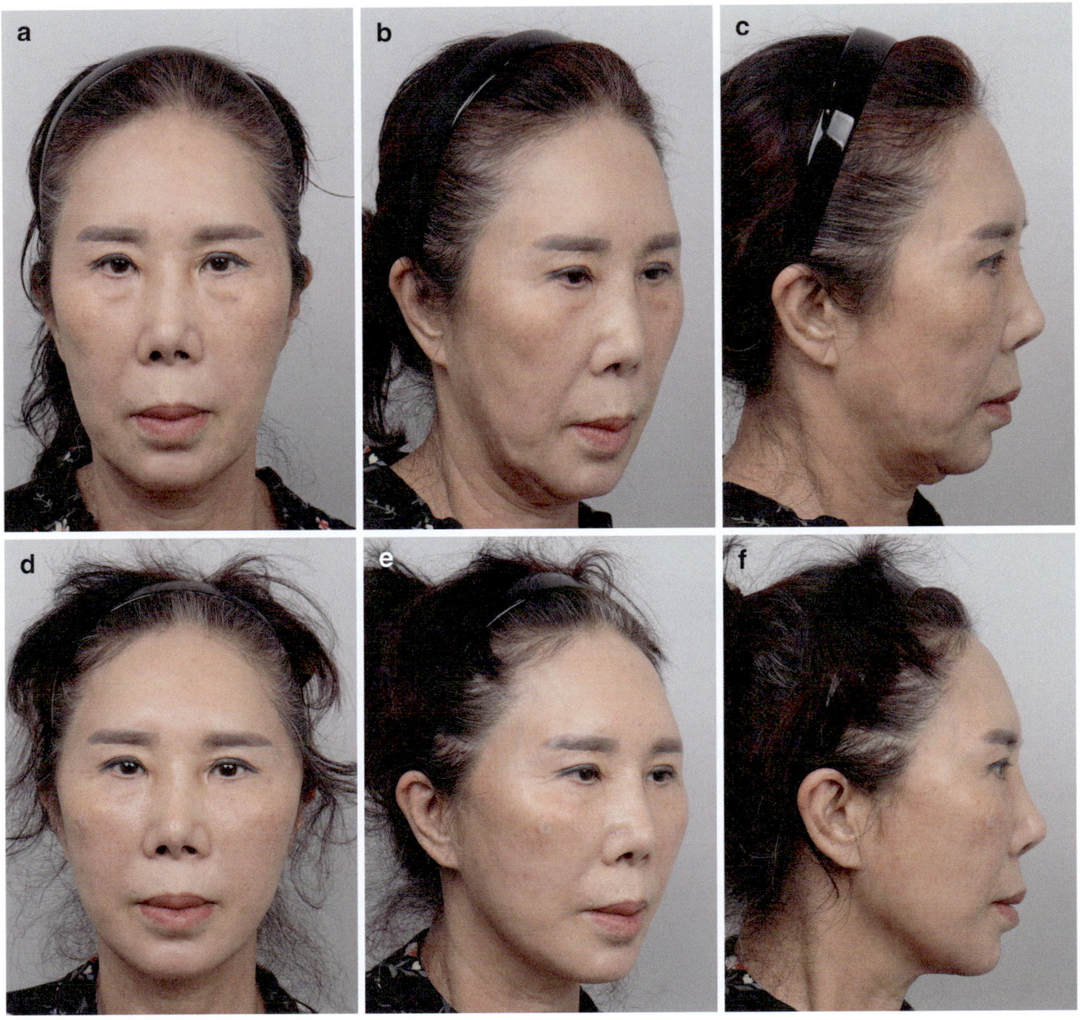

Fig. 7.6 Mini-lifting in a 66-year-old female patient. (**a**) Preoperative frontal view. (**b**) Preoperative three-quarter view. (**c**) Preoperative lateral view. (**d**) Postoperative 1-month frontal view. (**e**) Postoperative 1-month three-quarter view. (**f**) Postoperative 1-month lateral view

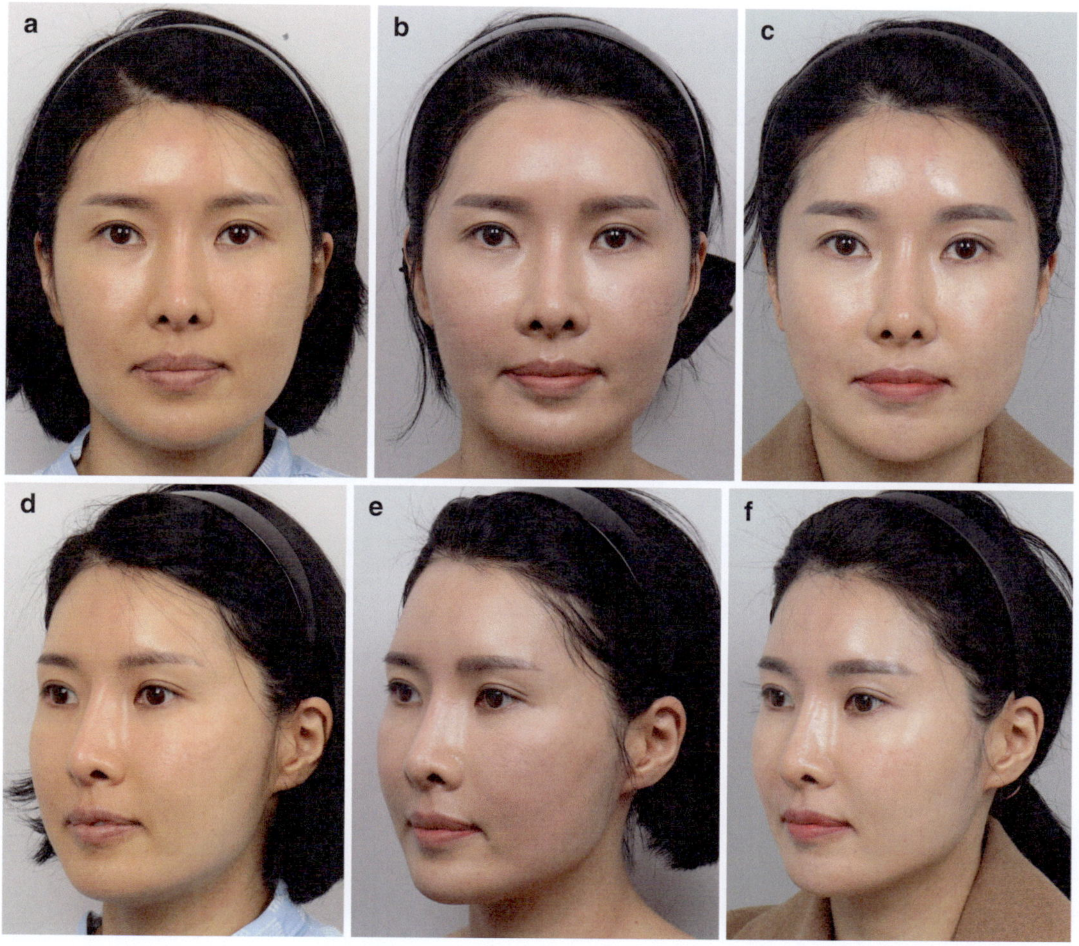

Fig. 7.7 Mini-lifting in a 42-year-old female patient. (**a**) Preoperative frontal view. (**b**) Postoperative 2 weeks frontal view. (**c**) Postoperative 6 months frontal view. (**d**) Preoperative three-quarter view. (**e**) Postoperative 2 weeks three-quarter view. (**f**) Postoperative 6 months three-quarter view

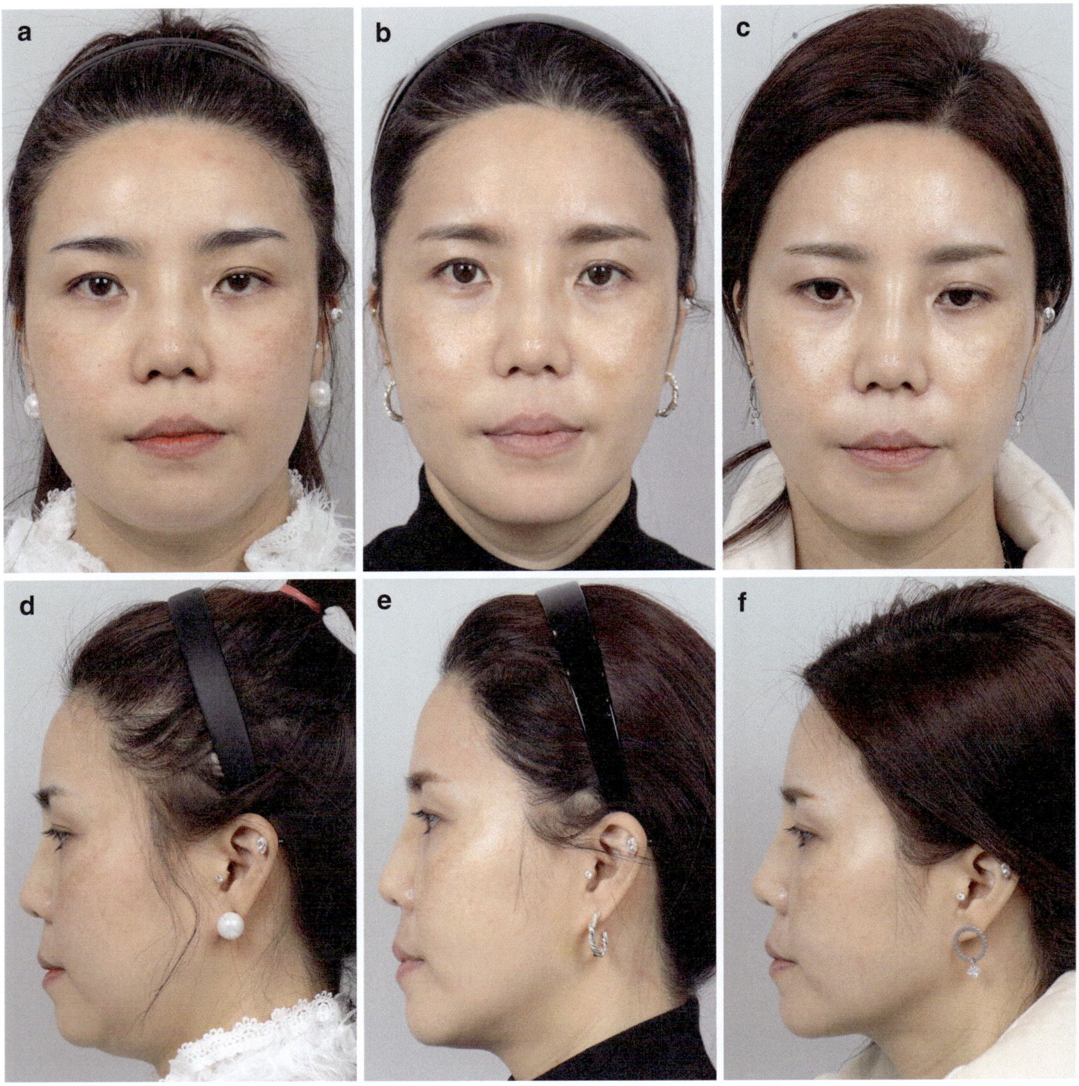

Fig. 7.8 Mini-lifting in a 47-year-old female patient. (**a**) Preoperative frontal view. (**b**) Postoperative 2 weeks frontal view. (**c**) Postoperative 1-month frontal view. (**d**) Preoperative lateral view. (**e**) Postoperative 2 weeks lateral view. (**f**) Postoperative 1-month lateral view

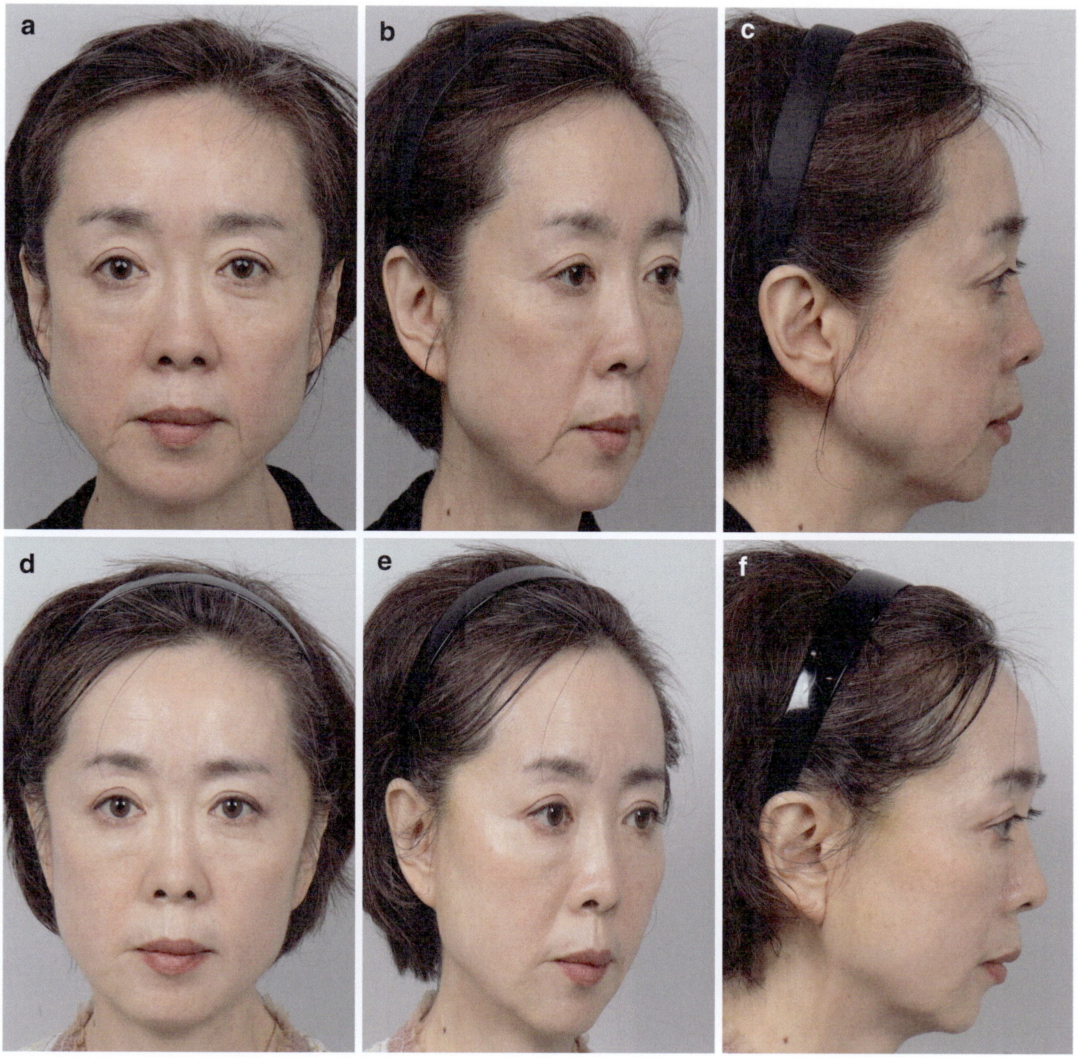

Fig. 7.9 Mini-lifting in a 60-year-old female patient. (**a**) Preoperative frontal view. (**b**) Preoperative three-quarter view. (**c**) Preoperative lateral view. (**d**) Postoperative 2 weeks frontal view. (**e**) Postoperative 2 weeks three-quarter view. (**f**) Postoperative 2 weeks lateral view

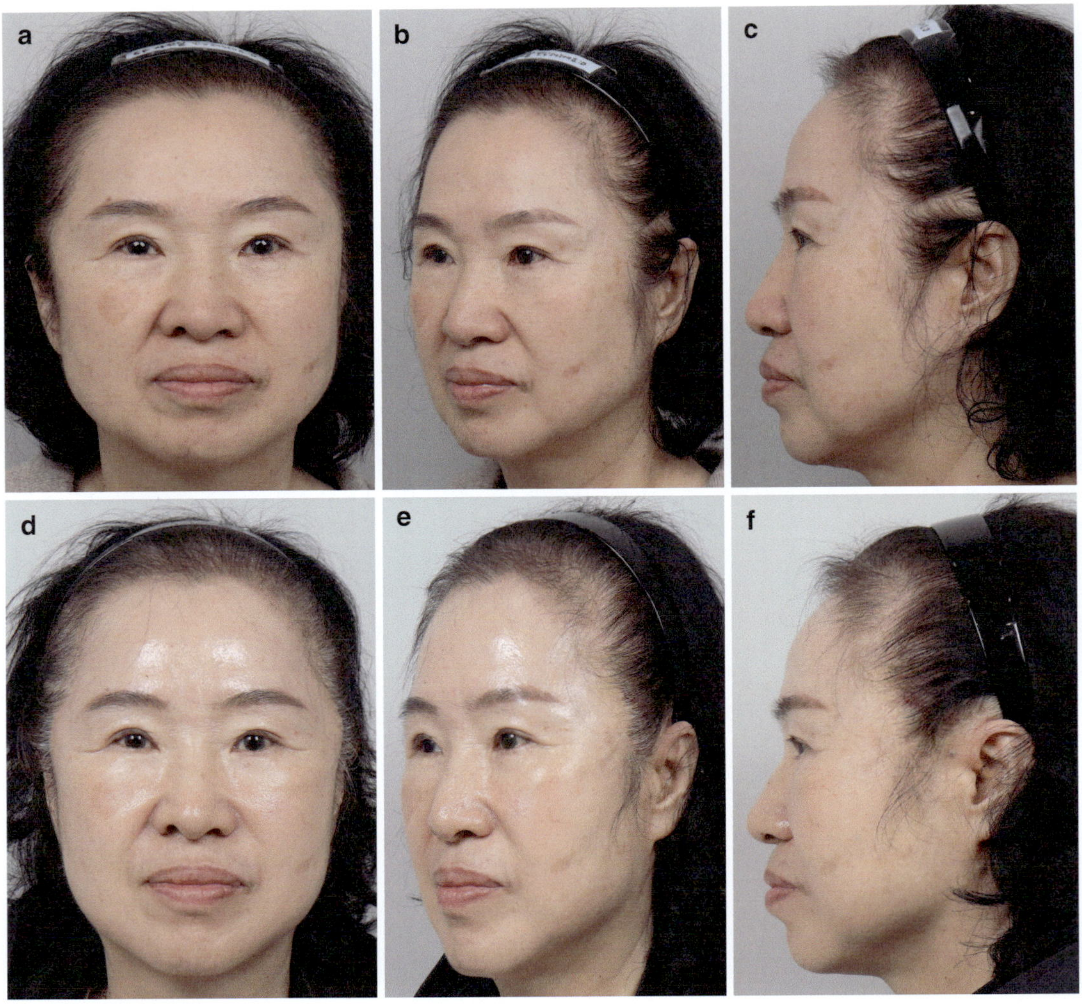

Fig. 7.10 Mini-lifting in a 66-year-old female patient. (**a**) Preoperative frontal view. (**b**) Preoperative three-quarter view. (**c**) Preoperative lateral view. (**d**) Postoperative 2 weeks frontal view. (**e**) Postoperative 2 weeks three-quarter view. (**f**) Postoperative 2 weeks lateral view

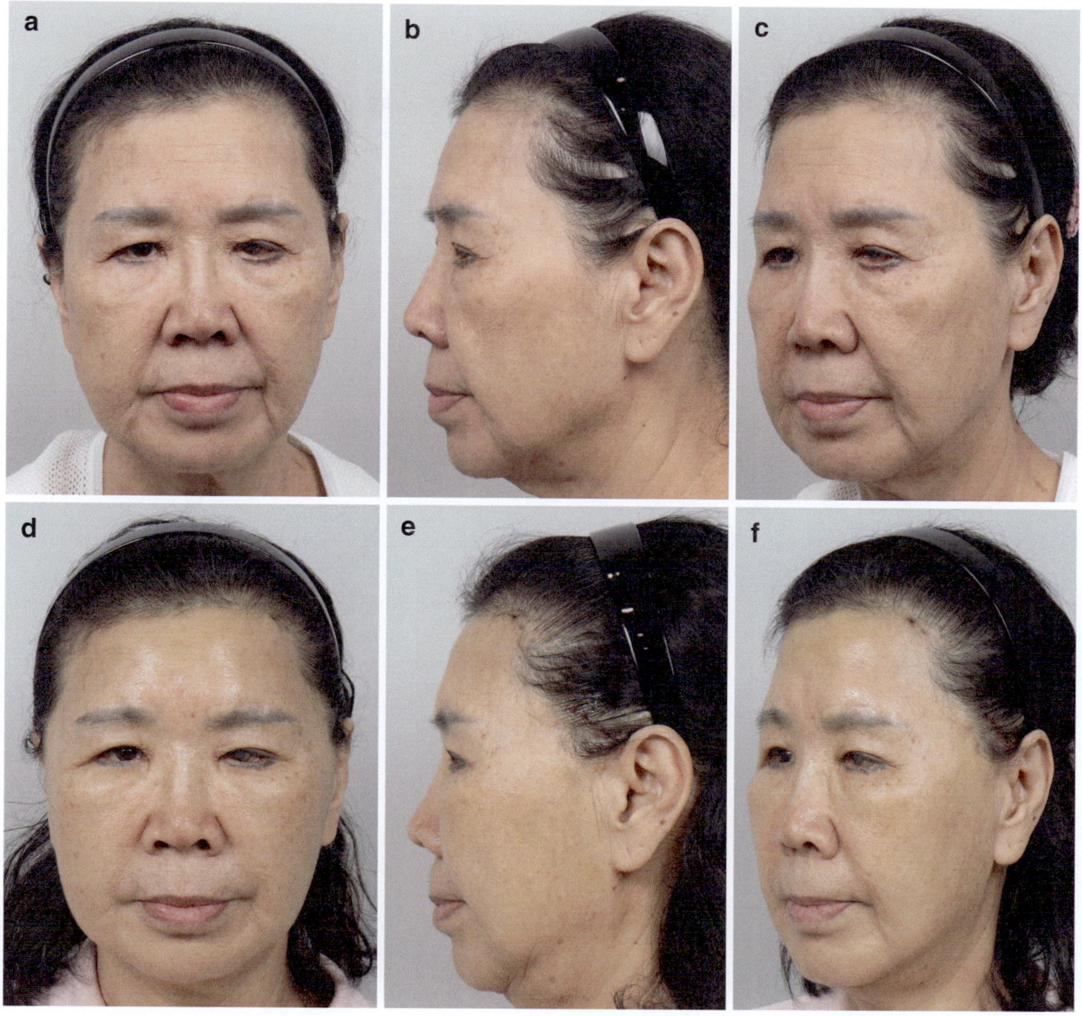

Fig. 7.11 Mini-lifting in a 68-year-old female patient. (**a**) Preoperative frontal view. (**b**) Preoperative lateral view. (**c**) Preoperative three-quarter view. (**d**) Postoperative 2 weeks frontal view. (**e**) Postoperative 2 weeks lateral view. (**f**) Postoperative 2 weeks three-quarter view

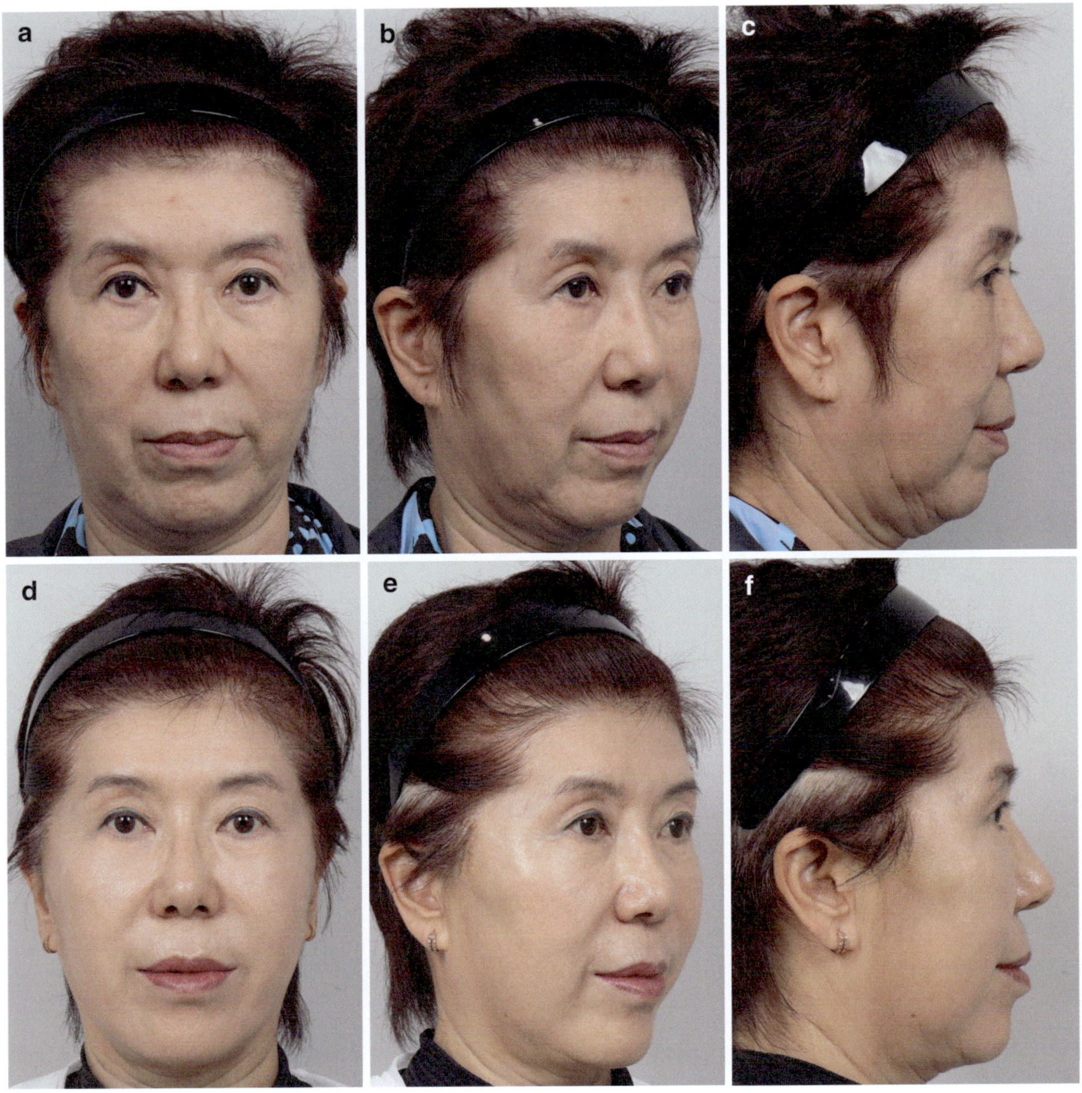

Fig. 7.12 Mini-lifting in a 59-year-old female patient. (**a**) Preoperative frontal view. (**b**) Preoperative three-quarter view. (**c**) Preoperative lateral view. (**d**) Postoperative 2 weeks frontal view. (**e**) Postoperative 2 weeks three-quarter view. (**f**) Postoperative 2 weeks lateral view

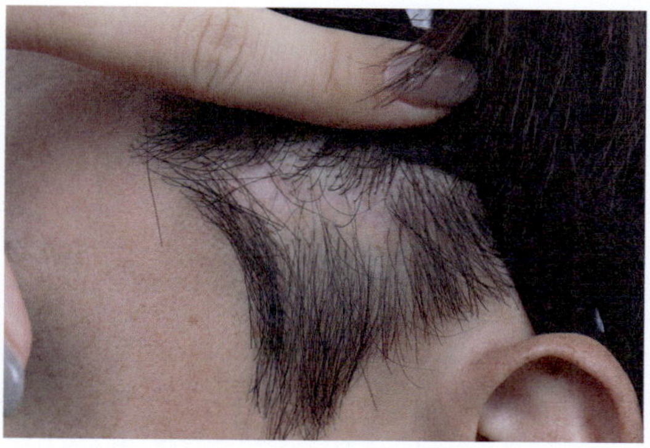

Fig. 7.13 A 42-year-old male patient, 1-month postoperative view. Scar revision surgery was performed after

7.5 Complications

As mentioned in Chap. 6 on the side effects of thread lifting, complications such as asymmetry and skin dimpling may occur. However, similar to the side effects of thread lifting, most of these issues tend to improve naturally over time. Temporal pain is also mostly temporary. The most significant complication associated with mini-lifting is thought to be alopecia at the incision site, which is believed to be related to tension. Alopecia can be improved through scar revision procedures (Fig. 7.13).

7.6 Conclusion

Facelift surgery has evolved over several decades and remains one of the most effective lifting procedures. However, in response to patient demands for less invasive options, methods that provide good lifting effects while being less invasive are being developed. Mini-lifting is one such method, applicable to a broader patient population than thread lifting, and serves as an additional option for patients who are considering the trade-offs between thread lifting and traditional facelift surgery.

References

1. Tran D, Townley JP, Barnes TM, Greive KA. An anti-aging skin care system containing alpha hydroxy acids and vitamins improves the biomechanical parameters of facial skin. Clin Cosmet Investig Dermatol. 2014;8:9–17.
2. Barrett DM, Casanueva FJ, Wang TD. Evolution of the rhytidectomy. World J Otorhinolaryngol Head Neck Surg. 2016;2(1):38–44. https://doi.org/10.1016/j.wjorl.2015.12.001.
3. Jost G, Levet Y. Parotid fascia and face lifting: a critical evaluation of the SMAS concept. Plast Reconstr Surg. 1984;74(1):42–51. https://doi.org/10.1097/00006534-198407000-00006.
4. Litner JA, Adamson PA. Limited vs extended face-lift techniques: objective analysis of intraoperative results. Arch Facial Plast Surg. 2006;8(3):186–90. https://doi.org/10.1001/archfaci.8.3.186.
5. Schmid M, Wolf RC, Freudenmann RW, Schönfeldt-Lecuona C. Tomophobia, the phobic fear caused by an invasive medical procedure – an emerging anxiety disorder: a case report. J Med Case Rep. 2009;3:131. https://doi.org/10.1186/1752-1947-3-131.
6. Caplin DA, Perlyn CA. Facelifts: a contemporary perspective. Mo Med. 2010;107(3):195–7.
7. Sulamanidze MA, Fournier PF, Paikidze TG, Sulamanidze GM. Removal of facial soft tissue ptosis with special threads. Dermatologic Surg. 2002;28(5):367–71. https://doi.org/10.1046/j.1524-4725.2002.01297.x.
8. Lycka B, Bazan C, Poletti E, Treen B. The emerging technique of the antiptosis subdermal suspension thread. Dermatologic Surg. 2004;30(1):41–4; discussion 44. https://doi.org/10.1111/j.1524-4725.2004.30000.x.
9. Wu WT. Barbed sutures in facial rejuvenation. Aesthet Surg J. 2004;24(6):582–7. https://doi.org/10.1016/j.asj.2004.09.007.
10. Unal M, İslamoğlu GK, Ürün Unal G, Köylü N. Experiences of barbed polydioxanone (PDO) cog thread for facial rejuvenation and our technique to prevent thread migration. J Dermatolog Treat. 2021;32(2):227–30. https://doi.org/10.1080/09546634.2019.1640347.
11. Siliprandi M, Bandi V, Lisa A, Vinci V, Maione L, Klinger F. Minimally invasive face lifting and lipofilling. Plast Reconstr Surg Glob Open. 2018;6(2):e1663. Published 2018 Feb 21. https://doi.org/10.1097/GOX.0000000000001663.
12. Dayan S. Aesthetic evolution drives birth of minimally invasive surgery subgroup. J Cosmet Dermatol. 2019;18(5):1182–5. https://doi.org/10.1111/jocd.13057.

13. Stephenson KL. The "mini-lift," an old wrinkle in face lifting. Plast Reconstr Surg. 1970;46(3):226–35. https://doi.org/10.1097/00006534-197009000-00003.
14. Little JW. Three-dimensional rejuvenation of the midface: volumetric resculpture by malar imbrication. Plast Reconstr Surg. 2000;105(1):267–85; discussion 286–9. https://doi.org/10.1097/00006534-200001000-00044.
15. Stuzin JM, Baker TJ, Baker TM. Refinements in face lifting: enhanced facial contour using vicryl mesh incorporated into SMAS fixation. Plast Reconstr Surg. 2000;105(1):290–301. https://doi.org/10.1097/00006534-200001000-00046.
16. del Campo AF. Update on minimally invasive face lift technique. Aesthet Surg J. 2008;28(1):51–61; discussion 62. https://doi.org/10.1016/j.asj.2007.06.006.
17. Sasaki GH, Cohen AT. Meloplication of the malar fat pads by percutaneous cable-suture technique for midface rejuvenation: outcome study (392 cases, 6 years' experience). Plast Reconstr Surg. 2002;110(2):635–54; discussion 655–7. https://doi.org/10.1097/00006534-200208000-00042.
18. Pontius AT, Williams EF 3rd. The extended minimal incision approach to midface rejuvenation. Facial Plast Surg Clin North Am. 2005;13(3):411–9. https://doi.org/10.1016/j.fsc.2005.04.002.
19. Keller GS, Namazie A, Blackwell K, Rawnsley J, Khan S. Elevation of the malar fat pad with a percutaneous technique. Arch Facial Plast Surg. 2002;4(1):20–5. https://doi.org/10.1001/archfaci.4.1.20.
20. Laferriere KA, Castellano RD. Experience with percutaneous suspension of the malar fat pad for midface rejuvenation. Facial Plast Surg Clin North Am. 2005;13(3):393–9. https://doi.org/10.1016/j.fsc.2005.05.002.
21. Gualdi A, Cambiaso-Daniel J, Gatti J, Bertossi D, Pietramaggiori G, Scherer SS, Wurzer P, Lumenta DB. Minimal undermining suspension technique (MUST): combined eyebrow and mid-face lift via temporal access. Aesth Plast Surg. 2017;41(1):40–6. https://doi.org/10.1007/s00266-016-0745-3.
22. Hamra ST. A study of the long-term effect of malar fat repositioning in face lift surgery: short-term success but long-term failure. Plast Reconstr Surg. 2002;110(3):940–51; discussion 952–9. https://doi.org/10.1097/00006534-200209010-00035.

Rhytidectomy

8

Contents

The non-incisional or minimally invasive lifting methods mentioned earlier are all based on surgical facelift techniques (rhytidectomy), and the ultimate goal of these procedures is to achieve results comparable to those of rhytidectomy. Rhytidectomy was first introduced over 100 years ago with skin excision, and the technique of only subcutaneous facelift through skin flap undermining became widely utilized; however, it had limitations in effecting changes in deeper tissues. The significant advancement in rhytidectomy came with the discovery of the SMAS (superficial

W. Lee, K. H. Jung, *Lifting Techniques in Plastic Surgery*,
https://doi.org/10.1007/978-981-96-4820-7_8

muscular aponeurotic system) structure. It was revealed that the SMAS and platysma are connected in the same layer, and separating this layer for movement apart from the skin led to better outcomes, establishing a standard for surgical rhytidectomy. Subsequent research on retaining ligaments further deepened the surgical approach to rhytidectomy.

8.1 Thread Lifting, Mini-Lifting, vs. Rhytidectomy

Recently, many terms associated with rhytidectomy (e.g., mini-lifting, minimal lifting, vertical lifting, midfacial lifting, lower facial lifting) have been used indiscriminately, leading to confusion among patients in clinical practice. Therefore, it is necessary to make clearer distinctions, and the author proposes to categorize rhytidectomy as follows: In the case of thread lifting, there should be no skin incision, and lifting that utilizes a limited skin incision confined to the temple without an incision extending down along the ear is classified as mini-lifting. If there is a skin incision line that extends down along the front of the ear, it is classified as rhytidectomy. If this incision line is limited to within the earlobe, it is defined as a minimal access cranial suspension (MACS) incision, while extending the incision along the postauricular sulcus is defined as a traditional facelift incision.

The differences between thread lifting, mini-lifting, and rhytidectomy can be summarized in two main points:

Is it possible to adequately excise remnant skin?
Is it possible to release the retaining ligaments?

Even if a certain amount of skin can be excised in mini-lifting, it is limited to the vertically loosened skin, and attempting excessive skin excision can lead to skin distortion (puckering) or an increased risk of scar widening, thus limiting the amount of excision (see Chap. 7). In contrast, rhytidectomy allows for sufficient skin excision by pulling the skin vertically along all RSTLs (relaxed skin tension lines), achieving a more natural lifting effect.

Additionally, since mini-lifting cannot perform retaining ligament release, it is akin to having a brake on the upward movement of tissues. Ignoring this and attempting to pull forcibly can result in dimpling or accentuating existing submalar hollowness (especially at the superoanterior border). On the other hand, rhytidectomy allows for the release of retaining ligaments, enabling more movement of the SMAS and facilitating smooth repositioning of the fat compartments as a single unit.

8.2 Types of Rhytidectomy

Rhytidectomy can be broadly classified into three categories based on whether and how the SMAS is manipulated:

1. Subcutaneous facelift without SMAS manipulation
2. SMAS suspension technique with simple SMAS manipulation
3. Deep plane rhytidectomy technique with sub-SMAS dissection

The subcutaneous facelift is a traditional method that has been performed since the 1900s, prior to the anatomical confirmation of the "SMAS" structure, and it had limitations in effectiveness and longevity. To achieve greater effects, new attempts were made to target deeper tissues, leading to the SMAS suspension technique (see Table 8.1). Initially, the simplest methods, such as plication and imbrication, were employed. However, to address issues such as widening malar distance or limited effectiveness, more aggressive methods were introduced, including SMASectomy, and a stacking method was developed for patients with less volume [1–5].

Table 8.1 Types of rhytidectomy

Type	Management layer: Skin (range of dissection)	Management layer: SMAS (method)	Operation name	The year of publication
1	Wide	–	Subcutaneous facelift	
2	Wide	Plication	SMAS suspension technique	1976
		Imbrication		
		SMASectomy		
		Stacking		
3	Limited	Sub-SMAS dissection	Deep plane	1990
	Less limited	Sub-SMAS dissection Including OOM	Composite	1992
	Wide	Sub-SMAS dissection (lower to high)	Extended	1995
	Wide	Sub-SMAS dissection (High)	High SMAS	2002

After it was established that the SMAS is a distinct structure, it was found that dissection in the sub-SMAS plane through a traditional SMASectomy incision could yield greater lifting effects, leading to the term “deep-plane facelift” [6].

However, when accessing the sub-SMAS through the traditional SMASectomy incision, improvements in the midface were limited. To address this, a method was devised to extend the SMAS incision upward to include the orbicularis oculi muscle in the SMAS flap, resulting in the composite facelift (Fig. 8.1a) [7, 8].

Both the “deep-plane” and “Composite facelift” techniques were highly evolved; however, they had the drawback of only achieving a vertical (perpendicular) vector from the SMASectomy incision. A method was developed to pull the midface and lower face with different vectors. This method starts the SMAS incision below the zygomatic arch and involves elevating a triangular flap that includes the orbicularis oculi muscle for fixation, termed the extended facelift (Fig. 8.1b) [9].

In both deep-plane and composite facelift procedures, the SMAS incision line is placed more anteriorly than the Pitanguy line, and in the extended facelift, the incision is made at the lower SMAS (below the zygomatic arch) to avoid damage to the frontal branch of the facial nerve. However, after it was discovered that the frontal branch runs superficially about 1.5 cm above the zygomatic arch, surgical methods began to be introduced that initiate the SMAS incision above the zygomatic arch or along it, known as the high SMAS technique [10, 11].

The author believes that while the term “deep-plane facelift” has become familiar to patients through social media, it has led to confusion as the same term is interpreted and explained in different ways, hindering a comprehensive understanding of rhytidectomy. Therefore, by examining the evolution of rhytidectomy, it is believed that a more comfortable approach can be achieved.

Recently, “deep plane” has been used as a term encompassing all surgical methods involving sub-SMAS dissection, and consequently,

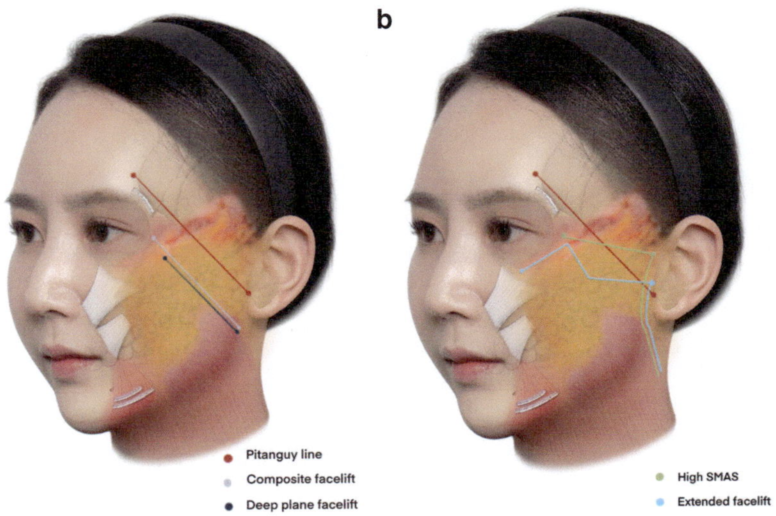

Fig. 8.1 Types of rhytidectomy and the location of each SMAS incision. (**a**) Composite and deep plane rhytidectomy. (**b**) High SMAS and extended facelift

composite facelift, extended facelift, and high SMAS facelift are all included within the same category.

8.3 Rhytidectomy Skin Incision

One of the primary concerns for patients undergoing facelift surgery is how noticeable the scars will be. During preoperative consultations, it is crucial to thoroughly explain the rationale behind the chosen incision locations, as this significantly impacts immediate satisfaction and the maintenance of the patient relationship. When determining incision lines, considerations can be divided into three main categories (Fig. 8.2).

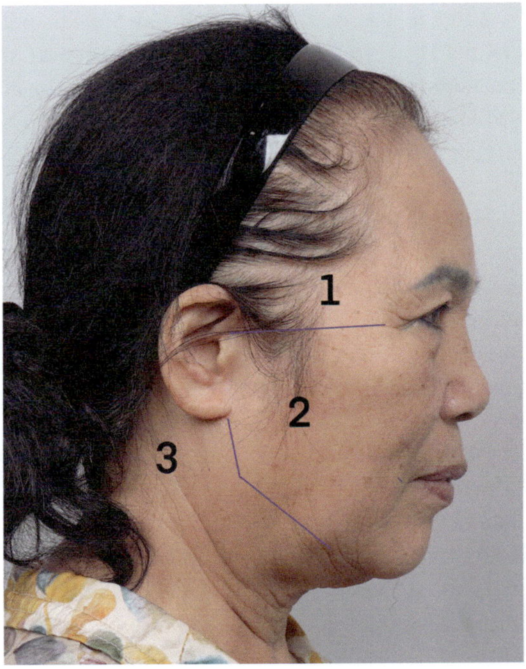

Fig. 8.2 Incision line locations. A (1) Temple area—inside the hairline vs. along the hairline. B (2) Preauricular area—pretragal vs. retrotragal. C (3) Postauricular—in the hairline (Lazy S) or along the hairline

8.3.1 Temple Area Incision: Hairline Inside vs. Along the Hairline

The hairline incision is performed inside the hairline if the distance between the hairline and the lateral canthus is within 4–5 cm; otherwise, the incision is made outside along the sideburn. However, the specific numbers are less important than the fact that using an incision inside the hairline can effectively conceal scars, but it may shorten the sideburn and cause the hairline to move backward, resulting in an aesthetically unfavorable outcome due to a relatively wider facial proportion.

The method of making an incision along the hairline maintains the shape of the hairline while creating the effect of a shorter distance between

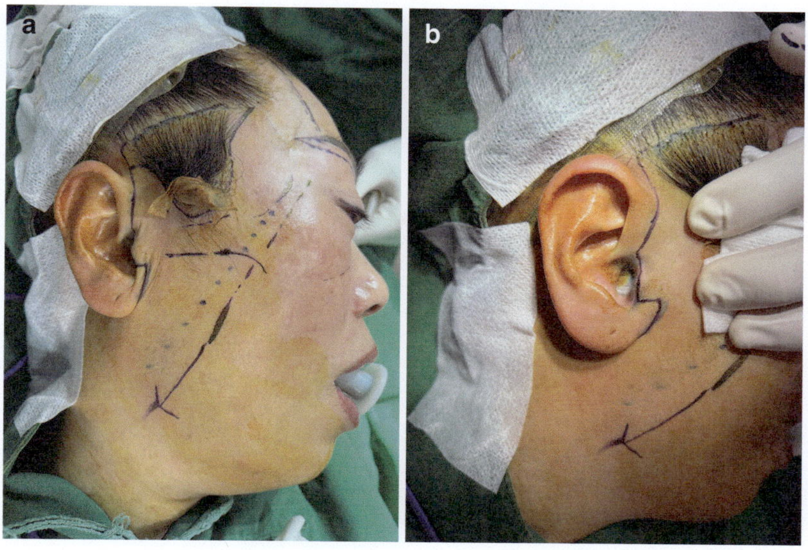

Fig. 8.3 Rhytidectomy skin incision line. (**a**) In the temple area, methods of incision along the hairline and inside the hairline. (**b**) Retrotragal incision method in the preauricular area

the hairline and lateral canthus (Fig. 8.3). Therefore, this is a good surgical option for patients with very short sideburns, and it is particularly preferred among Asian patients with wider cheekbones, as the face occupies a relatively larger proportion when viewed from the front or at a 45° angle. However, it may be difficult to conceal the wound immediately after surgery, and over time, there is a higher risk of visibility compared to Western patients. Technically, more time must be spent on trimming when making an incision inside the hairline compared to along it.

8.3.2 Preauricular Area Incision: Pretragal vs. Retrotragal Incision

When making an incision along a curved line following the helix, the incision will meet the tragus. The choice between a pretragal incision and a retrotragal incision should be made considering the skin color, thickness, and distribution of hair follicles. If hair follicles are densely distributed in the cheek (especially in cases where the sideburn extends downwards), and if the skin is thick or there is a significant contrast in color between the tragus and the cheek, a pretragal incision is recommended.

On the other hand, while the retrotragal incision has the clear advantage of concealing scars, it requires additional time and effort for skin flap elevation. To prevent distortion of the tragus and maintain a rectangular shape, the incision should be made by advancing approximately 5 mm horizontally from the bottom of the tragus and then sharply changing direction at a 90° angle to continue the incision along the earlobe. Below the earlobe, the incision should be made 1–2 mm away from the facial skin attachment to facilitate management during closure and minimize distortion of the earlobe shape.

8.3.3 Postauricular Area Incision: Inside the Occipital Hairline vs. Along the Hairline

The incision in the postauricular area is designed along the conchal groove. After marking this area, during the actual procedure, if the assistant bends the ear toward the face, it can be observed that the actual skin incision line shifts toward the ear compared to the groove. Therefore, caution is needed when placing the conchal groove incision after bending the ear, as this may result in the scar line being lower and more visible from the lateral view postoperatively.

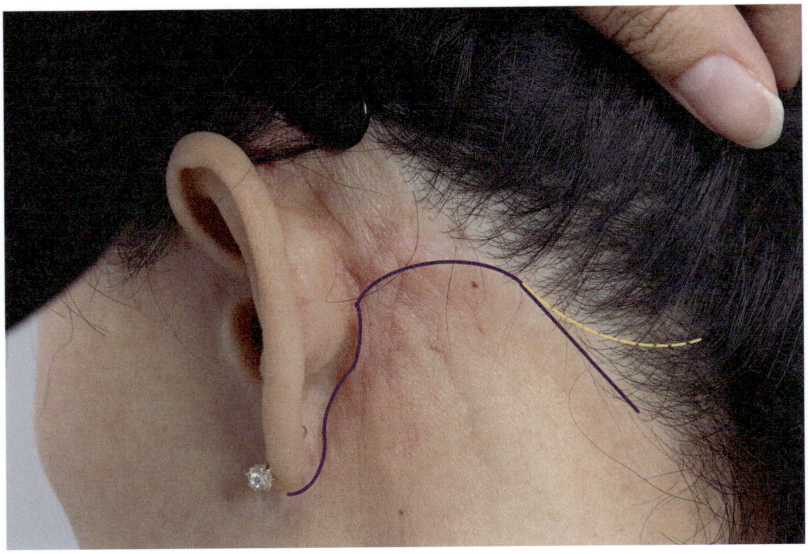

Fig. 8.4 Postauricular incision. The direction should change at the upper border of the external auditory canal to proceed towards the occipital hairline (purple), followed by a choice between incising along the hairline (purple) or hiding the incision inside the hairline (yellow) depending on the patient

The incision line that ascends along the conchal groove should smoothly change direction at the height of the upper margin of the antihelix or external auditory canal, advancing toward the occipital hairline. At the occipital hairline, there are two options: to enter more horizontally inside the hairline or to make the incision along the occipital hairline (Fig. 8.4). For patients with significant skin redundancy in the neck area, making the incision along the occipital hairline is more effective, and the length of the incision can be adjusted based on the amount of remnant skin.

8.4 Rhytidectomy Dissection

8.4.1 Subcutaneous Fat Dissection Range

After making the incision with a scalpel, the first step is to perform skin flap elevation, which raises questions about how and to what extent to dissect. The choice of surgical method affects the range of subcutaneous fat dissection, but generally, a minimum dissection of subcutaneous fat should extend to the line connecting the lateral canthus and the mandible angle to facilitate access to the sub-SMAS (superficial muscular aponeurotic system) (Fig. 8.5). For example, in a deep plane facelift, sufficient subcutaneous fat dissection is necessary to secure a robust cuff for SMAS fixation, and for an extended facelift, a greater range of subcutaneous fat dissection is required.

The dissection method involves using a scalpel to make the skin incision, followed by elevating the skin flap to a thickness of about 1 cm with a scalpel, sharp Metzenbaum scissors, or electronic cautery to find the appropriate depth. Subsequently, using facelifting scissors, blunt dissection is performed while maintaining tension towards the surgeon, continuing the subcutaneous fat dissection to the boundary of the lateral orbital rim and mandible border (Fig. 8.6). However, if attempting to progress further inward beyond this line with blind dissection, there is a

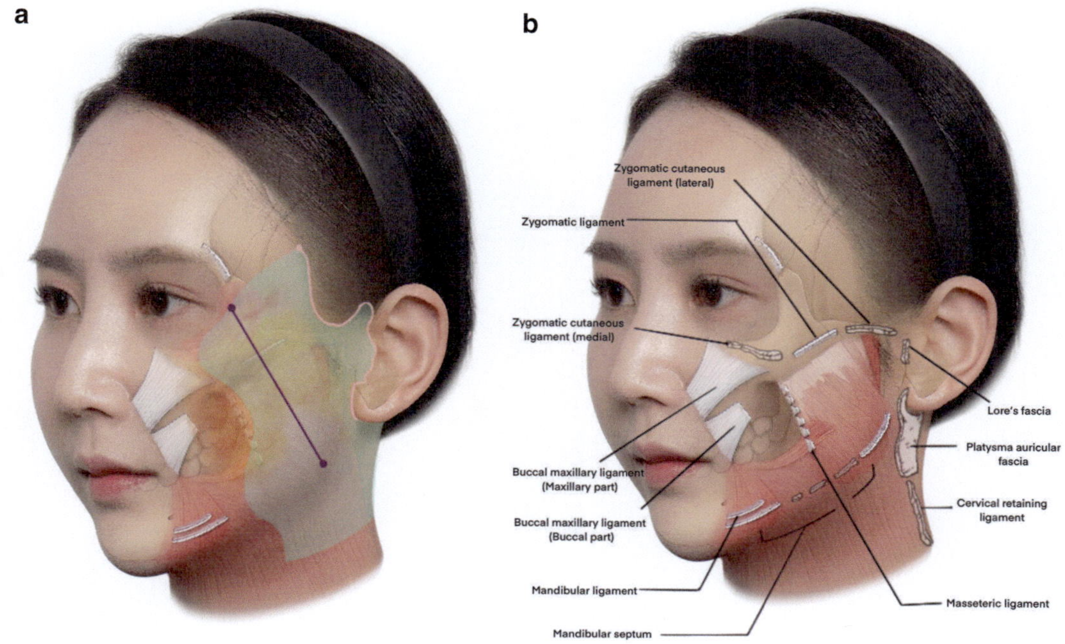

Fig. 8.5 Range of subcutaneous fat dissection. (**a**) Range of subcutaneous fat dissection (green) and reference line (lateral orbital rim—mandible angle: purple line). (**b**) Facial retaining ligaments encountered during rhytidectomy dissection

high likelihood that subcutaneous fat will be included in the skin flap in the zygomatic ligament area, which can often result in tearing in that area during subsequent SMAS elevation. Therefore, for more meticulous dissection, it is recommended to perform dissection visually when going inward beyond the lateral orbital rim and mandible border.

Once the skin flap is sufficiently elevated, the lateral belly of the orbicularis oculi muscle should be visible (Fig. 8.7). In the midface area, the perforator artery of the transverse facial artery, which penetrates through the SMAS, should be identified and ligated. It is crucial to release a portion of the zygomatic cutaneous ligament to ensure sufficient skin redundancy. In the lower face, it is recommended to elevate the dissection to the midpoint of the mandible border (facial artery and vein). In the neck area, at least down to the first transverse crease should be dissected, connecting naturally with the dissection range in the lower face. In cases where there is significant neck wrinkling, it may be necessary to dissect to the extent that both sides are tunneled.

8.4.2 Thickness of the Dissection Flap

There is considerable debate regarding the depth of skin flap elevation. When the skin flap is elevated thinly, a sturdier SMAS flap can be secured; however, this increases the risk of skin necrosis and may lead to more visible irregularities immediately after surgery. Conversely, elevating the skin flap thicker can result in a relatively thinner SMAS, and some superficial fat may adhere to the skin flap, making it difficult to achieve the desired fat repositioning effect. However, the author believes that the level of skin flap dissection is predetermined. The fat layer between the skin flap and the SMAS can be broadly divided into hypodermal fat (dermal white adipose tissue, dWAT) and subcutaneous fat (subcutaneous white adipose tissue, sWAT), with a paper-thin fascia separating the two layers. This fascia, however, is not clearly defined in all areas and is difficult to distinguish visually.

As discussed in Chap. 1, dWAT is found within a distinct collagen network, appearing

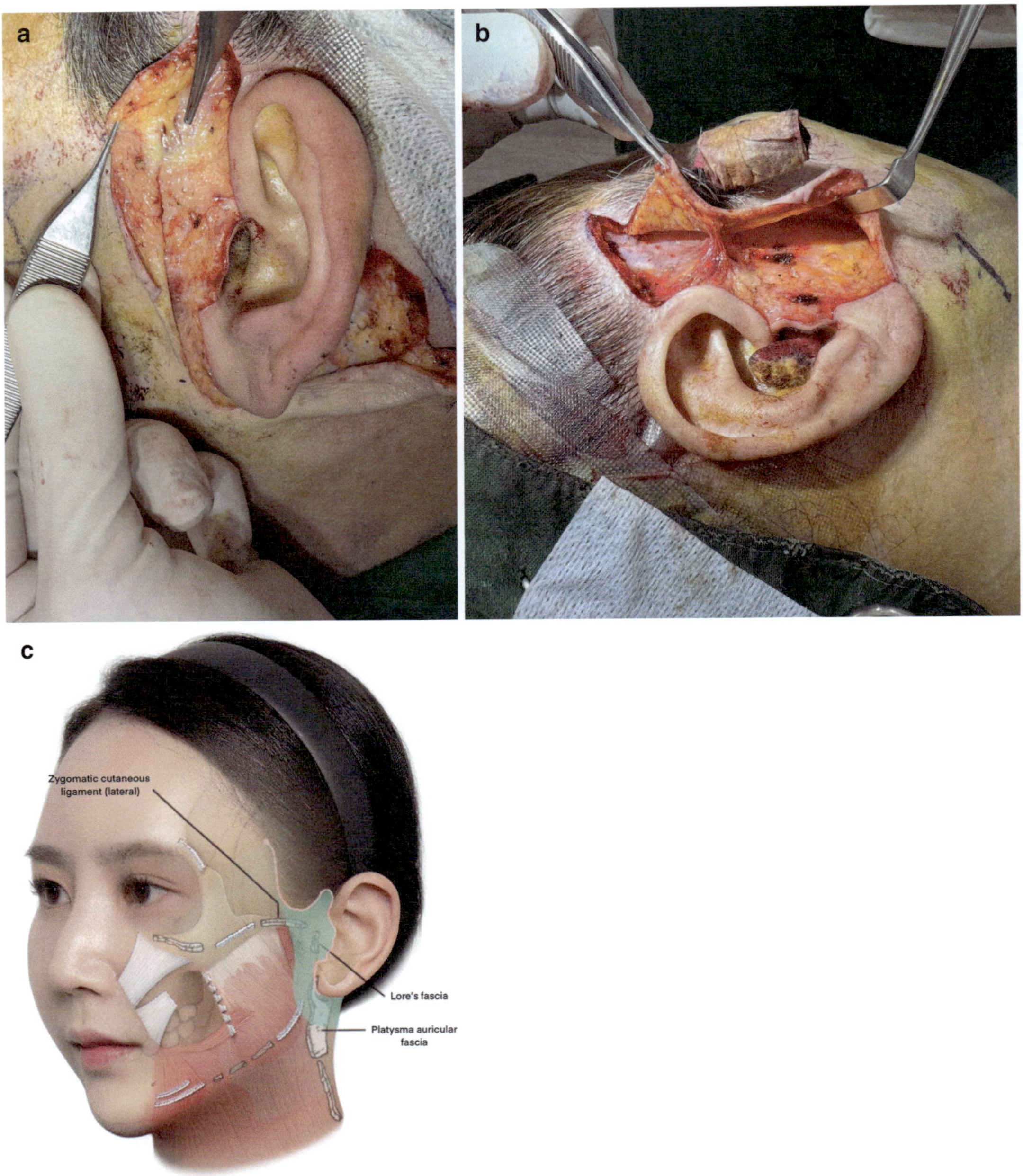

Fig. 8.6 Rhytidectomy subcutaneous dissection. (**a**) Skin flap elevated using a scalpel. (**b**) Observing the lateral zygomatic cutaneous ligament while switching to scissors for subcutaneous dissection. (**c**) Schematic diagram of subcutaneous dissection and the position of the lateral zygomatic ligament

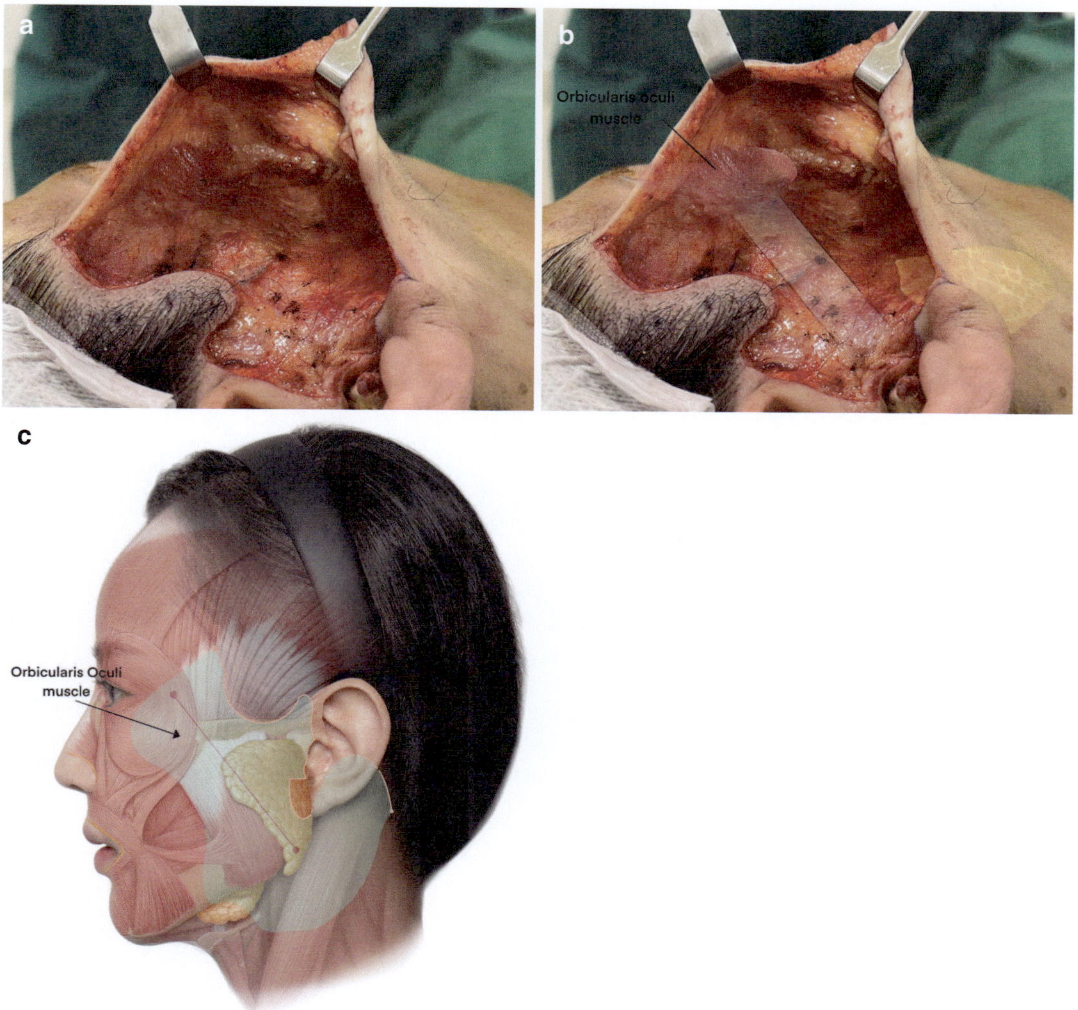

Fig. 8.7 Range of subcutaneous fat dissection. Elevation until the orbicularis oculi muscle is identified in the temple area and midface during subcutaneous flap elevation. (**a**) Surgical findings. (**b**) Schematic diagram of the orbicularis oculi muscle. (**c**) Diagram of the operation field. Dissection range (green)

smaller and firmer than sWAT, which is round and elastic, protruding from the dermal layer. Therefore, once the appropriate layer is identified early on, it is possible to perform subcutaneous fat dissection easily within a clean surgical field with minimal bleeding (Fig. 8.8).

8.4.3 Deep-Plane SMAS Elevation

Accessing the sub-SMAS layer varies depending on the preferred surgical method. The author employs a modified approach that combines the advantages of high SMAS and extended facelifts, which will be described here.

SMAS Incision First, the incision line advances along the edge of the zygomatic arch, transitioning to an oblique incision towards the cephalic direction along the fibers of the orbicularis oculi muscle belly as it reaches the orbital rim and lateral canthus. In front of the ear, the incision is made vertically down to the mandible angle, starting 1 cm away from the incision line, and then approaches the sub-SMAS layer along the posterior end of the platysma in the neck area (Fig. 8.9).

Lower-Face Sub-SMAS Dissection SMAS dissection begins by locating the end belly of the platysma from the zygomatic arch down to the earlobe. This area is preferred because the parotid gland covers the facial nerve, minimizing the risk of nerve damage. Additionally, the parotid gland

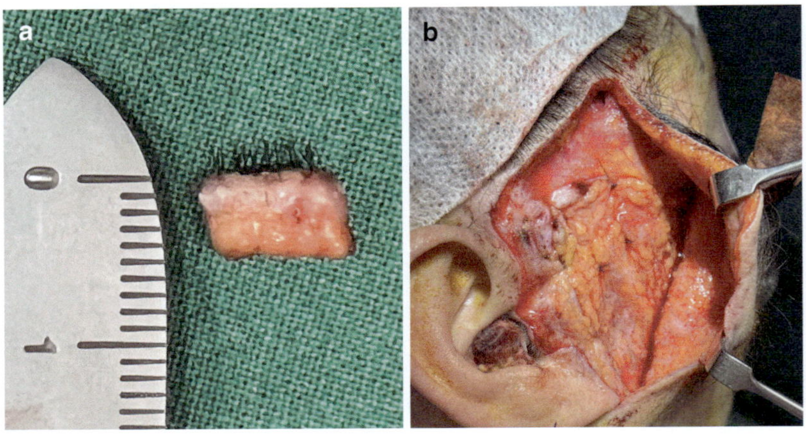

Fig. 8.8 Thickness of the skin flap. (**a**) Appropriate thickness of the skin flap, with approximately 2 mm of fat tissue adhering to the dermis during elevation. (**b**) dWAT is small and firmly attached to the dermis, while sWAT appears as relatively larger lobules and has a softer appearance

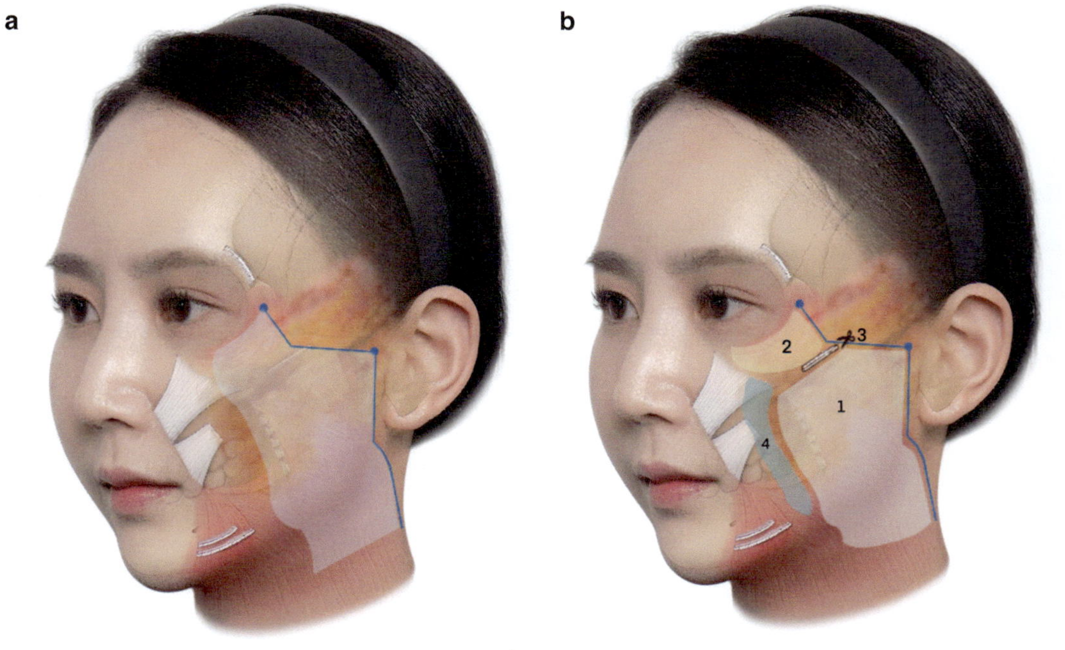

Fig. 8.9 SMAS incision and sub-SMAS dissection sequence. (**a**) Horizontal incision along the zygomatic arch and a vertical incision 1 cm anterior to the skin incision (blue line). (**b**) Dissection sequence. (**c**) Overall sub-SMAS dissection sequence

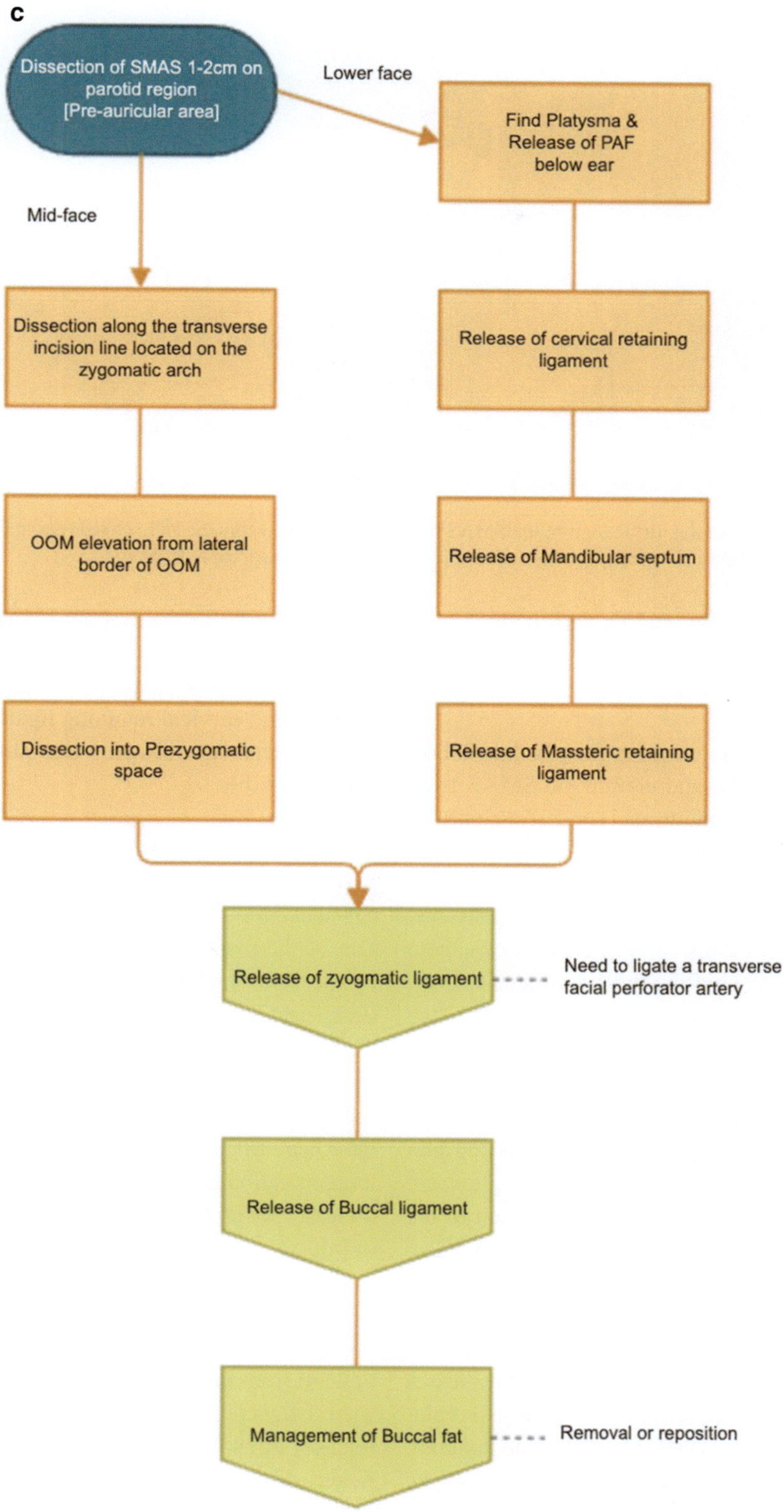

Fig. 8.9 (continued)

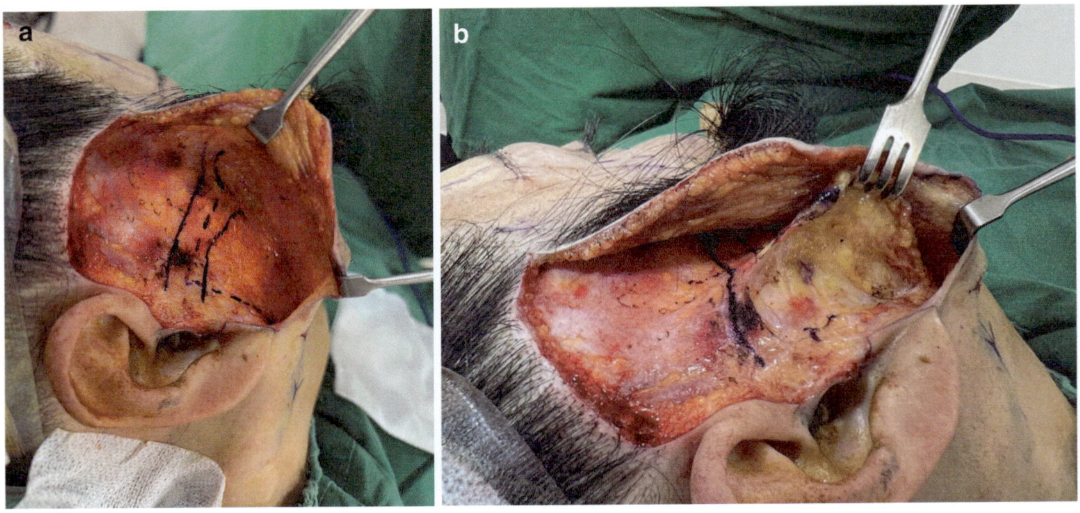

Fig. 8.10 SMAS elevation. (**a**) Design of the SMAS incision along the zygomatic arch. (**b**) Elevating the SMAS from the parotid region allows for relatively easy and safe identification of the appropriate layer

is enveloped in fascia, and its dark yellow color and glandular structure are easily distinguishable from adipose tissue (Fig. 8.10).

While there is a method to find the lateral border of the platysma and elevate the SMAS from the neck area, if the platysma is underdeveloped or strongly attached to the sternocleidomastoid muscle fascia, it may be challenging to find the appropriate layer, risking tearing of the platysma. Furthermore, if the dissection goes too deep, there is a risk of damaging the greater auricular nerve. Once the platysma is located in the neck, the SMAS can be elevated with forceps while applying tension, and dissection can be performed using electric cautery. To prevent excessive depth, cauterization should be performed closer to the platysma rather than the deep fascia, allowing for safe and natural dissection. Notably, dissection in the lower face is generally easier than in the midface, so it is recommended to start with the lower face.

Lower Face: Release of PAF and Cervical Retaining Ligament As dissection progresses with the platysma positioned superiorly, the platysma auricular fascia (PAF) will be encountered, which is firmly attached to the gland below the ear. Continuing dissection further down will reveal a strong structure located between the anterior border of the sternocleidomastoid muscle and the platysma, known as the cervical retaining ligament. Sufficient dissection of both the PAF and cervical retaining ligament is essential to achieve optimal neck lifting effects (Fig. 8.11a, b).

Lower Face: Release of Mandibular Septum Changing the dissection position from the neck to the lower face allows for identification of the mandibular septum along the mandible border, which is relatively less firm than the ligament and can be easily released (Fig. 8.11c, d). Dissection should extend to the midpoint of the mandible border where the facial artery ascends. Since the patient is lying supine with their head tilted upward during surgery, the marginal mandibular nerve is located below the mandible border up to the midpoint, reducing the risk of injury.

Lower Face: Release of Masseteric Ligaments As the sub-SMAS dissection is naturally extended upward from the neck to the lower face, the masseteric ligament will be encountered. Complete release of this ligament is essential because insufficient dissection can restrict movement of the SMAS and may lead to wrinkle reorientation (Fig. 8.12). However, this tissue is relatively

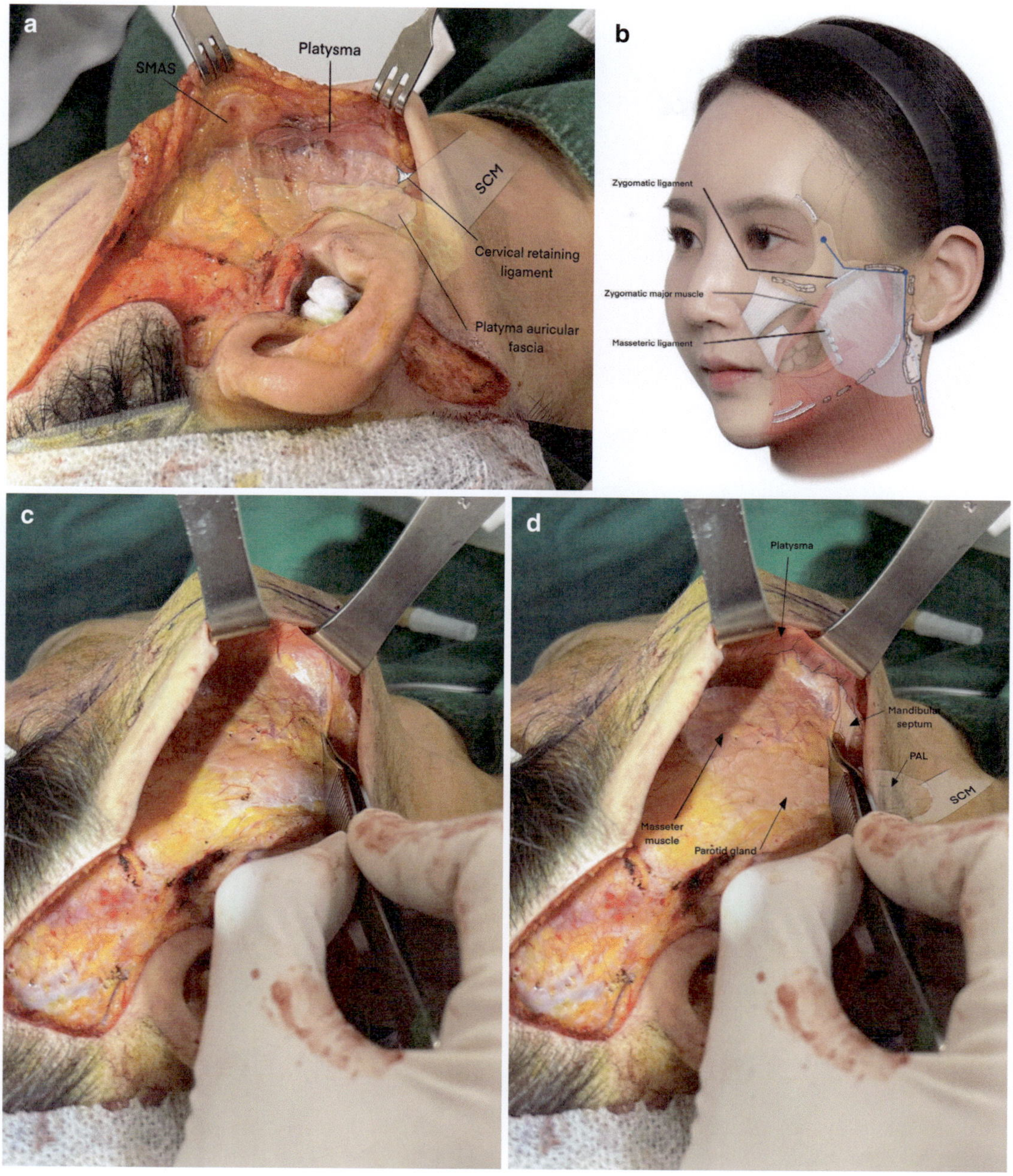

Fig. 8.11 Sub-SMAS dissection of the lower face. (**a**) Structures that need to be released during lower face dissection. (**b**) Area of sub-SMAS dissection. (**c**) Mandibular septum observed during lower face dissection. (**d**) Schematic explanation

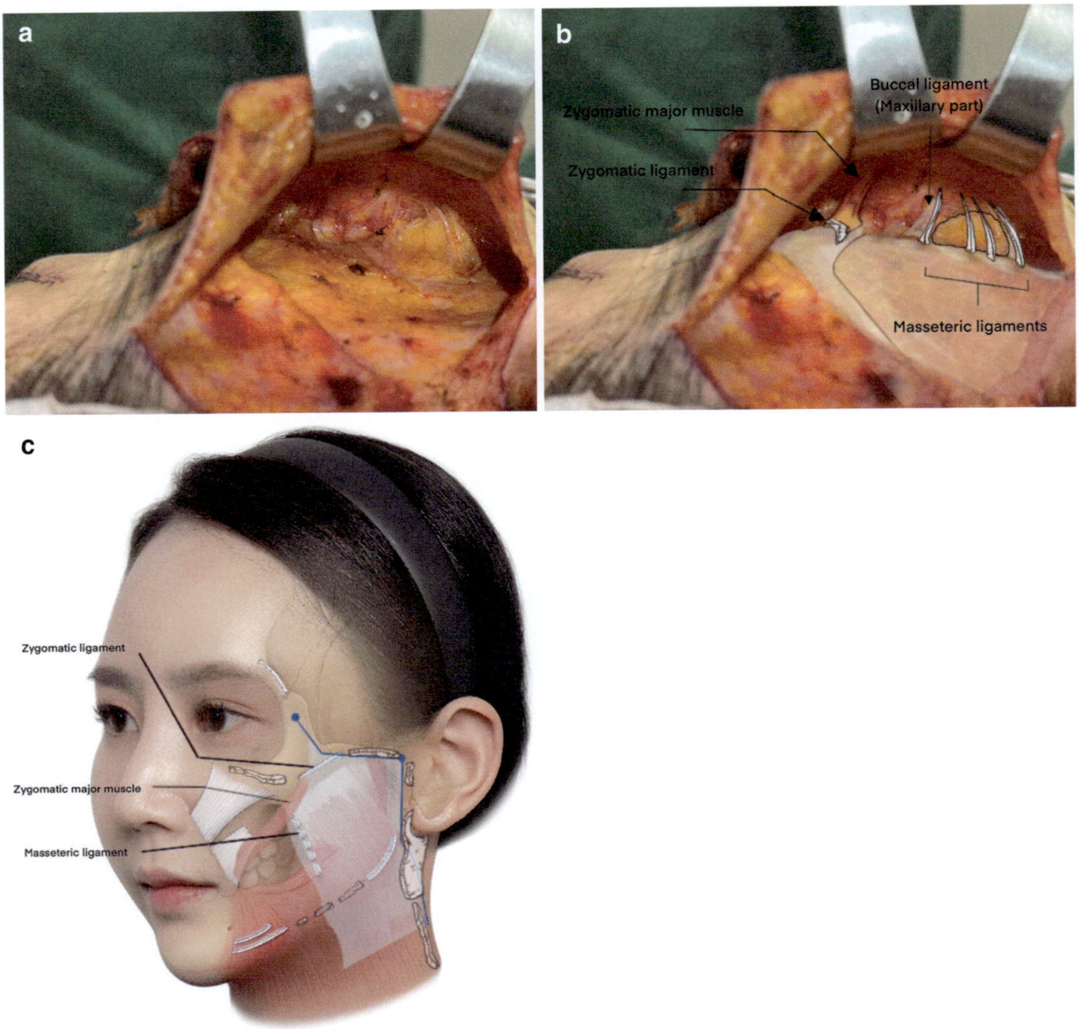

Fig. 8.12 Masseteric ligament. Multiple vertical fibrous bands can be observed along the anterior border of the masseter muscle. (**a**) Surgical findings. (**b**) Schematic diagram of surgical findings. (**c**) Illustration of retaining ligaments and surgical findings. Sub-SMAS dissection area (white)

weaker than the zygomatic ligament, making dissection straightforward. Many beginners often struggle to distinguish between some fibrous bands and nerves, leading them to halt further dissection. By applying vertical traction to the SMAS and palpating with the second finger, the fibrous bands can be easily identified due to their firmness.

Midface Sub-OOM Dissection

Continuing dissection from the lower face into the midface, a strong ligamentous structure can be identified at the superoanterior edge of the submalar hollowness, known as the zygomatic ligament (Fig. 8.13). This ligament is relatively loose, and if the layer distinction is clear, it can be released directly; however, this area is generally the most challenging. If the correct layer is not identified and dissection is performed too superficially, there is a risk of tearing the SMAS. Conversely, if dissection goes too deep, there is a risk of damaging branches of the zygomatic nerve that run over the zygomatic major muscle. In such cases, it is advisable to move to the area above the zygomatic ligament for dissection and then reassess. Above the zygomatic liga-

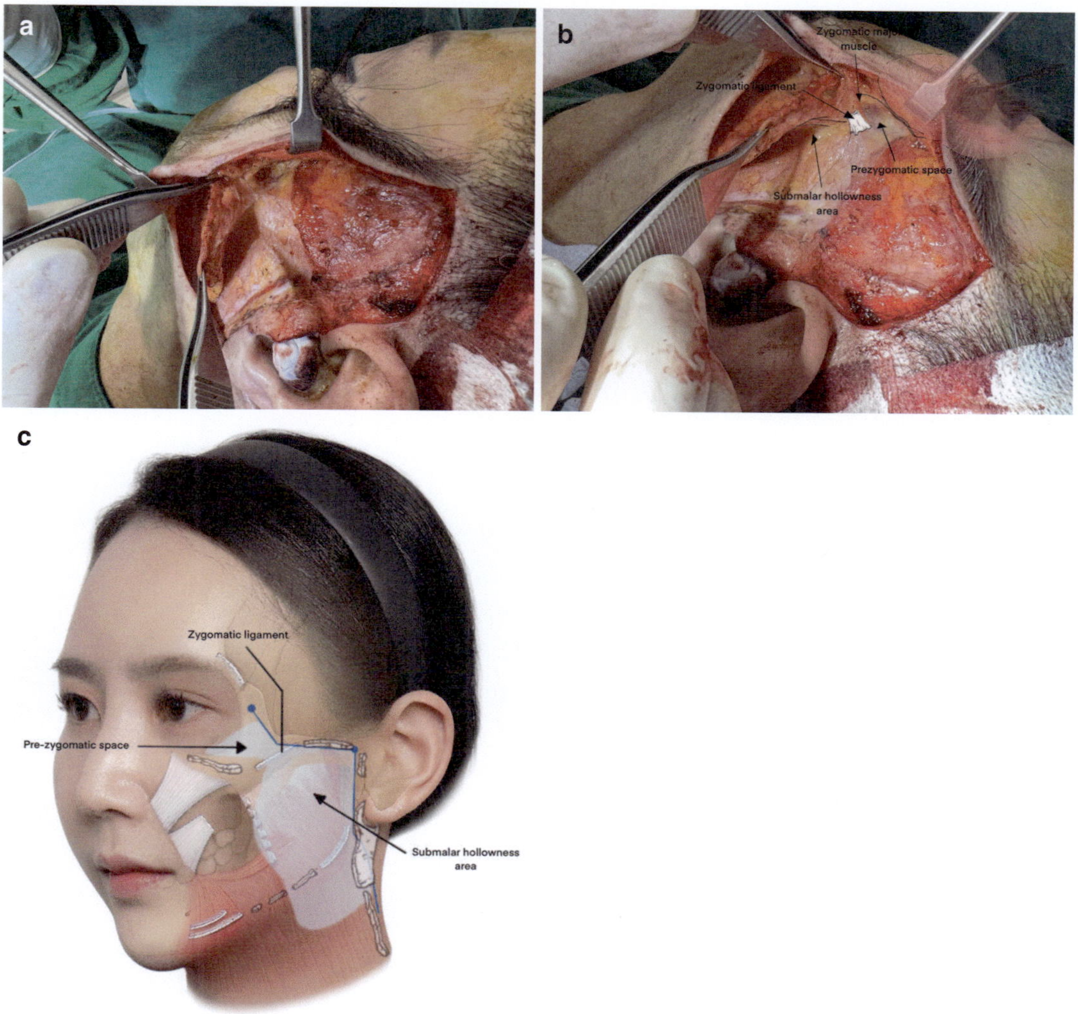

Fig. 8.13 Zygomatic ligament. A strong adhesion between the SMAS and deeper tissue near the origin of the zygomatic major muscle. (**a**) Surgical findings. (**b**) Schematic diagram of surgical findings. (**c**) Illustration of surgical findings and retaining ligaments. Sub-SMAS dissection area (white)

ment, the orbicularis oculi muscle can be identified, and by keeping the OOM superior, dissection of 0.5–1 cm can lead to the prezygomatic space, allowing for easy advancement to the mid-pupil level.

Release of Zygomatic Ligament

Once sufficient dissection of the lower and midface has been performed based on the zygomatic ligament, vertical traction on the SMAS will make it easier to visualize the zygomatic ligament. Adequate release of the zygomatic ligament allows for observation of the medial zygomatic cutaneous ligament, which is strongly attached to the skin along the medial margin of the zygomatic major muscle, as well as the lower edge of the OOM. Both areas must be sufficiently released; if the medial zygomatic cutaneous ligament is not adequately released, the mid-cheek groove may become more pronounced. Additionally, if the lower edge of the OOM is left intact while pulling the SMAS, it can lead to malar bulging.

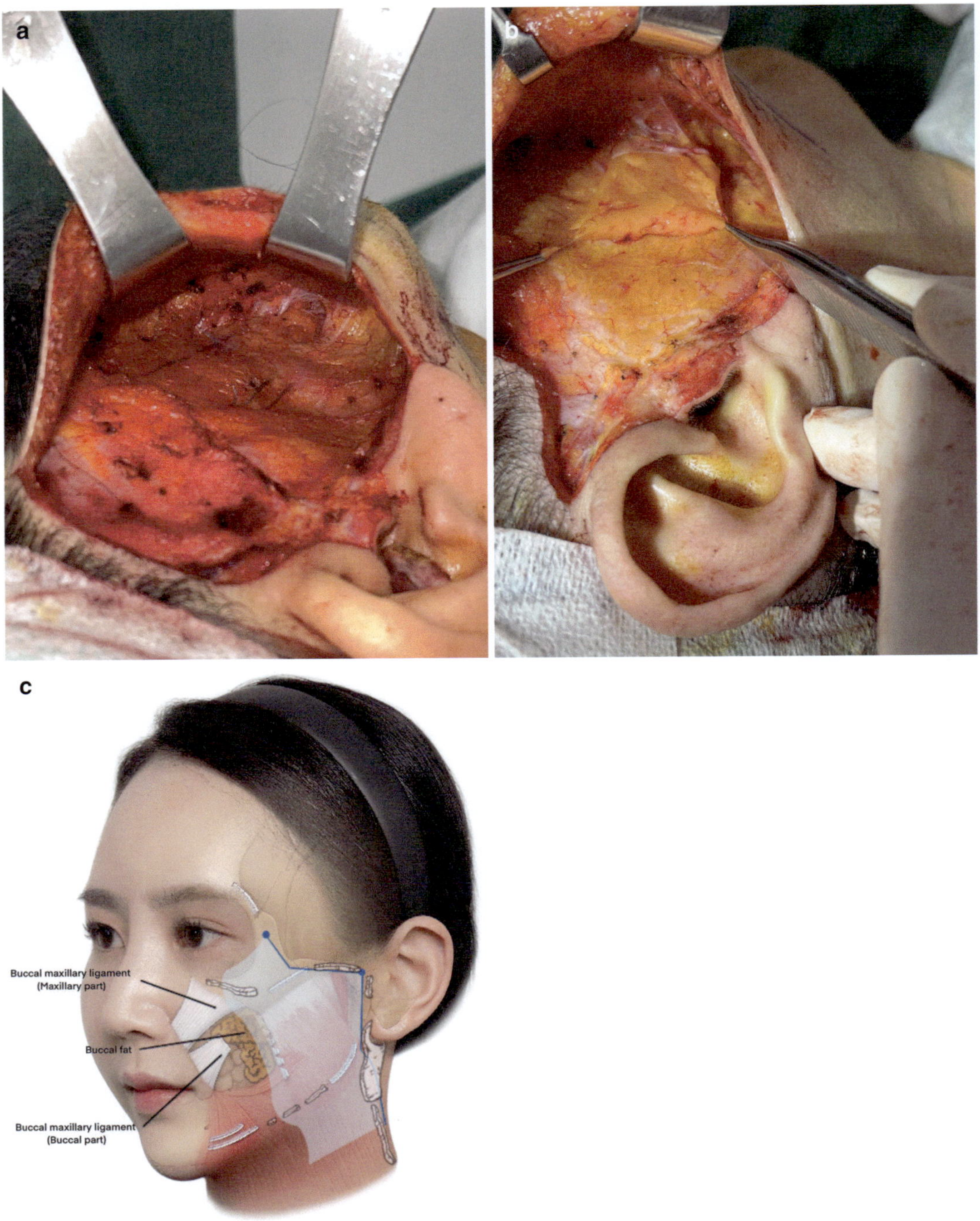

Fig. 8.14 Buccal maxillary ligament. (**a**) The buccal maxillary ligament encountered after releasing all masseteric retaining ligaments. (White arrow: maxillary part, sky blue arrow: buccal part) Buccal fat can be observed between them. (**b**) Buccal fat in an extracted state after capsulotomy. (**c**) Schematic diagram

Release of Buccal Ligament

After releasing both the zygomatic and masseteric ligaments, the dissection will encounter areas of strong adhesion between the SMAS and deep fascia, specifically the buccal maxillary ligament (Fig. 8.14). Between the maxillary part and buccal part of the buccal maxillary ligament, a gel-like adipose tissue that is distinctly separated from surrounding tissues can be found, known as buccal fat. Since the patient is lying on the operating table with their face turned to the opposite side, this fat is positioned superolaterally, making it easy to locate.

Management of Buccal Fat

Buccal fat can be divided into four extensions (pterygopalatine, pterygoid, temporal, buccal extension). In cases where there is an excess of buccal fat, it should be removed, but care should be taken not to remove the other extensions aside from the buccal extension. When removing buccal fat, it can be easily extracted using mosquito forceps after capsulotomy. By gently pulling the buccal fat in a tension-free manner, the feeding vessels that hold the buccal fat can be observed, and ligating these vessels can help prevent delayed hematoma in the buccal area. In patients with severe submalar hollowness or significant lateral cheek fat deflation, repositioning of the buccal fat can be effective. Capsulectomy is not recommended because the parotid duct and facial nerve buccal branch may be variably attached to or even penetrate the buccal fat, posing a risk of neuropraxia or duct damage during removal.

8.5 Fixation

The methods for fixing the freely elevated SMAS flap can be broadly divided into three areas: temple, preauricular, and neck. First, the SMAS is pulled to overlap with the superficial temporal fascia (STF) under sufficient tension, targeting the deep temporal fascia (DTF) for fixation. At the zygomatic arch, fixation is performed at two points targeting the periosteum to compress the fascia and deeper tissues. This is done for two reasons: first, to distribute tension due to the potential for cheese-wiring of the DTF from the movement of the temporalis, and second, to prevent widening of the zygoma distance by compressing the SMAS.

Once the superior vector fixation is complete, the procedure moves to the neck, where the SMAS, including the platysma, is pulled laterally to select fixation points. There are two methods for fixation: creating a strip SMAS flap and fixing it to the mastoid fascia or fixing it to the fascia of the posterior border of the sternocleidomastoid muscle (SCM).

After completing both superior and lateral fixation, the SMAS is fixed to Lore's fascia in the preauricular area without tension, using an approximation concept. Notably, leaving the Lore's fascia at the height of the tragus free without fixation minimizes the risk of deformity in the tragus postoperatively (Fig. 8.15).

Once all fascial fixations are complete, irrigation and meticulous bleeding control are performed before skin suturing. Appropriate tension is applied to three key points at the front and back of the ear during anchoring suture, followed by tension-free skin trimming for closure. The author first trims and closes along incision lines other than the tragus and earlobe to prevent pixie ear and tragus deformation, addressing the tragus and earlobe trimming and closure afterward.

The use of a Hemovac is recommended because negative pressure wound therapy can enhance skin survival rates through improved venous circulation and reduce swelling caused by seroma during the inflammatory phase. The author typically uses a 100 cc Hemovac, as an average drainage volume of 10–15 cc per day is commonly observed. Even in patients with a high bleeding tendency, it is rare for drainage to exceed 40 cc.

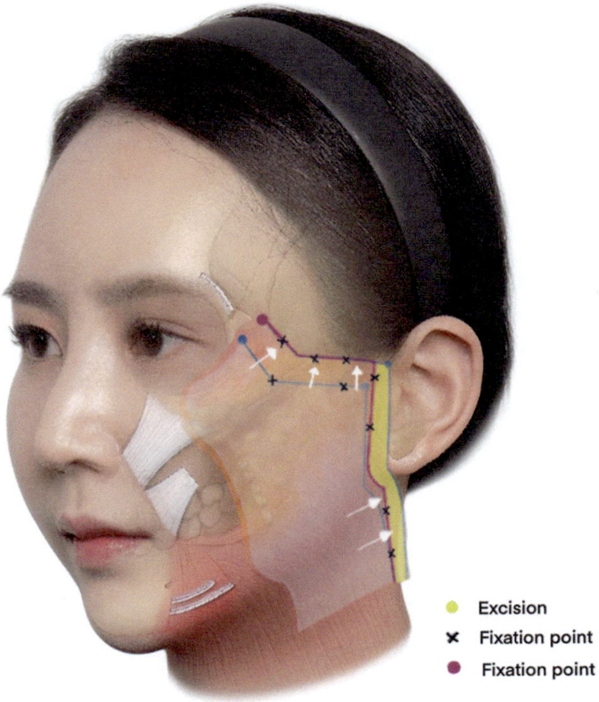

Fig. 8.15 Fixation points

8.6 Postoperative Care

If the Hemovac is inserted and negative pressure is confirmed, strong compression dressings are not necessary. A light dressing followed by the use of a garment is sufficient, and a garment that protects the neck and under the chin provides more stability. For the first 2–3 days post-surgery, patients should be educated to avoid positions that increase pressure on the facial area (such as bending forward or lifting heavy objects) because the risk of arterial bleeding leading to acute hematoma is highest within the first 24 hours postoperatively. Light daily activities are permitted, but patients should be cautioned against opening their mouths too wide. During sleep, it is important to avoid excessive pressure on the neck and to keep the face elevated above the heart. Therefore, patients should be advised to avoid high pillows and to sleep in a straight position with the upper body elevated at about 45°.

Since this surgery does not necessarily require hospitalization, patients managed on an outpatient basis should be instructed to return for Hemovac removal 2 days post-surgery. The Hemovac should be removed within at least 3 days because, as the inflammatory phase transitions to the proliferative phase, the Hemovac may react as a foreign body.

After the Hemovac is removed, patients should be educated to wear the garment for as much time as possible, as shearing forces can lead to delayed hematoma or seroma, which can delay skin flap healing. Sutures should be removed within 7–10 days. It is recommended to use scar ointment continuously for up to 3 months.

Physical activity should be restricted for the first 2 weeks, with light walking allowed after 2 weeks, jogging and running starting at 4 weeks, and more intense exercise beginning at 6 weeks. Swimming and sauna use should be restricted until after 6 weeks. Energy-based devices can be used without restriction after 6 weeks; however, high-intensity focused ultrasound (HIFU) should be avoided before 6 weeks, while radiofrequency devices can be started 4 weeks post-surgery. It should be noted that in some cases, swelling may be more pronounced or prolonged after these procedures.

8.7 Complications

8.7.1 Hematoma

Hematoma is the most common complication associated with facelift surgery. The incidence is known to be less than 2%, but it is a complication that requires immediate intervention when it occurs. Factors that increase the risk of hematoma include hypertension, male gender, use of aspirin or NSAIDs, smoking, and a BMI over 25, with hypertension being the most significant risk factor (Fig. 8.16).

Hematomas typically occur within 24 hours post-surgery. If a hematoma occurs, opening the wound for hemostasis and irrigation usually resolves the issue without sequelae. However, if a hematoma persists for an extended period, there is a risk of necrosis at the skin flap margin, and it can also reduce the skin tightening effect, leading to decreased initial satisfaction.

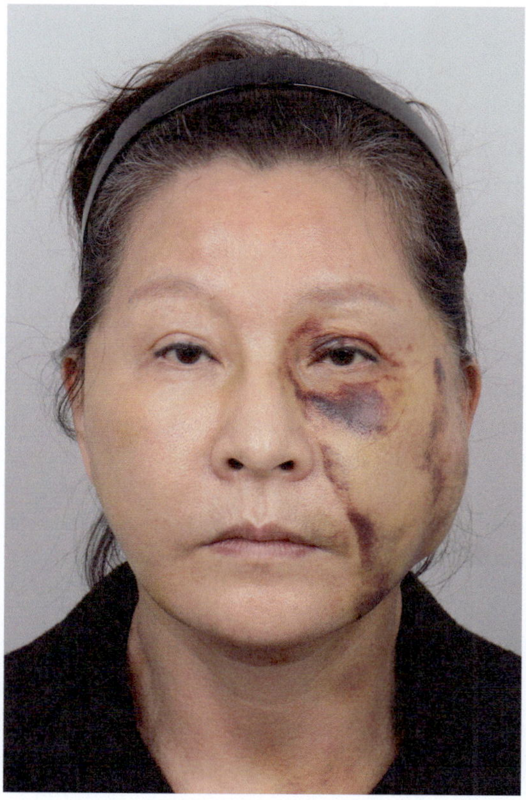

Fig. 8.16 A 59-year-old female patient with a systolic BP of 160 before surgery, presenting with a hematoma on postoperative day one

Patients with bleeding tendencies may experience delayed hematomas, which are small hematomas caused by venous bleeding. These can usually be resolved easily through aspiration, and it is advisable to prescribe ciprofloxacin afterward to prevent anaerobic infection.

8.7.2 Skin Necrosis

Extensive skin necrosis is very rare, but small areas of skin necrosis and delayed healing are common. Small areas of skin necrosis often occur at the tips of skin flaps and around the malar eminence. Necrosis at the tips of skin flaps is primarily due to circulation issues, with risk factors including extensive skin undermining, smoking, or conditions that affect blood circulation (e.g., diabetes). Shear forces can also lead to poor adhesion between the skin flap and fascia.

There are two main causes of skin necrosis around the malar eminence (Fig. 8.17). One is damage to the dermal plexus when the skin around the malar eminence is thinned during undermining. The other is due to compression dressing or overly tight garments post-surgery, which can restrict blood supply.

When skin necrosis occurs, the principle is to manage it with dressings according to the wound. Injecting PDRN (polydeoxyribonucleotide) can promote angiogenesis and aid in faster recovery. Cases that can be resolved with dressings typically conclude treatment within one and a half to two months; however, additional management may be needed due to subsequent wound contraction.

If skin necrosis occurs in the full thickness of the dermis, more aggressive treatment is required. Treatment with full-thickness skin grafts (FTSG) followed by adjunctive treatments such as pigment lasers, fractional laser therapy, or microcoring can yield relatively good results.

8.7.3 Incisional Scar

Scarring at the incision site is a concern for both surgeons and patients following facelift surgery.

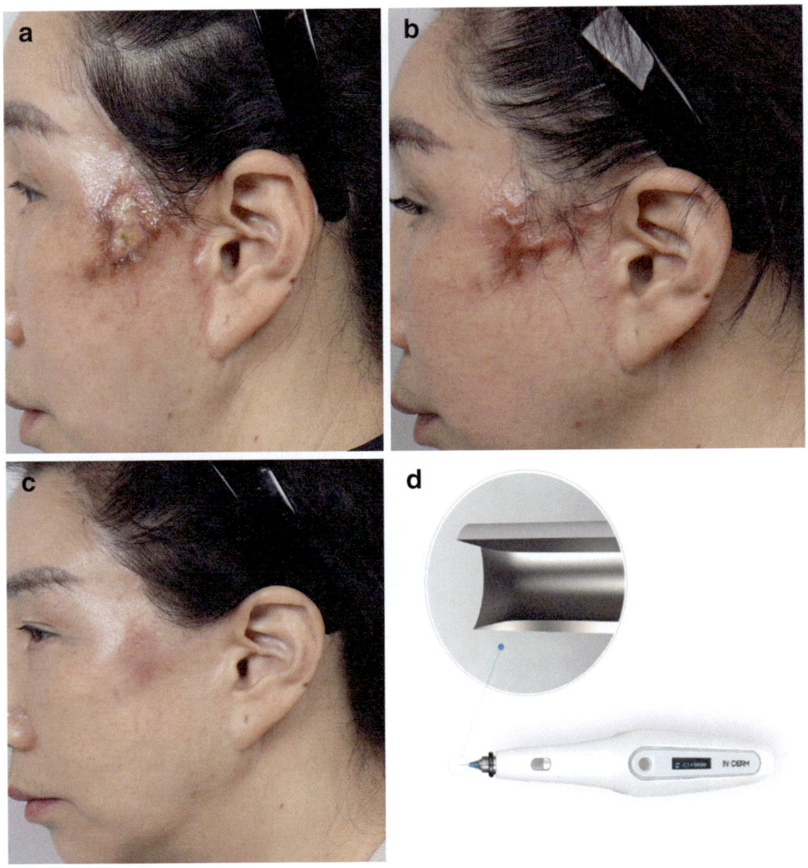

Fig. 8.17 Skin necrosis occurring after rhytidectomy in a 64-year-old female patient, with necrosis around the malar eminence. (**a**) One and a half months post-surgery. (**b**) Status after initial treatment with dressing. (**c**) Three treatments with a microcoring device (0.5 mm) 5 months post-surgery. (**d**) Schematic diagram of the microcoring device (NDerm, NFinder, Seoul, Korea)

Types of scars that can occur at the incision site include hypertrophic scars, widening scars, hyperpigmentation, and hypopigmentation.

Hypertrophic scars can cause persistent itching and pain, leading to long-term discomfort for patients, and require correction. These scars often occur along the postauricular sulcus line, likely due to the high density of sebaceous glands in the skin behind the ear. Excessive lateral vectoring during skin trimming behind the ear increases the risk of hypertrophic scars.

Widening scars occur due to excessive tension applied to the skin, leading not only to widening but also a tendency to become depressed scars. To prevent this, excessive skin excision should be avoided.

Pigmentation changes in scars can be observed particularly around 2 to 3 months post-surgery, with a higher likelihood in patients with darker skin tones (higher Fitzpatrick type scale). However, pigmentation often improves naturally over time, and laser treatment can expedite this process if necessary.

Hypopigmentation is often more noticeable in patients during cold winters or after alcohol consumption, and it is a type of scar that is difficult to correct. If it occurs along the facelift incision, scar revision may lead to increased tension and result in another scar, making it challenging to perform. Recently developed microcoring devices can achieve good results through partial removal, and partial tattooing can be used to make the discoloration less noticeable (Fig. 8.18).

8.7.4 Pixie Ear

Changes in the position and angle of the ear (deformation) occur in over 90% of patients after facelift surgery, although severe deformities often go unnoticed by patients. Pixie ear is one of the most concerning issues for patients. It is char-

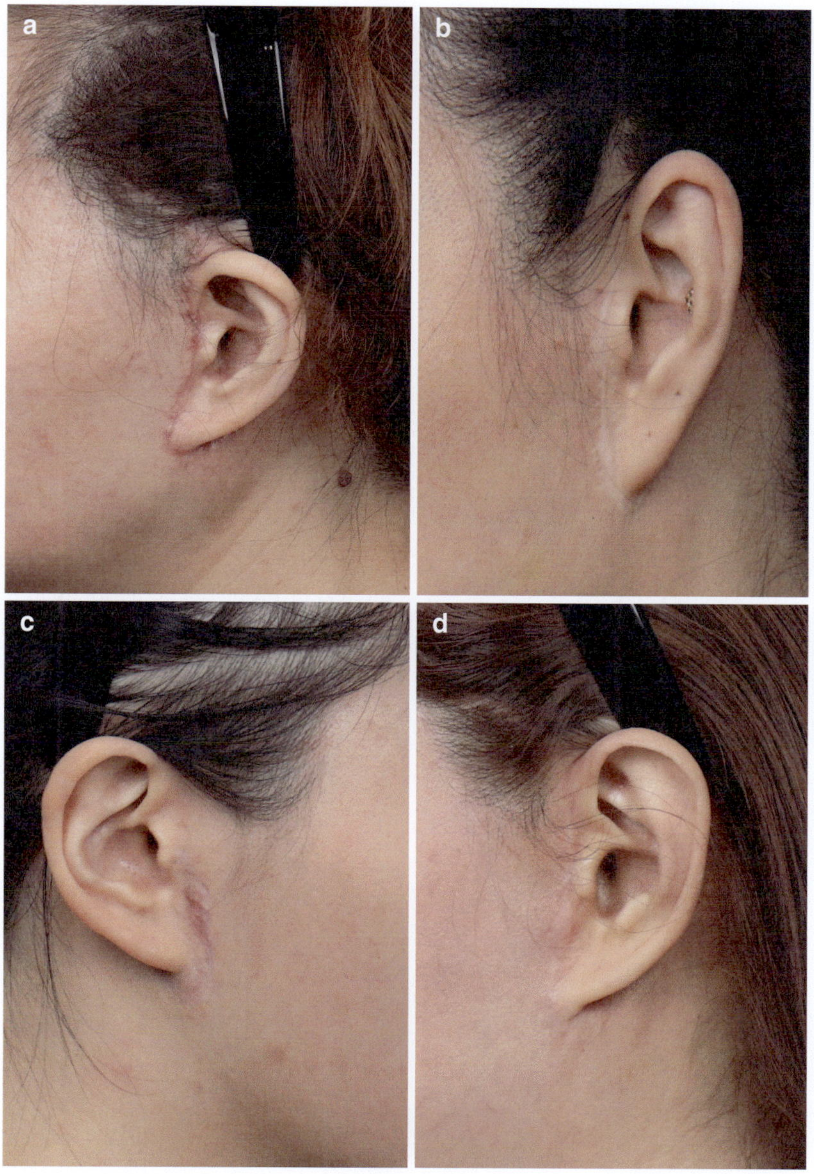

Fig. 8.18 Various incision site scars. (**a**) Hyperpigmentation. (**b**) Hypopigmentation. (**c**) Widening scar. (**d**) Hypertrophic scar

acterized by the otobasion, the point where the earlobe meets the face, being positioned lower than the lowest point of the earlobe, sometimes extending down to the angle of the mandible (Fig. 8.19).

The cause of pixie ear is excessive skin excision, which pulls the earlobe inferomedially. This issue may not be observed during surgery when the patient is lying down but can become apparent months later.

Traditional methods for correcting pixie ear include the V-Y advancement flap, but this can create another visible scar, making it less preferred by patients. The postauricular rotation flap can be used when there is sufficient skin laxity behind the ear, as it leaves less visible scarring.

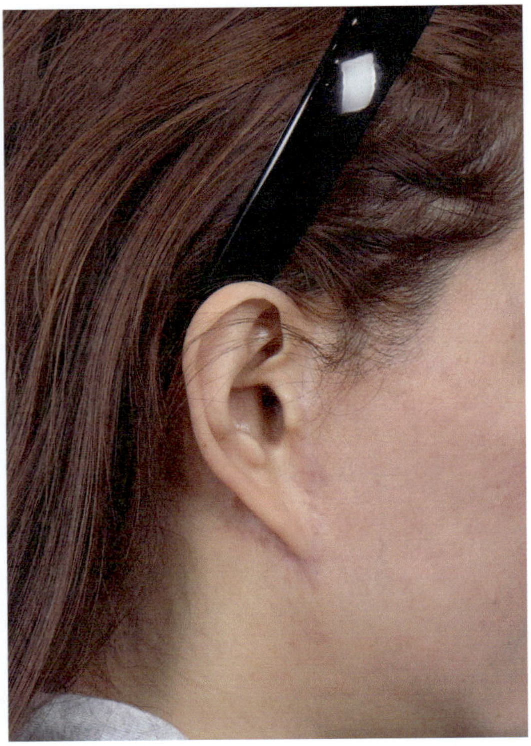

Fig. 8.19 A 42-year-old female patient with pixie ear after facelift surgery

Correction methods using cogged threads can also effectively shape the earlobe, but their duration is limited (Fig. 8.20). For fundamental improvement, a secondary facelift may be necessary to redistribute the load on the skin to the fascia, minimizing skin tension; however, if excessive skin was excised during the primary surgery, complete correction may be difficult.

8.7.5 Infection

The probability of infection following facelift surgery is extremely low, at less than 1%. The primary route of infection is usually through skin flora, particularly *Staphylococcus* species. Even in clean surgeries, prolonged surgical time warrants the use of prophylactic antibiotics; therefore, it is recommended to administer intravenous cephalosporin 30–60 minutes prior to incision. Although there is no evidence supporting the effectiveness of antibiotics post-surgery, it is common practice to prescribe a course of antibiotics for 3–5 days, similar to other surgical procedures.

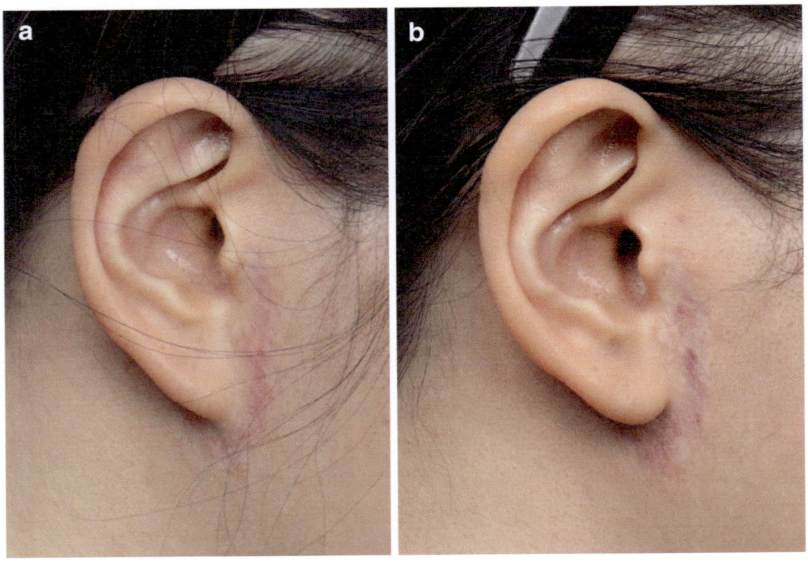

Fig. 8.20 A 29-year-old female patient who developed midface ptosis after a bone contouring operation 1 year ago. After undergoing rhytidectomy at another hospital, she developed pixie ear 6 months later. Although facelift scar revision and pixie ear correction were recommended, she only desired minimal correction of the pixie ear, which was achieved through thread lifting. (**a**) Before correction. (**b**) Two months after thread lifting correction

8.7.6 Motor Nerve Injury

Complete injury to the facial motor nerves is very rare. However, some patients may experience temporary neuropraxia symptoms, which are mostly due to indirect damage from electrocautery. The most commonly affected nerve is the buccal branch. During zygomatic ligament release, there is a risk of injury during dissection, especially in patients where layer distinction is difficult, and damage can also occur when removing buccal fat.

When the orbicularis oculi muscle is included in the SMAS (superficial musculoaponeurotic system) elevation, the zygomatic branch may also sustain some damage, but the symptoms are less pronounced compared to buccal branch injuries. This is thought to be because the function impairment due to damage is masked by the fixation of the SMAS that includes the orbicularis oculi muscle.

If the damage is not complete, patients may exhibit reduced movement of the facial muscles immediately after surgery, with natural recovery typically observed within 2–3 months, and nearly all symptoms resolving by 6 months. Facial exercises or steroid administration may help reduce the recovery time.

While most injuries to the buccal and zygomatic branches can recover naturally, there is a risk of synkinesis in some cases, necessitating caution during surgery. Rarely, patients may experience loss of function in the frontalis muscle due to frontal branch injury; however, if it is clear that the skin flap dissection was performed only from above the STF (superficial temporal fascia), gradual recovery can be expected over time. During the recovery period, administering botulinum toxin to the opposite side can help correct asymmetry.

8.7.7 Sensory Nerve Injury

Sensory loss in the surgical area is inevitable within the skin dissection zone. Damage to skin innervation gradually recovers over time, typically presenting as intermittent sharp pain and numbness for 2–3 months, with a decrease in the severity and frequency of these symptoms after 3 months, stabilizing by 6 months. However, even with recovery, it is unlikely that patients will regain 100% of their presurgery sensory function.

The greater auricular nerve is responsible for the sensation of the skin around the ear and parotid gland, ascending along the sternocleidomastoid (SCM) muscle (Fig. 8.21). It is enveloped in the fascia of the SCM, which poses a risk of injury during skin and fascia dissection. Complete damage to this nerve can lead to permanent loss of sensation in the earlobe, necessitating caution. If damage is confirmed during surgery, neurorrhaphy should be performed.

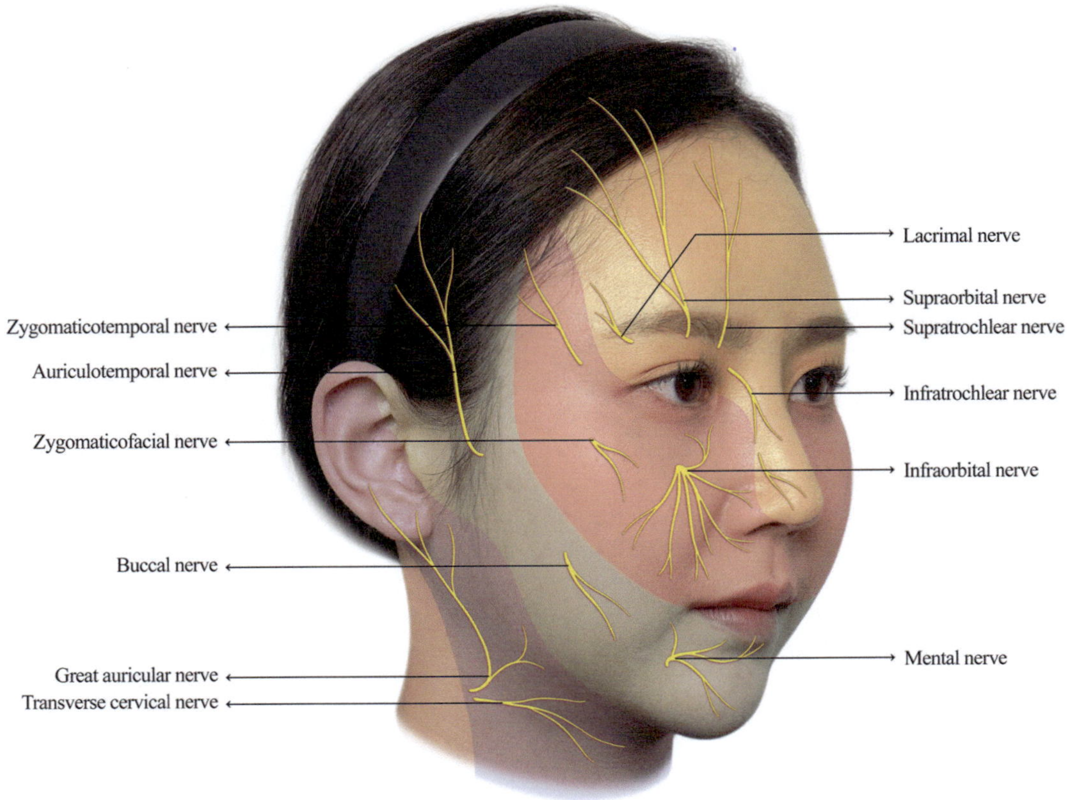

Fig. 8.21 Sensory nerve innervation of the face

References

1. Cannon B. Plastic surgery: new methods and refinements. JAMA. 1975;234(12):1273.
2. Mitz V, Peyronie M. The superficial musculo-aponeurotic system (SMAS) in the parotid and cheek area. Plast Reconstr Surg. 1976;58:80–8.
3. Barrett DM, Casanueva FJ, Wang TD. Evolution of the rhytidectomy. World J Otorhinolaryngol Head Neck Surg. 2016;2(1):38–44.
4. Baker DC. Lateral SMASectomy. Plast Reconstr Surg. 1997;100:509–13.
5. Chaudhry O, Levine S. Lateral SMASectomy. Clin Plast Surg. 2019;46(4):523–32. https://doi.org/10.1016/j.cps.2019.06.003.
6. Hamra ST. The deep-plane rhytidectomy. Plast Reconstr Surg. 1990;86(1):53–61; discussion 62–3.
7. Hamra ST. Composite rhytidectomy and the nasolabial fold. Clin Plast Surg. 1995;22(2):313–24.
8. Hamra ST. Building the composite face lift: a personal odyssey. Plast Reconstr Surg. 2016;138(1):85–96. https://doi.org/10.1097/PRS.0000000000002310.
9. Mendelson BC. Extended sub-SMAS dissection and cheek elevation. Clin Plast Surg. 1995;22(2):325–39.
10. Stuzin JM, Wagstrom L, Kawamoto HK, Wolfe SA. Anatomy of the frontal branch of the facial nerve: the significance of the temporal fat pad. Plast Reconstr Surg. 1989;83(2):265–71. https://doi.org/10.1097/00006534-198902000-00011.
11. Trussler AP, Stephan P, Hatef D, Schaverien M, Meade R, Barton FE. The frontal branch of the facial nerve across the zygomatic arch: anatomical relevance of the high-SMAS technique. Plast Reconstr Surg. 2010;125(4):1221–9. https://doi.org/10.1097/PRS.0b013e3181d18136.

Forehead Lifting

9

Contents

Most antiaging surgeries aim for aesthetic and psychological improvement. Forehead lifting, in addition to these goals, is a procedure that provides additional functional improvements, making it necessary for a broader range of patients. The changes in the eyebrows due to aging not only create a negative appearance but also exacerbate eyelid drooping, obstructing vision, causing dermatitis, and leading to pigmentation issues. Since forehead lifting effectively addresses these functional problems, it should be performed more proactively. Ultimately, forehead lifting is a process aimed at achieving two effects: improving the shape of the eyebrows and reducing forehead wrinkles.

9.1 Changes in the Forehead Due to Aging

Like other facial tissues, the forehead undergoes significant height increase due to resorption of the medial superior orbital rim with aging, along with a bony absorption process that widens the floor of the orbit inferiorly and laterally [1, 2].

W. Lee, K. H. Jung, *Lifting Techniques in Plastic Surgery*,
https://doi.org/10.1007/978-981-96-4820-7_9

There are three superficial fat compartments and three deep fat compartments in the forehead (Fig. 9.1).

As one ages, fat deflation occurs, leading to the descent of tissues that have lost tension. Unlike the face, the forehead tends to develop fewer deep wrinkles due to this descending process. Instead, bulging occurs as the fat compartments descend and accumulate along the boundary of the middle frontal septum (MFS), making the area between the MFS and inferior frontal septum (IFS) appear recessed. Additionally, skin loosening and laxity contribute to the descent of the eyebrows (Fig. 9.2).

The lowered eyebrow area can lead to visual discomfort due to upper eyelid skin laxity or lateral hooding, further exacerbating crow's feet. Patients with weakened levator palpebrae superioris muscle due to aging may hyperactivate the frontalis muscle to compensate, leading to the formation of forehead wrinkles. Consequently, the eyebrows become more arched, and the appearance of eyebrow ptosis is artificially corrected. This repetitive expression exacerbates skin laxity, and once it exceeds a certain threshold, it results in a state that cannot be compensated by the frontalis, leading to static eyebrow ptosis.

Furthermore, increased activation of the frown muscle due to aging pulls the medial area of the eyebrows downward, deepening the arch of the eyebrows. This creates an appearance of a frowning or angry face. If the frontalis is further hyperactivated to resolve this, the middle third of the eyebrow is raised, while the lateral third descends relatively, and the medial third is pulled down by the frown muscle, resulting in a distorted appearance of the eyebrows that looks very angry (Fig. 9.3).

Thus, the shape (Fig. 9.4) and height of the eyebrows, as well as the degree of forehead wrinkles, are determined by the degree and balance of activation of the frown and frontalis muscles. Judging the patient's condition accurately and correcting the shape of the eyebrows alongside appropriate surgery is an important aspect of forehead lifting.

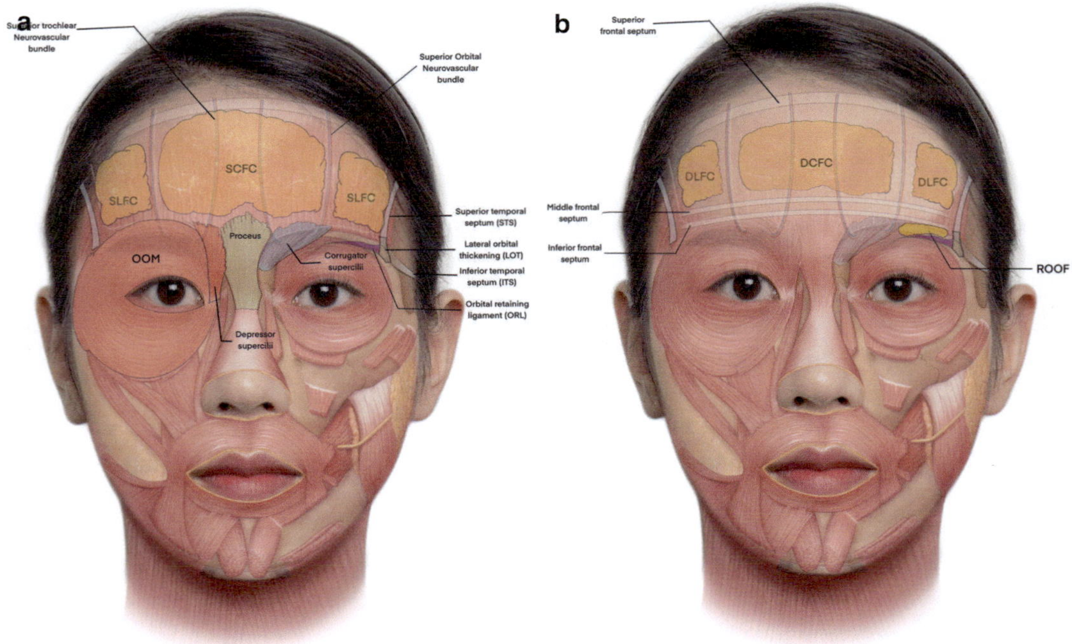

Fig. 9.1 Fat compartments of the forehead. (**a**) Superficial fat compartment. (**b**) Deep fat compartment (SCFC superficial central fat compartment, SLFC superficial lateral fat compartment, OOM orbicularis oculi muscle, DCFC deep central fat compartment, DLFC deep lateral fat compartment)

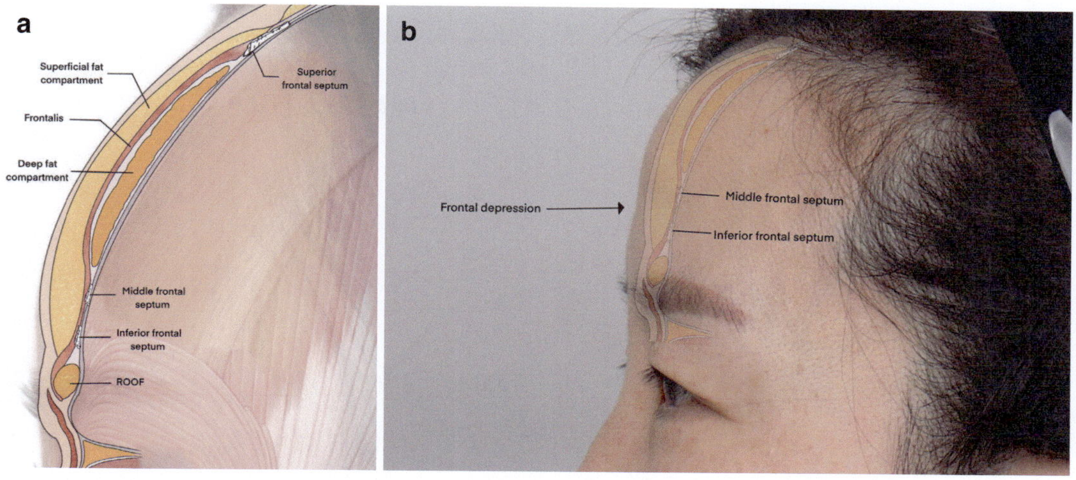

Fig. 9.2 Causes of frontal depression. (**a**) Anatomy. (**b**) Depressed area

Fig. 9.3 Changes in the shape of the forehead and eyebrows due to aging. (**a**) Normal. (**b**) Eyebrow ptosis due to mild fat descending. (**c**) Hyperactivation of the frontalis to compensate for eyebrow ptosis. (**d**) State with added hyperactivation of the frown muscle

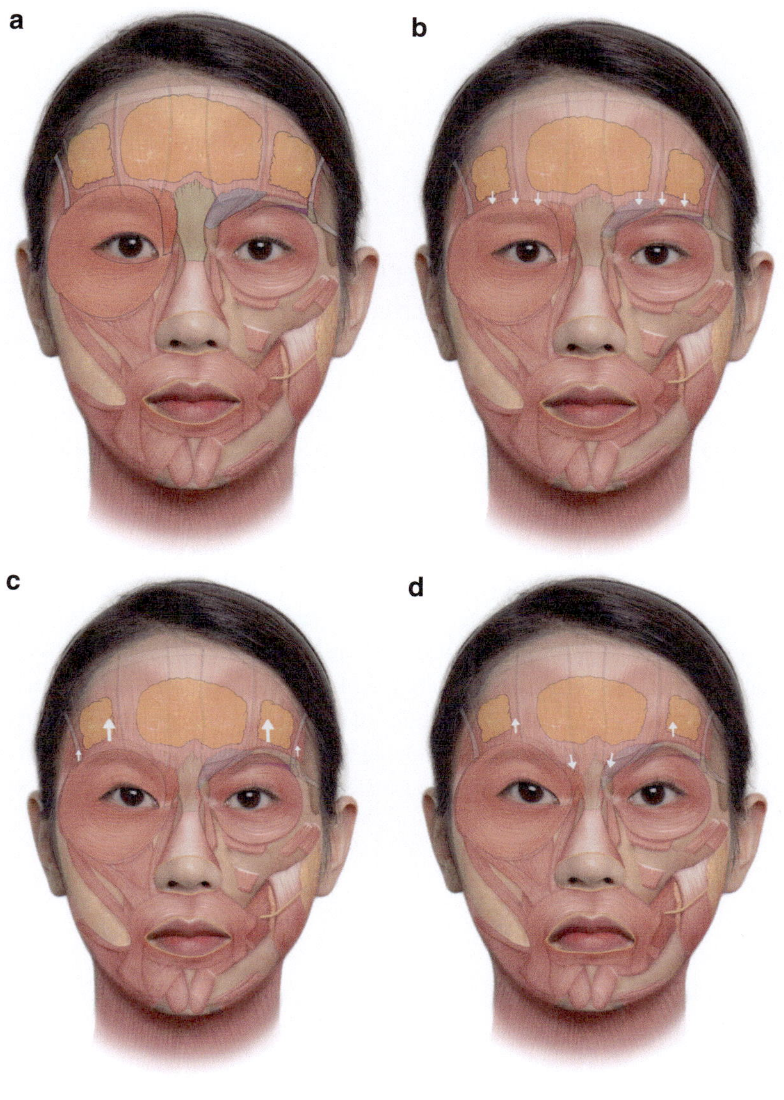

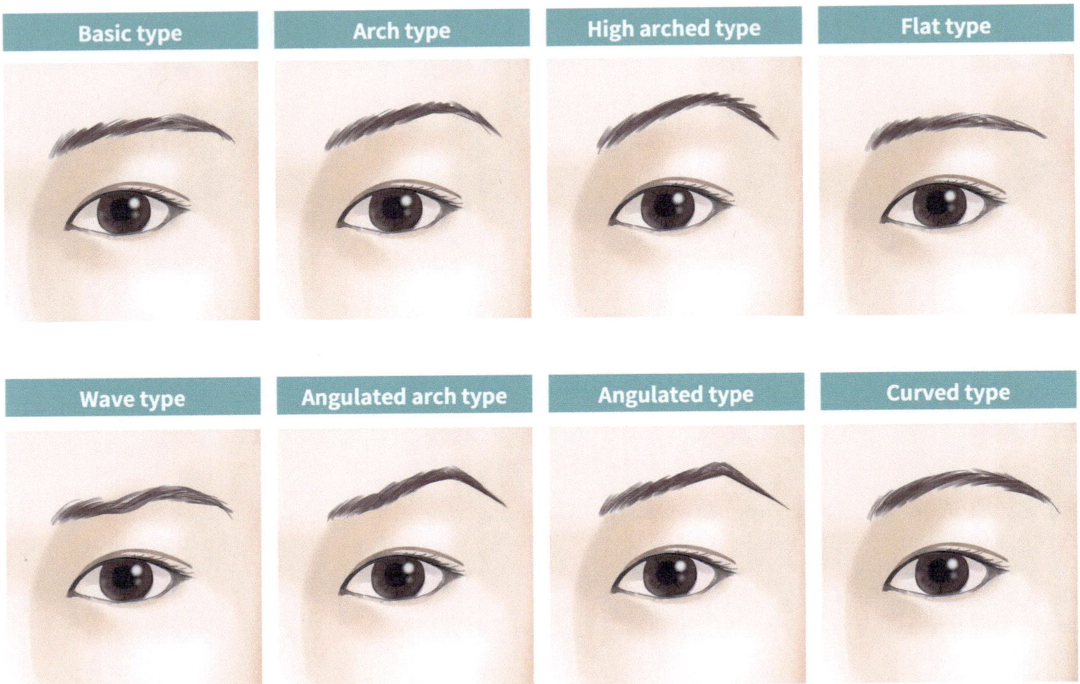

Fig. 9.4 Types of eyebrow shapes

9.2 Thread Lifting vs. Endoscopic Forehead Lift vs. Incisional Forehead Lift

There are various approaches to forehead lifting. The less invasive thread lifting method tightens loosened skin and repositions fat compartments [3]. This technique is particularly suitable for patients with mild skin laxity, minimal fat deflation, and those who are averse to invasive surgery.

Endoscopic forehead lifting involves accessing the sub-periosteal plane through incisions made within the scalp, allowing for the lifting of the forehead tissues as a single unit (en bloc), which has the advantage of a longer duration of effect. However, there is a risk of slightly moving the hairline backward, which can widen the forehead, and symptoms due to sensory nerve damage may persist for a long time. Additionally, since this procedure involves lifting a periosteal flap en bloc, it yields good results when skin laxity is moderate or less, and when the skin is firmly attached to the periosteum. In cases of severe skin laxity, the lower incisional forehead lift may be more effective.

The most significant difference with the incisional forehead lift is that it lifts multiple layers, reduces excess skin, and can directly improve already deep wrinkles. In some cases, it can also reduce a widened forehead, making it the most invasive option but one that offers substantial benefits. Therefore, it is effective for patients with severe skin laxity, deep static forehead wrinkles, and those with a wide forehead accompanied by eyebrow drooping.

9.3 Forehead Thread Lifting

The goal of forehead thread lifting is to insert threads between the hairline and the eyebrows, restoring fullness to the forehead and improving the shape of the eyebrows. While wrinkles caused by fat deflation can be improved, wrinkles due to hyperactivation of the frontalis muscle are difficult to address with thread lifting. Thus, the primary objective of forehead thread lifting is to correct eyebrow ptosis and enhance their shape.

Several thread lifting methods are known for correcting eyebrow ptosis, but even if the ptosis is corrected, patients may not feel younger if the shape remains unchanged. Therefore, the author emphasizes focusing on changes in eyebrow shape rather than merely lifting during the procedure.

In forehead thread lifting, a total of six bidirectional (multidirectional) cog threads and one double-arm bidirectional cog thread (21 gauge, 300 mm length) are used. Initially, three entry points are utilized. One hole is made at the center of the hairline, and two holes are created laterally, slightly outside the superior temporal septum (STS). The patient is instructed to activate the frown muscle to mark the positions of the transverse and oblique heads of the corrugator supercilii. An 18G needle is used to puncture the entry points, followed by widening with Metzenbaum scissors (Fig. 9.5).

First, the needle of the double-arm long thread is inserted through the center hole and exits through the lateral holes. The needle is then reinserted through the previously exited hole to emerge at the lower border of the eyebrow's halfway point, penetrating the STS (Fig. 9.6, no. 1).

Next, bidirectional cogged threads are inserted. The first step involves inserting two lines targeting the medial edge of the opposite eyebrow (corrugator oblique head) through the lateral hairline holes (Fig. 9.6, no. 2). The needle is then inserted from the center hairline hole to the marking point of the corrugator transverse head (Fig. 9.6, no. 3). Finally, the needle is inserted from the central entry point to the medial edge of the eyebrow (corrugator oblique head) (Fig. 9.6, no. 4).

After the procedure, changes in the angle of the eyebrows indicate an improvement in shape (Fig. 9.7).

When the focus is on the shape of the eyebrows rather than simply lifting them, older patients tend to prefer flatter eyebrows compared to younger patients, resulting in higher patient satisfaction (Figs. 9.8 and 9.9).

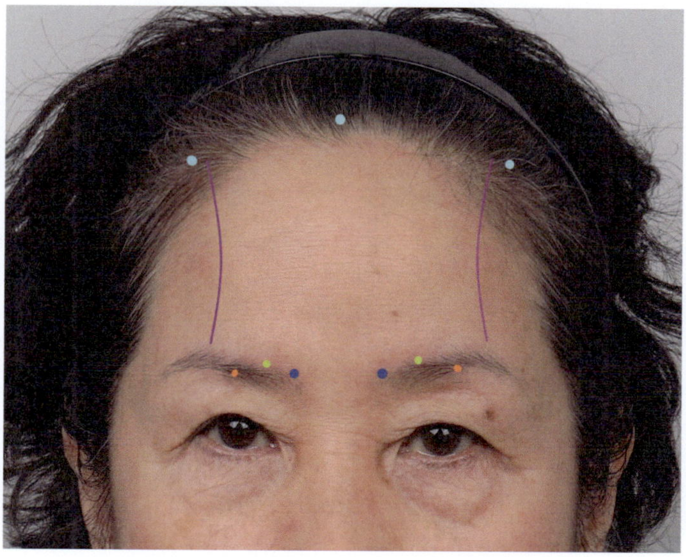

Fig. 9.5 Design for forehead thread lifting. Three fixation points are established above the superior frontal septum (SFS) and outside the superior temporal septum (STS) (light blue), with target points set at the halfway point of the lower border of the eyebrow (orange), the corrugator oblique head (blue), and the transverse head (light green)

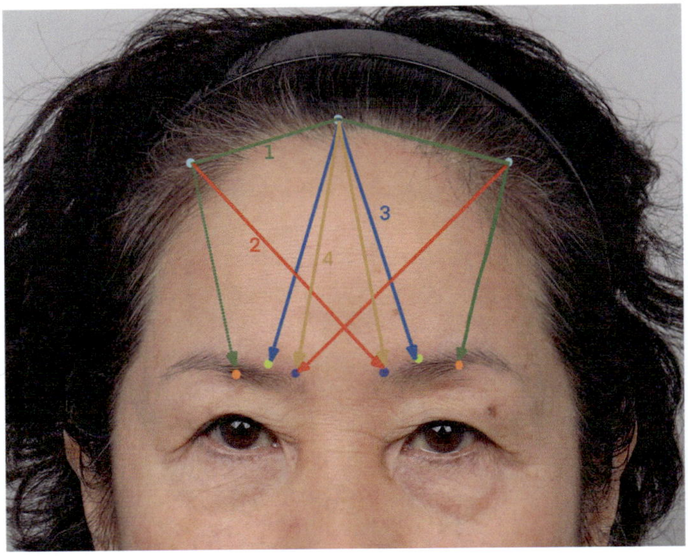

Fig. 9.6 Eyebrow thread lifting method. First, the long thread is inserted on both sides (green), followed by the sequential insertion of six bidirectional threads

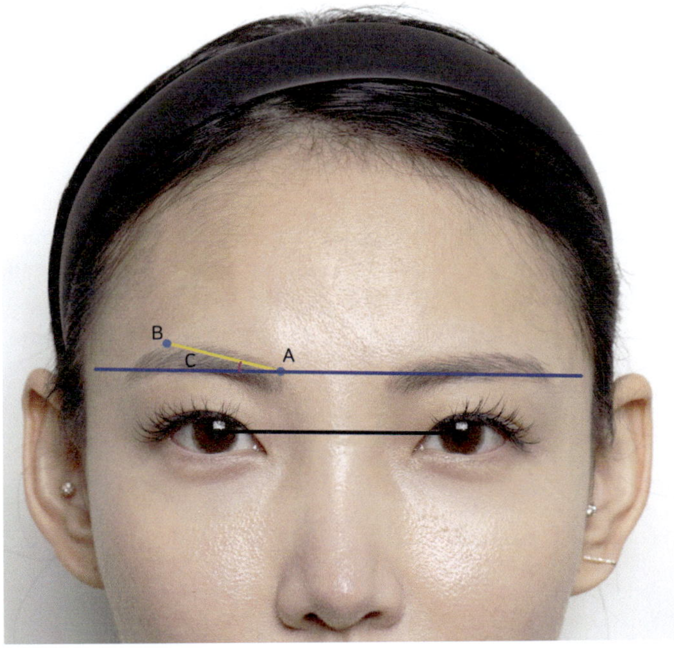

Fig. 9.7 Evaluation of the procedure. (**a**) Most medial part of the eyebrow. (**b**) Eyebrow tilt. (**c**) Angle of inclination extended from the horizontal line of the mid-pupil to the eyebrow area

For patients who desire more improvement in ptosis than in shape, a method using shorter threads to insert in reverse can be employed. In this case, two threads are inserted at a 45° angle through three or four entry points along the lower border of the eyebrow, providing an immediate eyebrow lifting effect (Fig. 9.10). However, since the cannula has difficulty passing through the superior frontal septum, fixation points cannot be utilized compared to previous surgical methods, leading to a shorter duration of effect (Figs. 9.11 and 9.12).

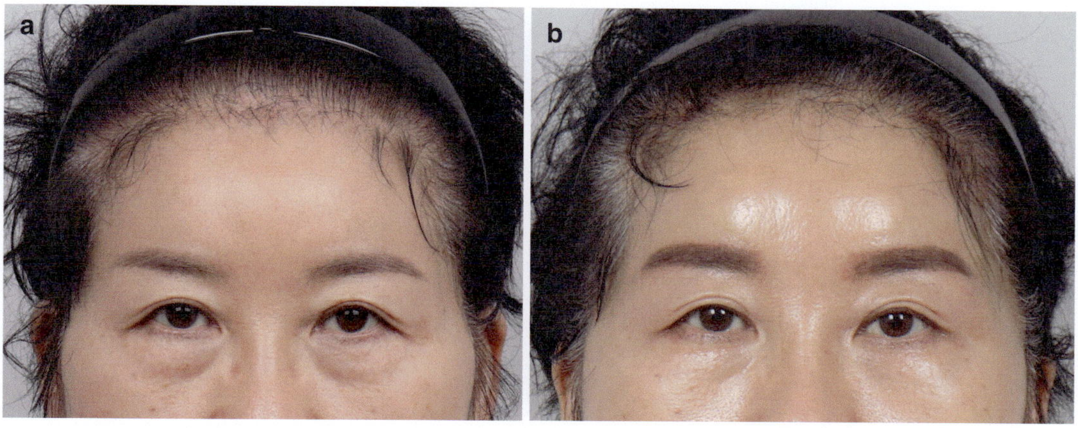

Fig. 9.8 61-year-old female patient. (**a**) Preoperative right angle: 13°, left angle: 12°. (**b**) Three months postoperative right angle: 9°, left angle: 10°

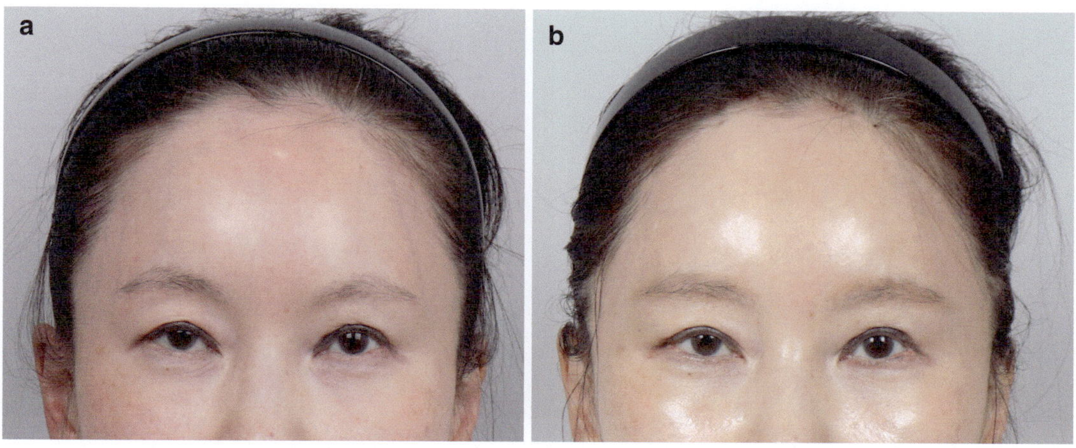

Fig. 9.9 53-year-old female patient. (**a**) Preoperative right angle: 27°, left angle: 25°. (**b**) Postoperative right angle: 19°, left angle: 15°

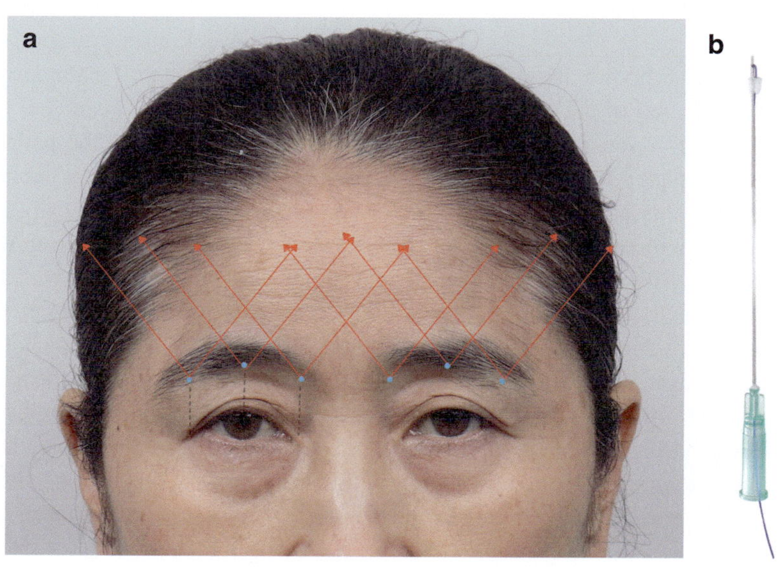

Fig. 9.10 Eyebrow thread lifting method. (**a**) Inserting two threads in reverse at a 45° angle from the lower border of the eyebrow at the lateral canthus, mid-pupil, and medial canthus. (**b**) N cog multi 21G 60 mm 2-0

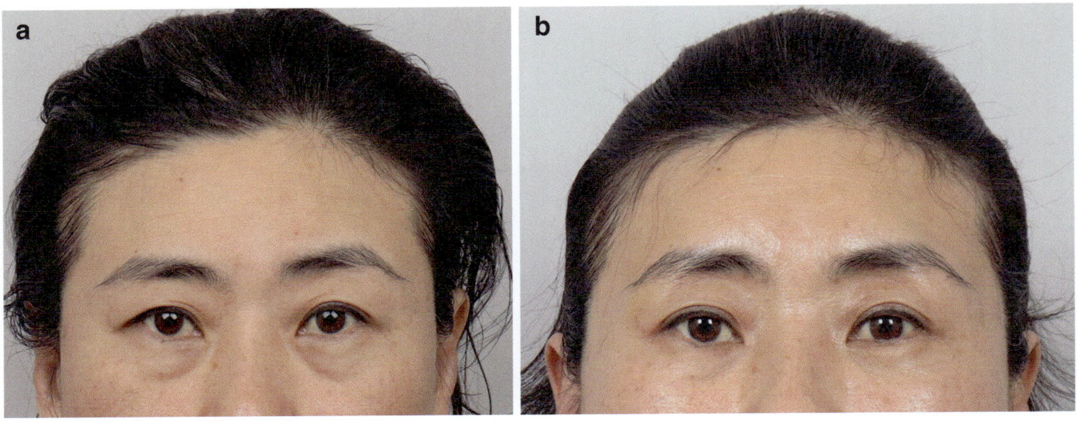

Fig. 9.11 52-year-old female patient undergoing eyebrow lifting with 12 threads. (**a**) Preoperative. (**b**) One month postoperative

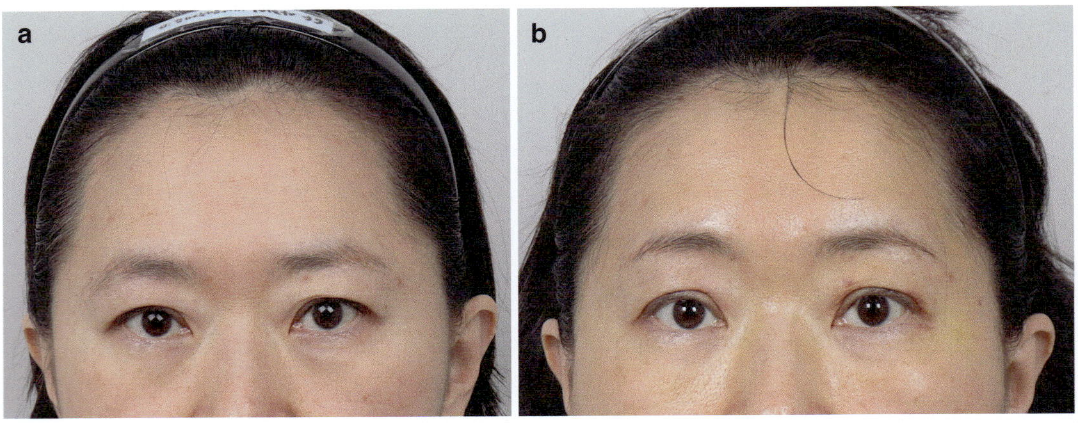

Fig. 9.12 47-year-old female patient. Eyebrow lifting with 12 threads. (**a**) Preoperative. (**b**) One month postoperative

9.4 Endoscopic Forehead Lift

For patients who are dissatisfied with the results of thread lifting or the duration of its effects, or for those seeking more fundamental improvements, an endoscopic forehead lift is necessary. This procedure can be performed on all patients with eyebrow ptosis. When performed on patients with minimal forehead wrinkles and mild skin laxity, it allows for eyebrow correction while minimizing the issue of forehead widening. However, in cases of moderate or greater skin laxity and significant wrinkles, avoiding forehead widening becomes challenging. It should also be explained to patients that deep static wrinkles are difficult to correct with an endoscopic forehead lift. While crow's feet may improve slightly with the forehead lift, complete resolution is difficult due to their dynamic nature.

Incisions can be made in 3–5 locations depending on the patient. A vertical incision of 2–3 cm is made at the hairline boundary or 5 mm behind it on the scalp. For the temporal incision, a line extending from the alar base to the lateral orbital rim is drawn, and the incision is made 1 cm inside the point where this line meets the hairline; a 1 cm incision is sufficient (Fig. 9.13).

First, through the scalp incision, the subperiosteal plane is dissected up to 1.5–2 cm above the eyebrows using an elevator without the endoscope (Fig. 9.14). Dissection should extend towards the vertex of the scalp. After this, the

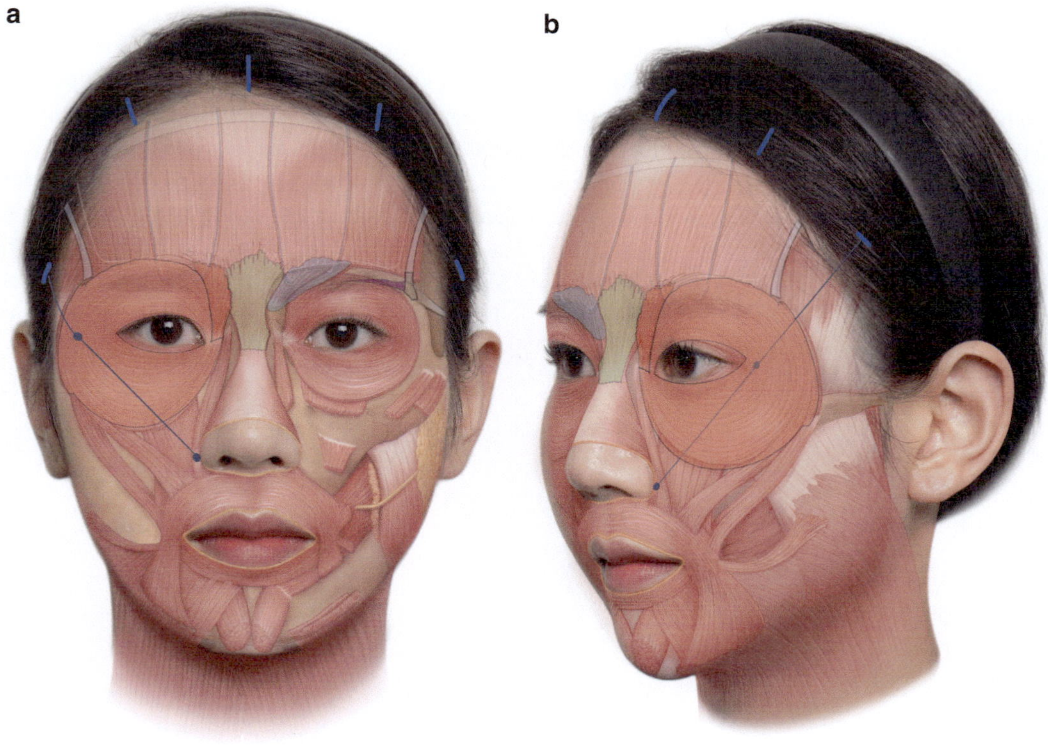

Fig. 9.13 Incision lines for endoscopic forehead lift. (**a**) Scalp incision line. (**b**) Temporal incision line

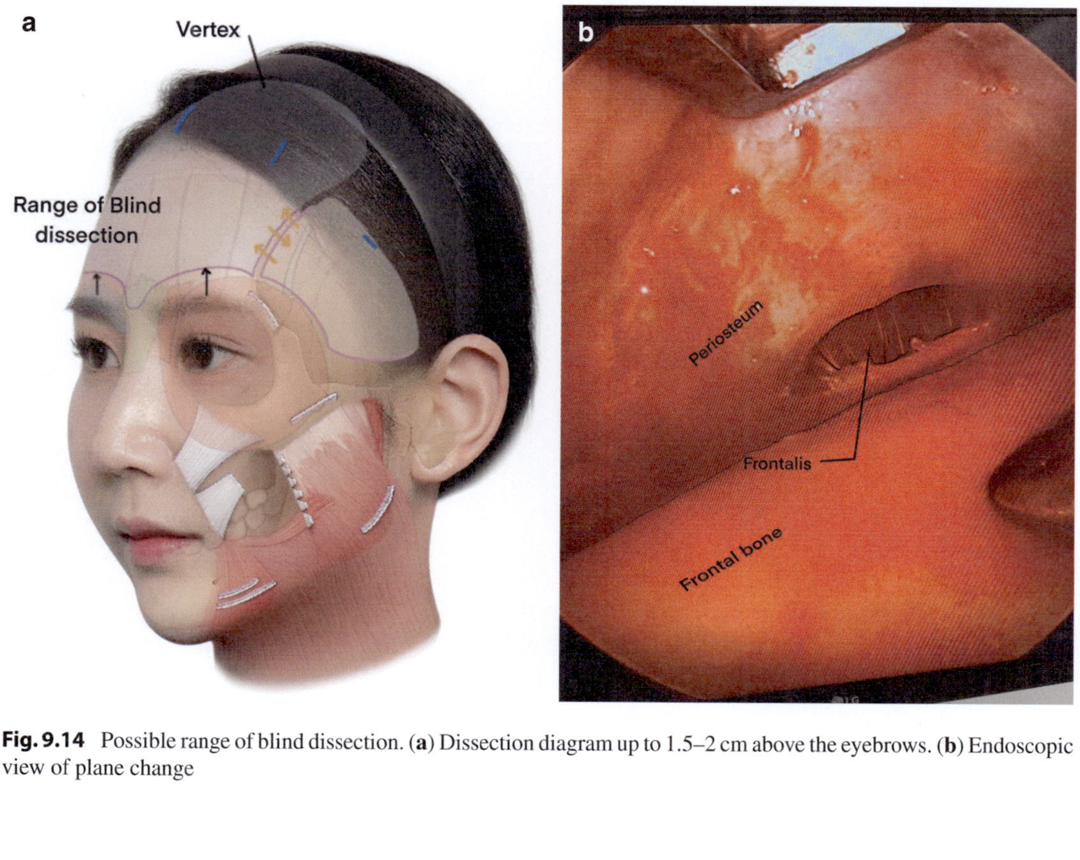

Fig. 9.14 Possible range of blind dissection. (**a**) Dissection diagram up to 1.5–2 cm above the eyebrows. (**b**) Endoscopic view of plane change

superior temporal septum must be released to connect the forehead and temporal areas. This can be done by approaching from the forehead side to the temporal area or vice versa, depending on the surgeon's preference. In the temporal area, dissection is performed with the DTF (deep temporal fascia) at the base, specifically in the area between the STF (superficial temporal fascia) and the DTF, where the innominate fascia is located.

Next, using the endoscope, an incision is made in the forehead periosteum, and the lower end of the frontalis muscle is cut to enter the superficial fat compartment layer. At this point, the insertion of the frown muscle can be observed, and further dissection downward will reveal the supratrochlear neurovascular bundle (STN). Care must be taken during corrugator muscle myotomy, as the STN penetrates the corrugator supercilii muscle (Fig. 9.15). After performing the corrugator mus-

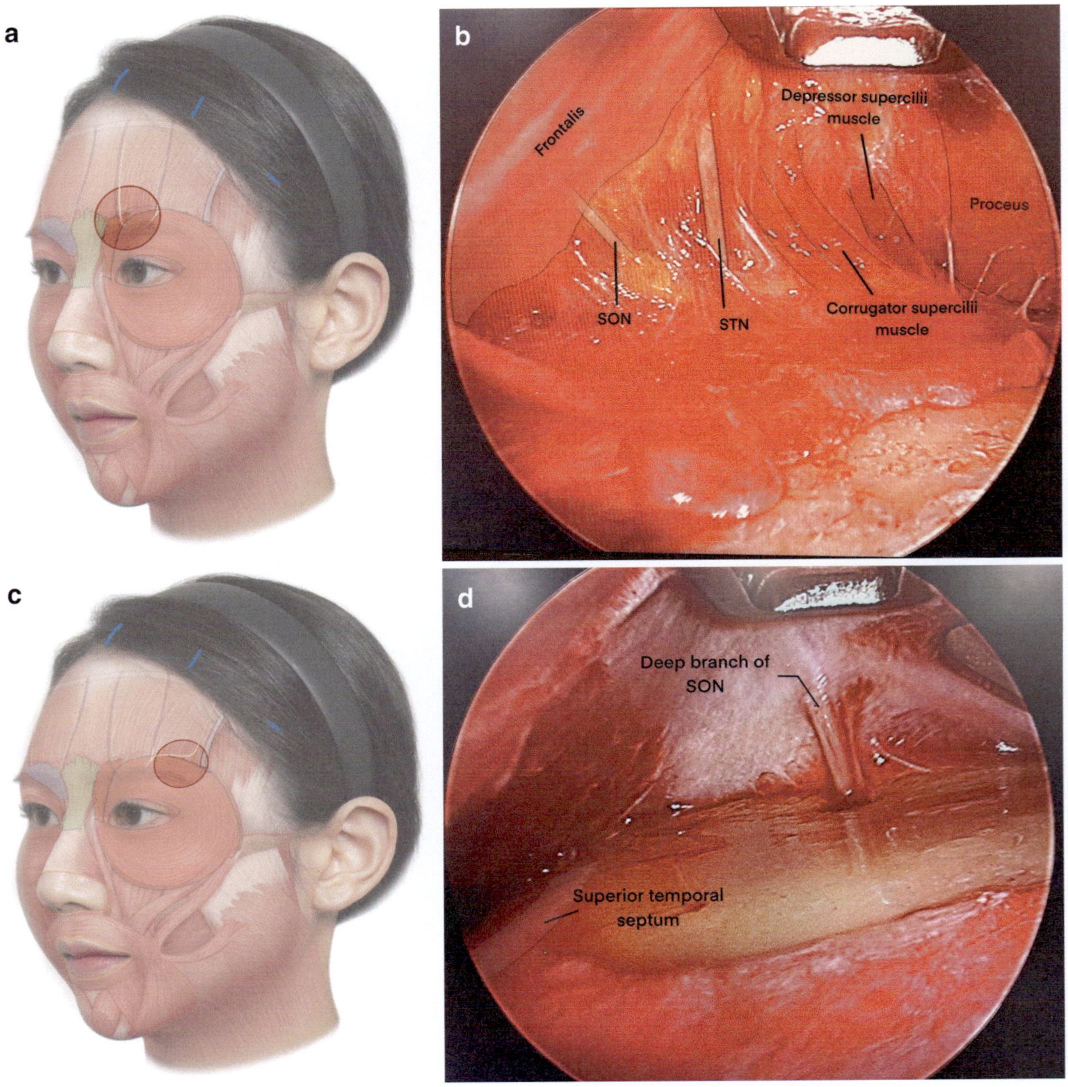

Fig. 9.15 Dissection range above the eyebrows. (**a**) Myotomy performed while skeletonizing the supratrochlear and supraorbital neurovascular bundles. (**b**) Endoscopic view of corrugator supercilii, depressor supercilii, and procerus myotomy. (**c**) Area of the superior temporal septum. (**d**) Endoscopic view

cle myotomy, the depressor supercilii muscle, which is located more superficially, should also be myotomized. Following the skeletalization of the STN (dissecting only the neurovascular structures), the procerus muscle in the center should be adequately myotomized, as there are no particularly critical structures in this area. Continuing the dissection laterally will lead to the supraorbital neurovascular bundle (SON), which should also be skeletalized.

Dissection in the temporal area begins with the release of the lateral orbital thickening, followed by the release of the inferior temporal septum. The dissection should progress further down to the area around the lateral canthal tendon to ensure sufficient mobility (Fig. 9.16). Care must be taken to avoid damaging the sentinel vein and the lateral zygomatico-temporal artery and vein (LZTA&V) during this process (Fig. 9.17).

Once all dissections are completed, the mobilized forehead tissue is pulled upward and fixed, checking the shape of the eyebrows and the amount of lift needed to determine the fixation points. There are two main methods for fixation. The first method involves bone tunneling followed by securing the periosteum with threads, which provides a more secure and robust fixation but makes it difficult to adjust the amount of lift. Therefore, recently, materials such as Endotine® have been widely used for fixation. The fixation site should be chosen so that the material is not exposed at the incision site when the skin is pulled, and fixing too far back may reduce the effectiveness. For patients with thin skin, it is advisable to use materials made with shorter spikes, as they may be palpable. These materials, made of polylactic acid (PLA), are designed to be naturally absorbed over approximately 10–12 months [4]. The following are the results of the endoscopic forehead lifting surgery (Figs. 9.18 and 9.19).

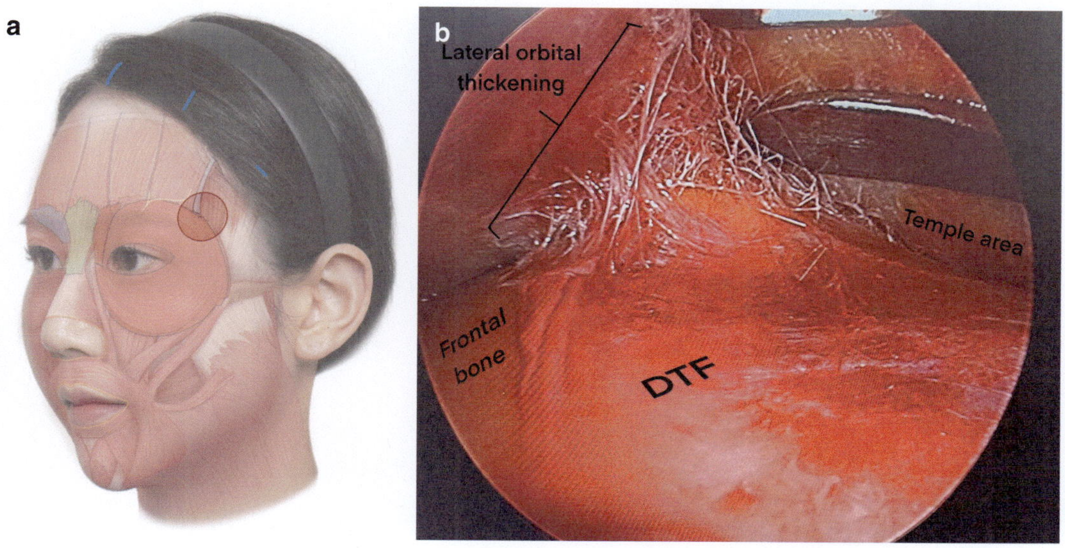

Fig. 9.16 Dissection in the temporal area. (**a**) Schematic diagram. (**b**) Endoscopic view of lateral orbital thickening dissection

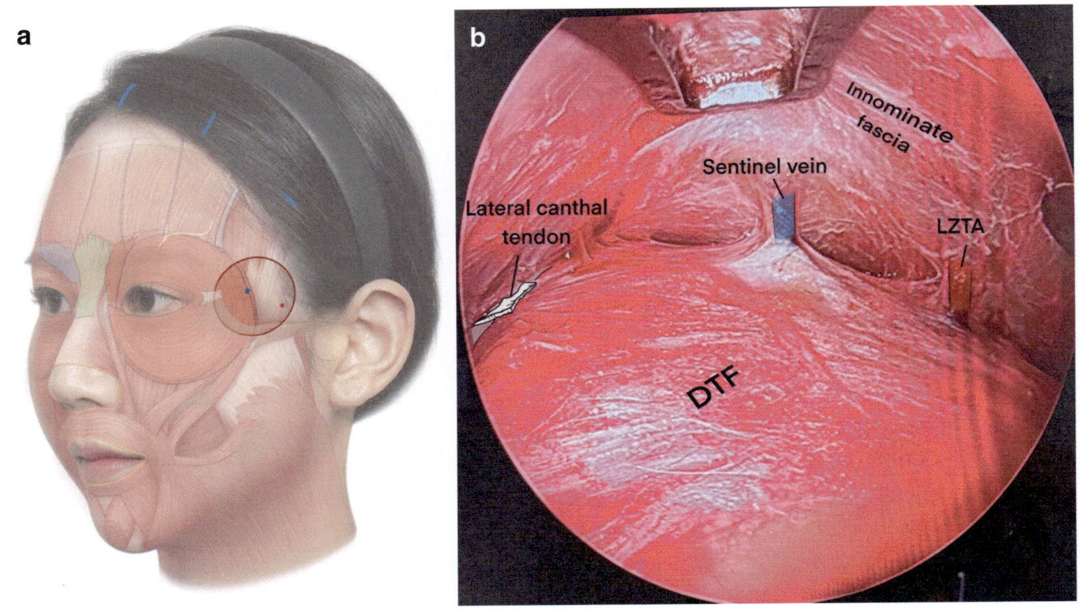

Fig. 9.17 Dissection in the temporal area. (**a**) Schematic diagram. (**b**) Sentinel vein and lateral zygomatico-temporal artery (LZTA) and vein

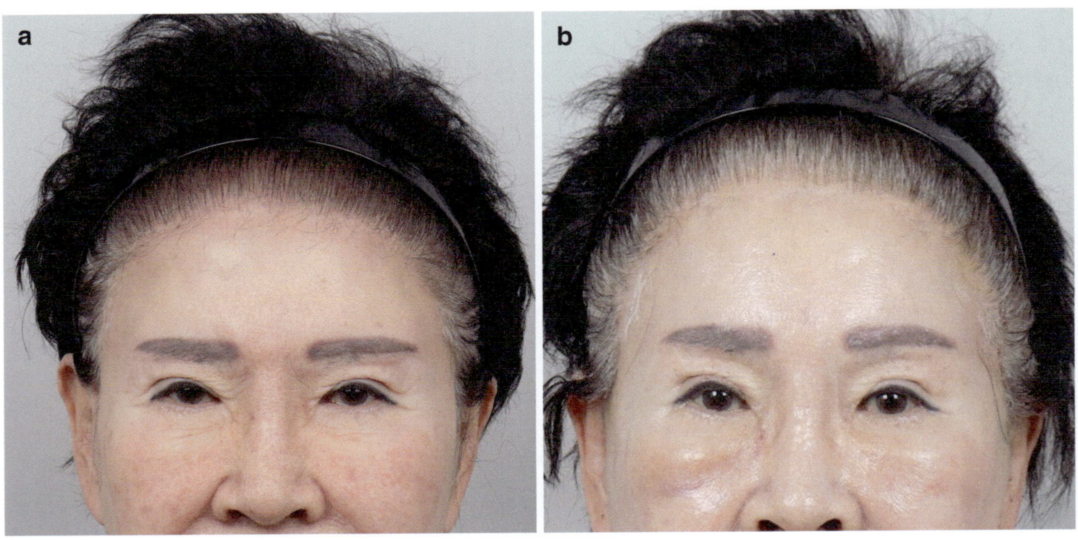

Fig. 9.18 68-year-old female patient undergoing endoscopic forehead lift. (**a**) Preoperative. (**b**) Postoperative 3 months

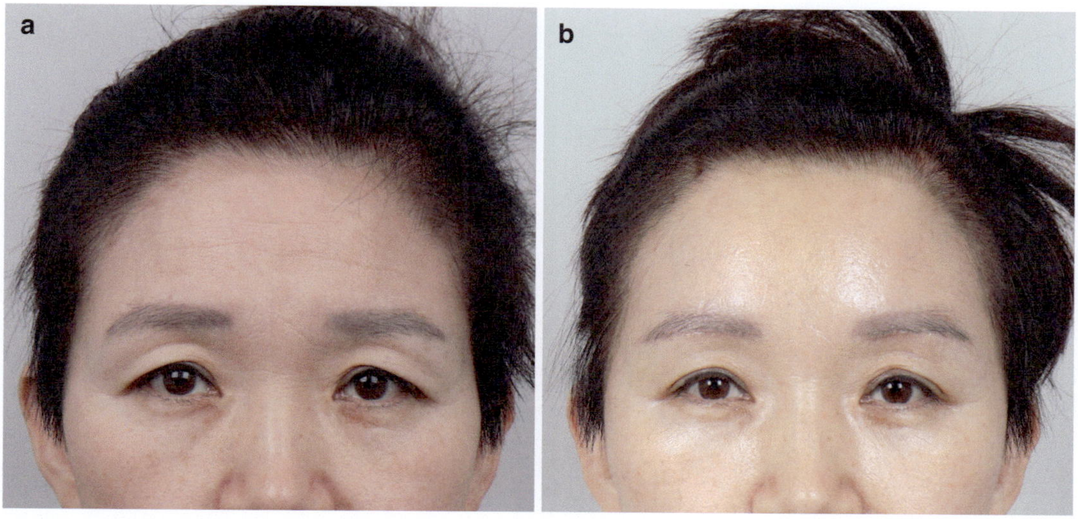

Fig. 9.19 50-year-old female patient undergoing endoscopic forehead lift. (**a**) Preoperative. (**b**) Postoperative 3 months

9.5 Incisional Forehead Lift

In cases of severe skin laxity or deeply etched static forehead wrinkles, there are limitations to what can be achieved with an endoscopic forehead lift. This is because the loose space between the periosteum, skin, and subcutaneous fat tissue means that even if the periosteum is pulled strongly upward, it cannot be adequately lifted. Therefore, in such cases, an incisional forehead lift is a more rational approach.

The incision is made along the hairline, and the incision should extend to the point where the temporal crest meets the vertical descent of the temporal hairline to also improve the sagging tissue in the temporal area (Fig. 9.20).

Skin dissection is performed up to 1.5 cm above the eyebrows using facelifting scissors, and the skin flap is elevated while continuing dissection downward until the dermal attachment of the frown muscle is released. Laterally, the superior temporal septum (STS) is released, but dissection should only extend above the Pitanguy line.

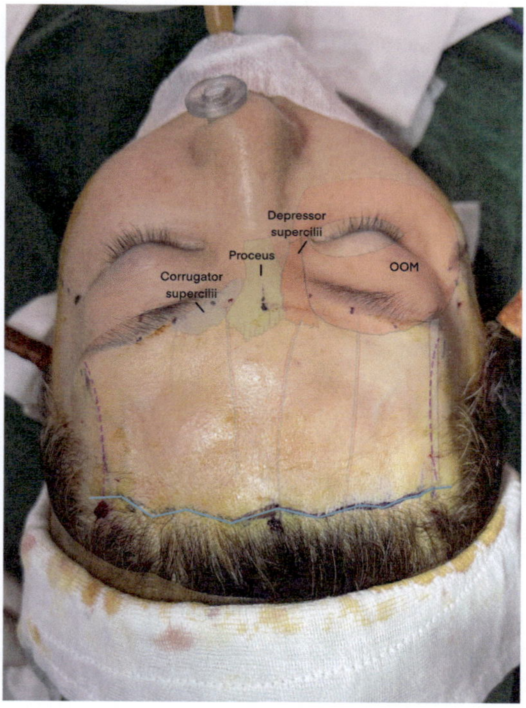

Fig. 9.20 Incision line for forehead lift. Incision line following the hairline (blue line)

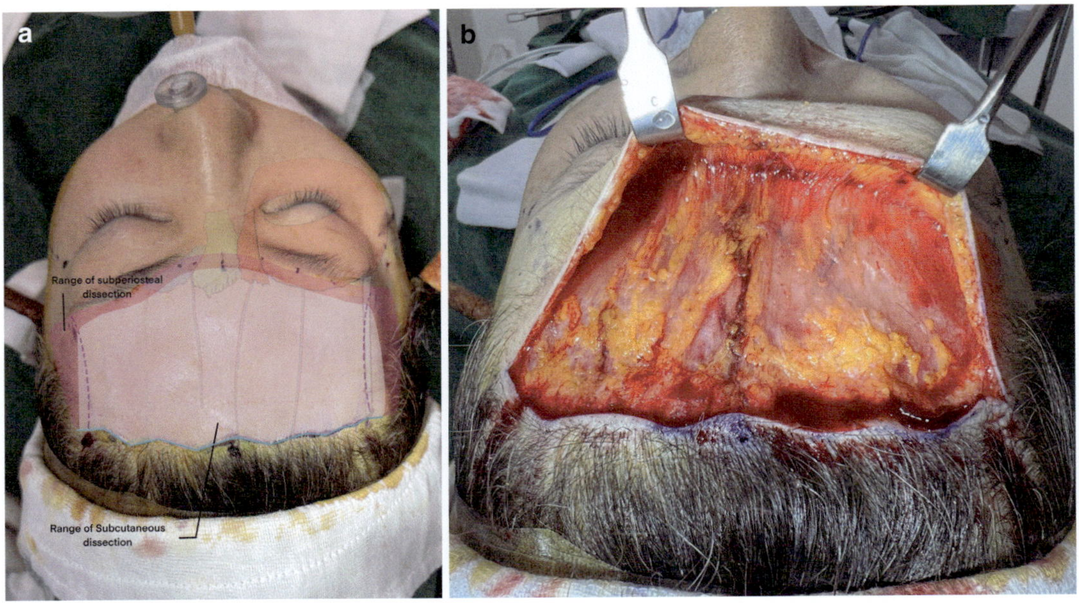

Fig. 9.21 Dissection range for forehead lift. (**a**) Schematic diagram of skin dissection and subperiosteal dissection range. (**b**) Subcutaneous fat dissection

Once the skin dissection is complete, a transverse incision of about 2–3 cm is made in the frontalis, inside the course of the STN, and access is gained to the subperiosteal plane, where blind dissection is performed up to 1.5–2 cm above the eyebrows (Fig. 9.21). If necessary, the dissection can be extended downward and laterally using an endoscope at this stage. After dissection is complete, the frontalis is plicated in 8–10 places, and the skin is pulled taut without tension, trimmed, and closed, concluding the surgery (Fig. 9.22). Suture removal should be performed within 10 days. Patients are encouraged to visit the hospital for scar evaluation up to 6 months postoperatively (Figs. 9.23 and 9.24).

In cases where the forehead needs to be reduced in width, after elevating the forehead skin flap, dissection should be performed toward the scalp instead of subperiosteal dissection toward the forehead, and the scalp flap can be pulled forward and secured.

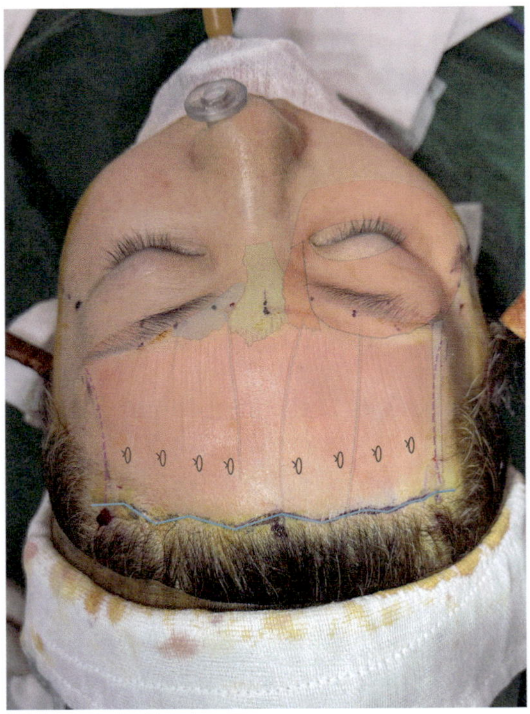

Fig. 9.22 Location of frontalis plication

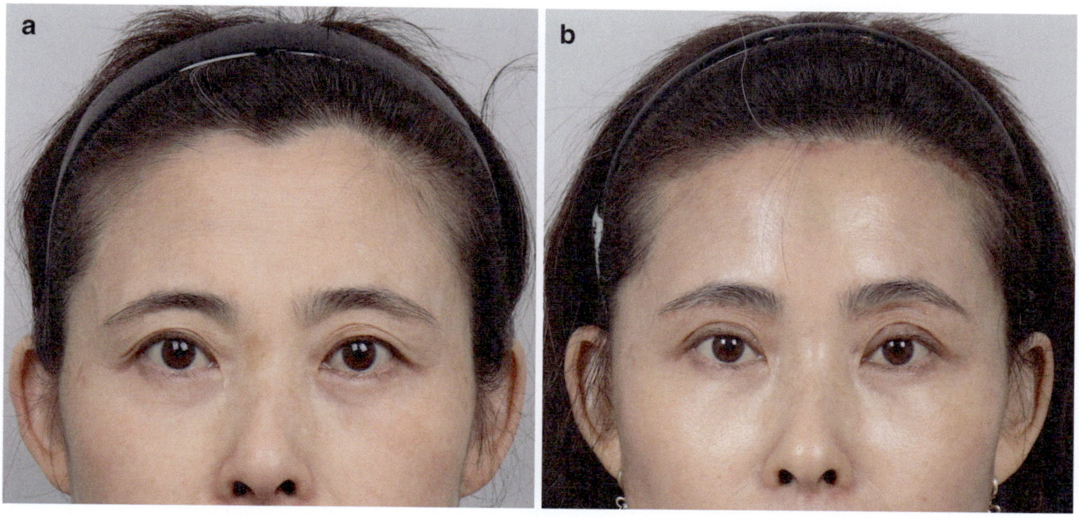

Fig. 9.23 53-year-old female patient undergoing incisional forehead lift. (**a**) Preoperative. (**b**) Postoperative 3 months

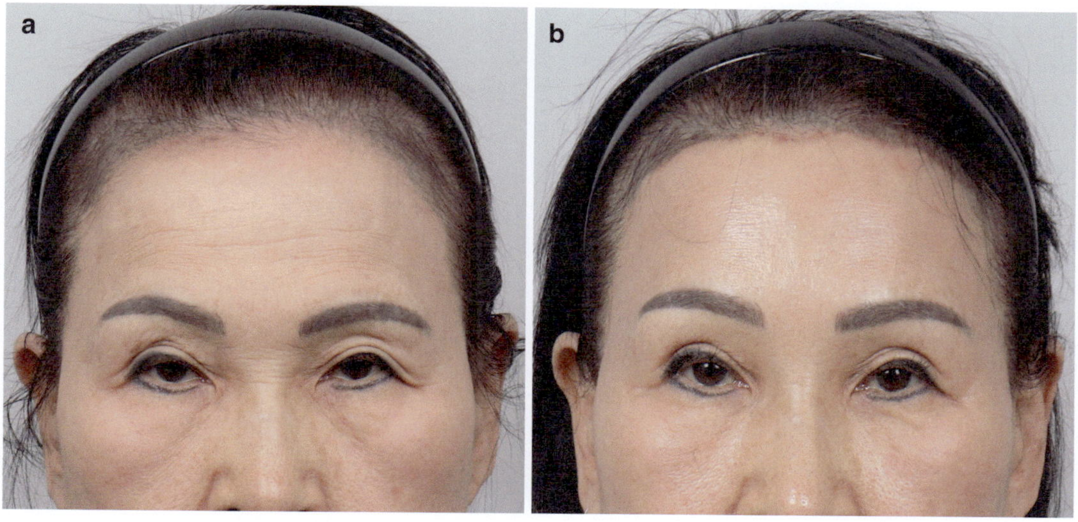

Fig. 9.24 71-year-old female patient undergoing incisional forehead lift. (**a**) Preoperative. (**b**) Postoperative 3 months

9.6 Complications

9.6.1 Swelling and Bruising

In forehead surgery, swelling and bruising due to bleeding immediately after the procedure can lead to the bruising descending around the eyes, which in severe cases may make it difficult for the patient to open their eyes or cause the orbital margin to become prominent due to the bruising. Therefore, it is essential to ensure adequate hemostasis and cleansing during both endoscopic and incisional forehead lifts, and the insertion of a Hemovac can significantly reduce these issues.

9.6.2 Alopecia

It is rare for patients to complain of hair loss in the surgical area after an endoscopic forehead lift [5]. Although the affected area is relatively small, vertical incisions can become noticeable when the hair is parted. To avoid this, the use of electrocautery on the scalp should be limited, and care should be taken to avoid traction injuries. If hair loss has already occurred and is extensive, partial hair transplantation may be beneficial, and injections that promote hair growth in the surrounding area can help improve the condition.

9.6.3 Sensory Nerve Injury

One of the most challenging issues following forehead surgery is sensory nerve injury. The causes can vary; direct damage to the nerve during surgery or excessive traction on the nerve without adequate skeletalization of the neurovascular bundle can lead to traction-induced neuropraxia. In severe cases, the nerve may be compressed against the margins of notches or the orbital foramen, resulting in compression syndrome. If only simple numbness is observed, a wait-and-see approach for 2–3 months is recommended, as natural symptom relief may occur, leading to recovery within 6 months to 1 year. For patients experiencing numbness along with hypersensitivity or pain, a similar observation period of 2–3 months is advised. If no significant improvement is noted, decompression of the affected nerve (STN, SON, or deep branch of SON) may be performed along its root, with non-cross-linked hyaluronic acid being helpful. Triamcinolone is not recommended as it can induce lipolysis, and if these treatments are ineffective, surgical decompression may be necessary.

9.6.4 Scarring

Scarring from incisional forehead lift surgery is rarely hypertrophic, but widening scars can occur, and in some cases, white scars may become noticeable due to excessive tension on the skin. For already formed scars, treatment with a microcoring device, similar to that used in face-lift surgery, is effective. Additionally, using polymer compounds or injectables known as skin boosters can facilitate rapid improvement in thinned dermis.

9.6.5 Skin Necrosis

Skin necrosis during incisional forehead lift surgery is very rare. However, some margins of the skin flap may heal slowly or experience partial necrosis. Full-thickness necrosis is uncommon, and most cases can recover within a month with simple hydrocolloid dressing.

References

1. Kahn DM, Shaw RB Jr. Aging of the bony orbit: a three-dimensional computed tomographic study. Aesthet Surg J. 2008;28(3):258–64.
2. Avelar LET, Cardoso MA, Bordoni LS, et al. Aging and sexual differences of the human skull. Plast Reconstr Surg Glob Open. 2017;5(4):e1297.
3. Kim H, Jung J, Choi SW, Yun CW, Lee W. Eyebrow lifting using multidirectional absorbable thread. J Cosmet Dermatol. 2023;22(10):2780–4. https://doi.org/10.1111/jocd.15771.
4. Berkowitz RL, Jacobs DI, Gorman PJ. Brow fixation with the Endotine forehead device in endoscopic brow lift. Plast Reconstr Surg. 2005;116(6):1761–7; discussion 1768–70. https://doi.org/10.1097/01.prs.0000187686.87209.5a.
5. Kashkouli MB, Abdolalizadeh P, Mansour S, Hamami P, Karimi N, Khademi B. Short- and long-term patient satisfaction and complications in 650 endoscopic forehead lift procedures. Ophthalmic Plast Reconstr Surg. 2022;38(2):138–45. https://doi.org/10.1097/IOP.0000000000002003.

Case Studies

10

Contents

Various lifting surgical techniques have been described thus far. One of the most important considerations is, "If the patient in front of me were my family, what surgery would I choose?" It is crucial to understand the advantages and disadvantages of each lifting procedure and to provide appropriate explanations to ensure high patient satisfaction post-surgery. In this chapter, we will review various cases and consider what procedures the reader might choose, followed by a case study of the surgical methods selected by the author.

10.1 Case 1

A 57-year-old female patient presented with subzygomatic hollowness observed in the frontal view preoperatively, and the lower face exhibited

W. Lee, K. H. Jung, *Lifting Techniques in Plastic Surgery*,
https://doi.org/10.1007/978-981-96-4820-7_10

sagging tissue with an irregular contour, with prominent marionette lines (Fig. 10.1).

Problem-Solving Solution: The patient was informed about the limitations of improving subzygomatic hollowness and the potential for symptom relief of the marionette lines with a thread lifting procedure. However, due to concerns about scarring, a mini-lift was decided upon. The incision was made in a zigzag pattern inside the hairline, and as described in Chap. 7, six multidirectional cogged threads were inserted using a reverse technique for fixation. Two weeks post-surgery, the lower facial tissues had migrated toward the midface, resulting in improvement of the subzygomatic hollowness, with the square-shaped face transforming into a more rounded appearance and a significant improvement in the irregular contour. The marionette lines also showed improvement (Fig. 10.2).

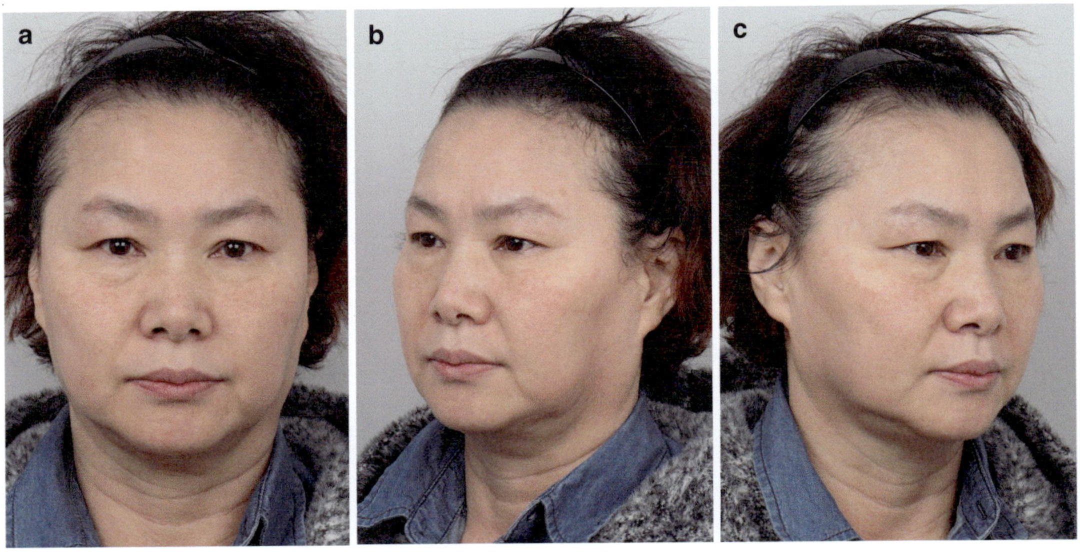

Fig. 10.1 Preoperative findings in a 57-year-old female patient (**a**) Preoperative frontal view. (**b**, **c**) Preoperative three-quarter view

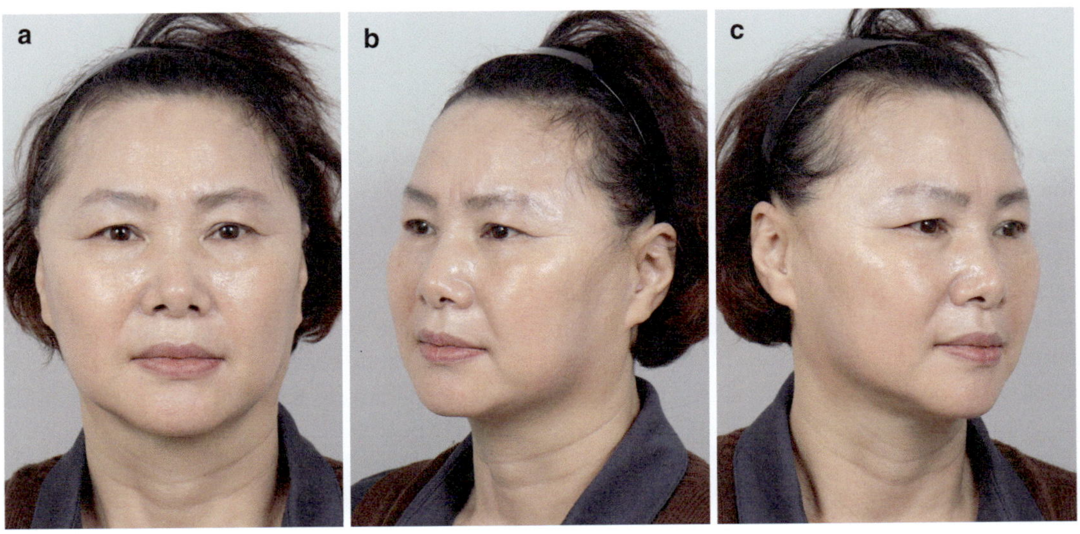

Fig. 10.2 Postoperative 2 weeks (**a**) Frontal view. (**b**, **c**) Three-quarter view

10.2 Case 2

A 51-year-old female patient presented with a relatively long midface, deep subzygomatic hollowness, and marionette lines, along with an unclear and irregular contour of the lower face (Fig. 10.3).

Problem-Solving Solution: The patient was informed about the limitations of improving subzygomatic hollowness and the potential for symptom relief of the marionette lines with a thread lifting procedure. Due to concerns about scarring, a mini-lift was decided upon. The incision was made in a zigzag pattern inside the hairline, and six bidirectional cogged threads were inserted using a reverse technique for fixation. Two weeks post-surgery, the lower facial tissues had migrated toward the midface, resulting in improvement of the subzygomatic hollowness, with a clearer and cleaner line along the mandible border. The marionette lines also showed improvement (Fig. 10.4).

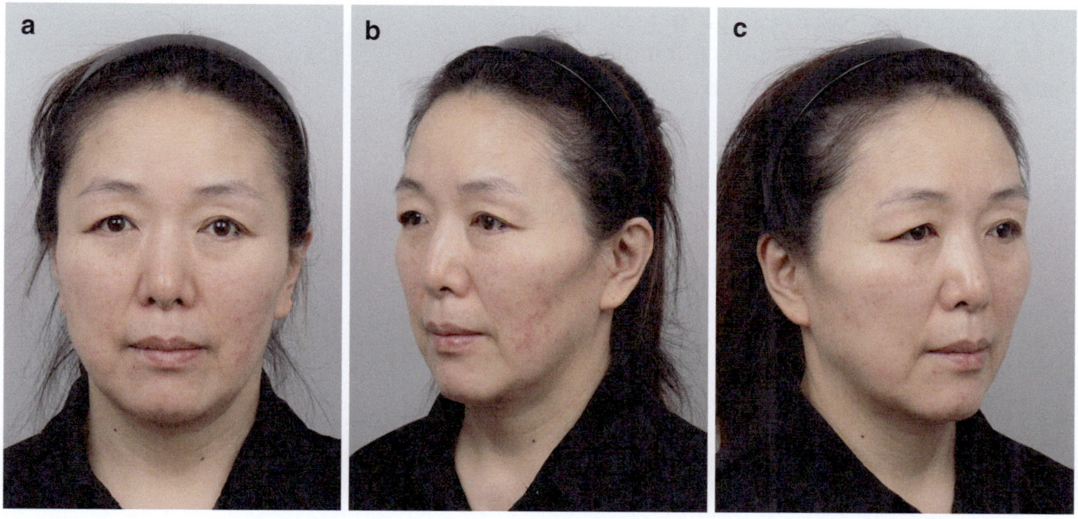

Fig. 10.3 A 51-year-old female patient. (**a**) Preoperative frontal view. (**b**, **c**) Preoperative three-quarter view

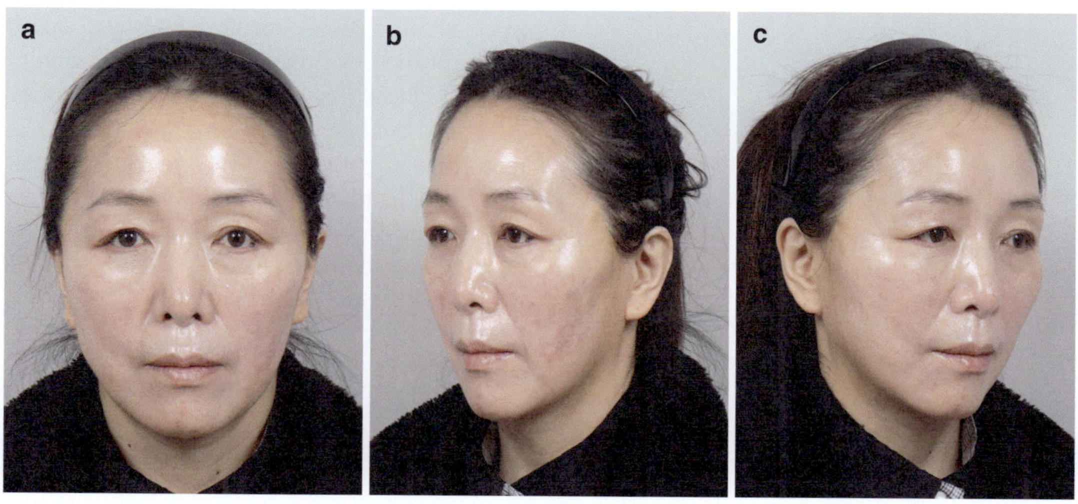

Fig. 10.4 Postoperative 2 weeks. (**a**) Frontal view. (**b**, **c**) Three-quarter view

10.3 Case 3

A 45-year-old female patient had undergone two previous thread lifting procedures with minimal effect and sought improvement in the contour of her lower face while achieving a lifting effect (Fig. 10.5).

Problem-Solving Solution: The patient had relatively mild skin laxity and was considered too young for rhytidectomy. She expressed a desire to avoid scarring and preferred a minimally invasive approach, leading to the decision to perform a mini-lift. After making an incision inside the hairline, the entire tissue was lifted using the reverse thread method, resulting in a dramatically sharper contour of the lower face, which the patient found very satisfying (Fig. 10.6).

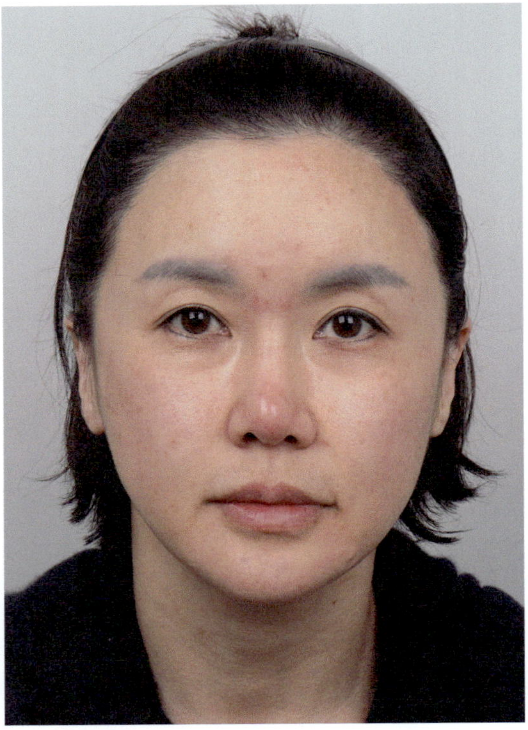

Fig. 10.5 Preoperative frontal view of a 45-year-old female patient

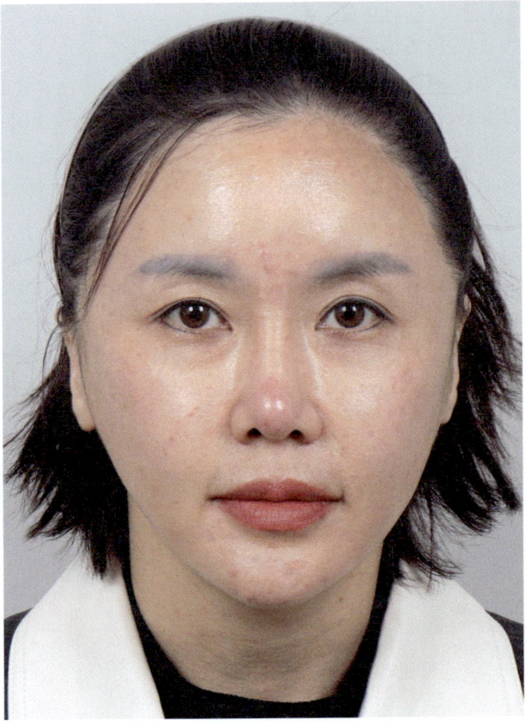

Fig. 10.6 Postoperative 2 weeks

10.4 Case 4

A 50-year-old female patient had previously undergone thread lifting procedure with minimal effect and sought further lifting (Fig. 10.7).

Problem-Solving Solution: The frontal photograph showed subzygomatic hollowness, and it was explained that maximizing the elevation of the lower facial tissues would improve the lifting effect and contour of the subzygomatic area. A mini-lift was performed. After making an incision in the hairline, the lower facial tissues were elevated using the reverse technique, and the results showed improvement in subzygomatic hollowness and contour (Fig. 10.8).

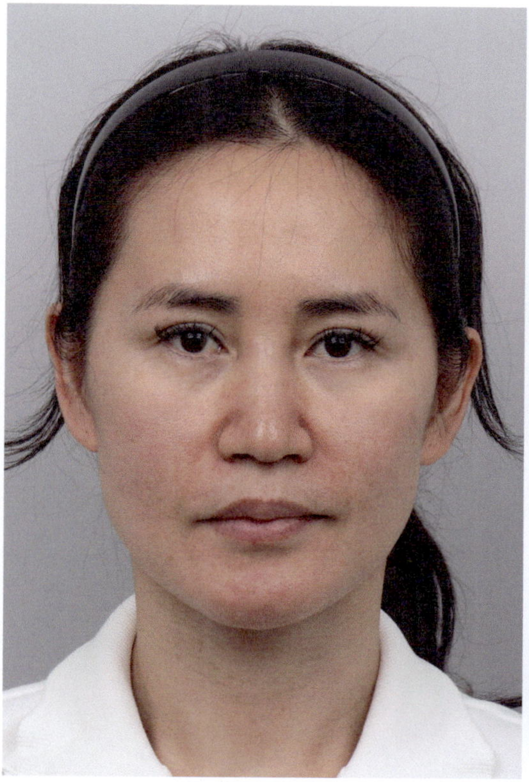

Fig. 10.7 Preoperative findings in a 50-year-old female patient

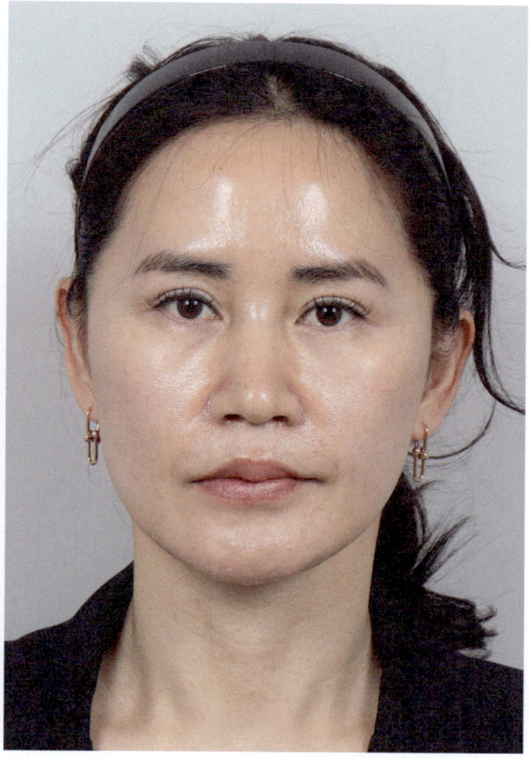

Fig. 10.8 Postoperative 2 weeks

10.5 Case 5

A 55-year-old female patient presented seeking improvement of the jawline and neckline (Fig. 10.9).

Problem-Solving Solution: The frontal photograph revealed marionette lines and irregularity of the jawline. Additionally, a medial platysma band and loosened skin were observed in the neck. Due to the absence of deep wrinkles caused by severe sagging, it was explained that repositioning the SMAS, including the platysma, while providing a lateral vector to the neck and lower face, along with the removal of deep fat pads that exacerbate the jawline irregularity, would improve the contour. A rhytidectomy was performed, with the incision hidden inside the hairline, and the possibility of future hair transplantation was discussed (Fig. 10.10).

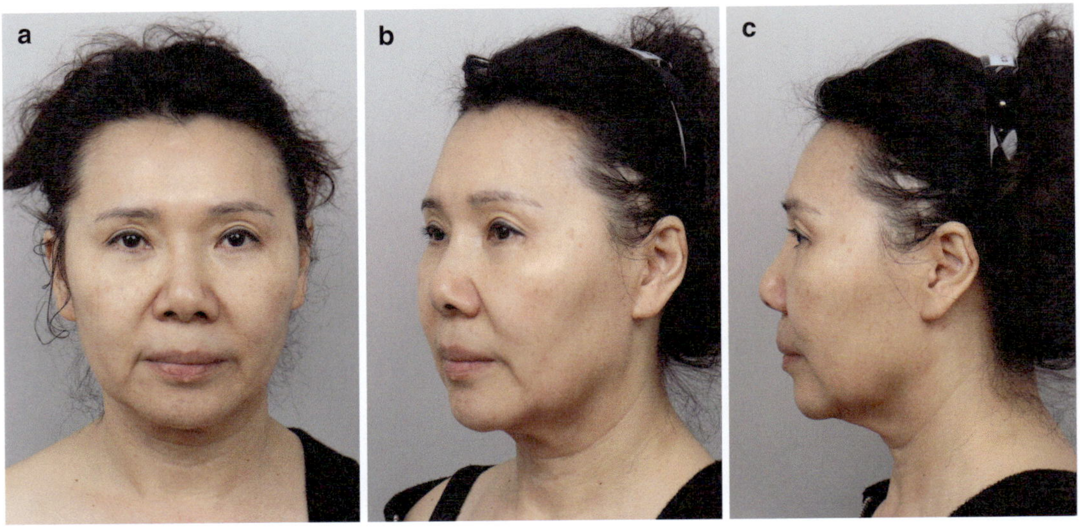

Fig. 10.9 Preoperative findings in a 55-year-old female patient (**a**) Preoperative frontal view. (**b**) Preoperative three-quarter view. (**c**) Preoperative lateral view

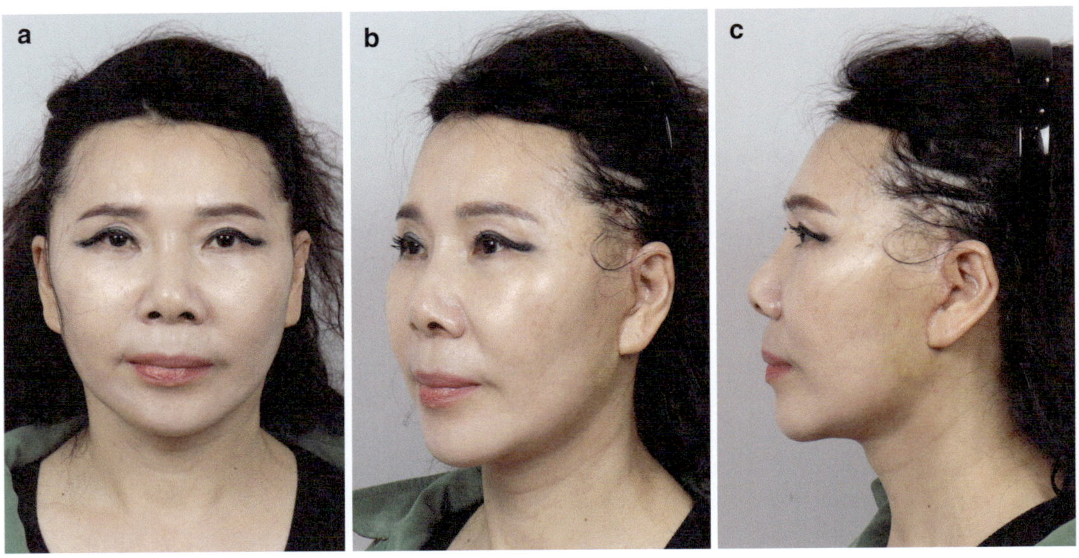

Fig. 10.10 Postoperative 2 months (**a**) Frontal view. (**b**) Three-quarter view. (**c**) Lateral view

10.6 Case 6

A 48-year-old female patient presented seeking improvement for looking older than her age (Fig. 10.11).

Problem-Solving Solution: The frontal photograph revealed deep marionette lines, with thin and loosened skin causing folds, and noticeable buccal fat extension on the right side. Additionally, a mid-cheek groove was observed, particularly more pronounced on the medial side than the mid-pupil. Given the thin and weak nature of her skin, rhytidectomy was recommended, and to avoid a sunken appearance in the cheeks, it was decided not to remove the deep fat pads. The plan included performing lower eyelid surgery while repositioning the fat from under the eyes to the anterior cheek [1] (Fig. 10.12).

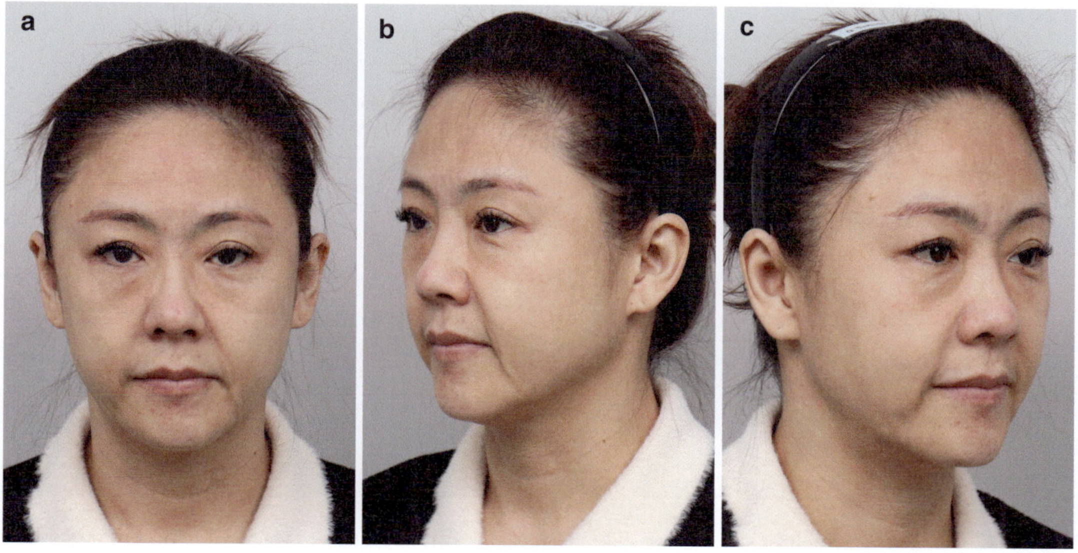

Fig. 10.11 Preoperative findings in a 48-year-old female patient (**a**) Preoperative frontal view. (**b**, **c**) Preoperative three-quarter view

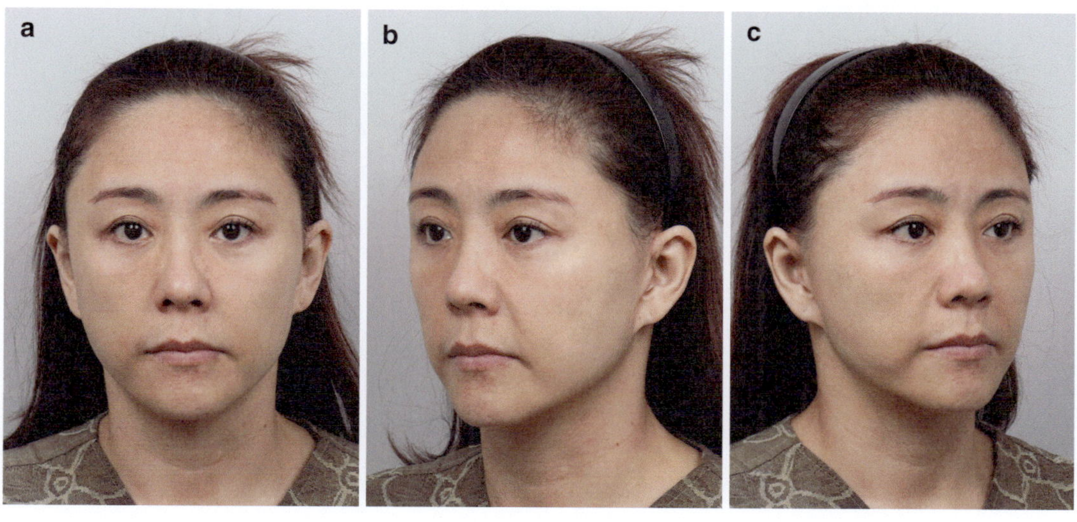

Fig. 10.12 Postoperative 6 months (**a**) Frontal view. (**b**, **c**) Three-quarter view

10.7 Case 7

A 53-year-old female patient presented to change the overall appearance of wrinkles on her forehead and around her mouth, which made her look older (Fig. 10.13).

Problem-Solving Solution: The frontal photograph showed deep marionette lines, with thin and loosened skin causing folds, and noticeable buccal fat extension on the right side. A mid-cheek groove was also observed, particularly more pronounced on the medial side than the mid-pupil. Due to the thin and weak nature of her skin, rhytidectomy was recommended for facial improvement, and to avoid a sunken appearance in the cheeks, it was decided not to remove the deep fat pads. The plan included performing lower eyelid surgery while repositioning the fat from under the eyes to the anterior cheek. For the forehead, an incision was made to perform a forehead lift to address the fine wrinkles, while also improving upper orbital fat bulging and correct-

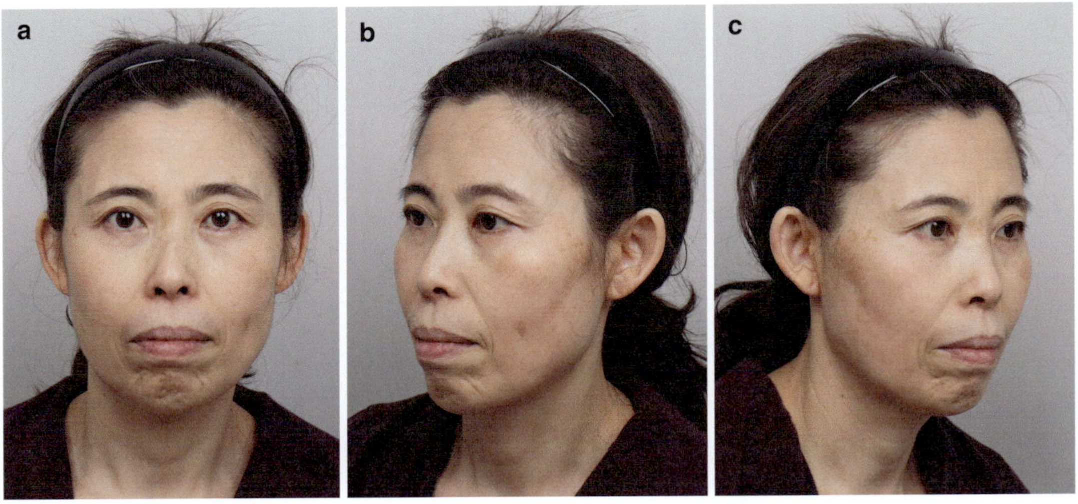

Fig. 10.13 Preoperative findings in a 53-year-old female patient (**a**) Preoperative frontal view. (**b**, **c**) Preoperative three-quarter view

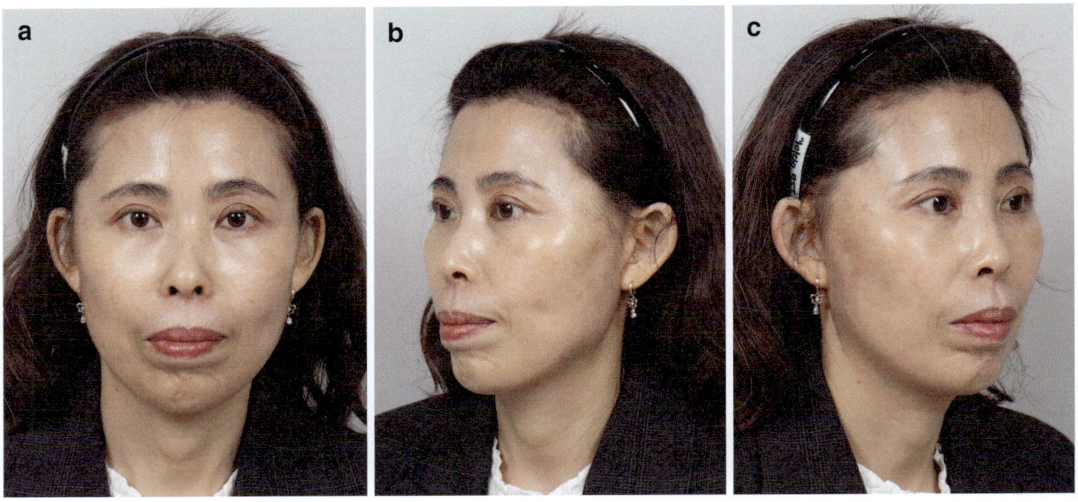

Fig. 10.14 Postoperative 3 months (**a**) Frontal view. (**b**, **c**) Three-quarter view

ing the double eyelid line through a brow lift and non-incisional double eyelid surgery (Fig. 10.14).

10.8 Case 8

A 69-year-old female patient presented with complaints about changes in her facial shape (Fig. 10.15).

Problem-Solving Solution: The frontal photograph revealed a square-shaped face, with deep marionette lines on the right side and moderate asymmetry. Additionally, jawline irregularity due to buccal fat extension was noticeable, and the mid-cheek groove was more pronounced on the right side. Multiple vertical wrinkles in front of the ear indicated excess skin, and considering her age, rhytidectomy was deemed appropriate. Although she could not return for a month due to residential issues, significant improvements in facial shape were observed post-rhytidectomy, along with improvements in the sagging platysma band (Fig. 10.16).

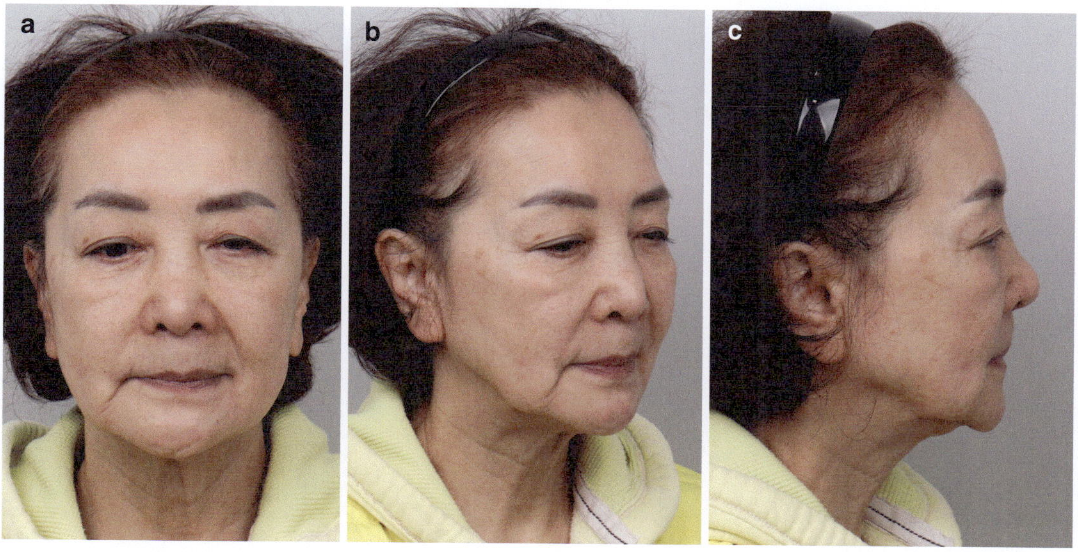

Fig. 10.15 Preoperative findings in a 69-year-old female patient. (**a**) Preoperative frontal view. (**b**) Preoperative three-quarter view. (**c**) Preoperative lateral view

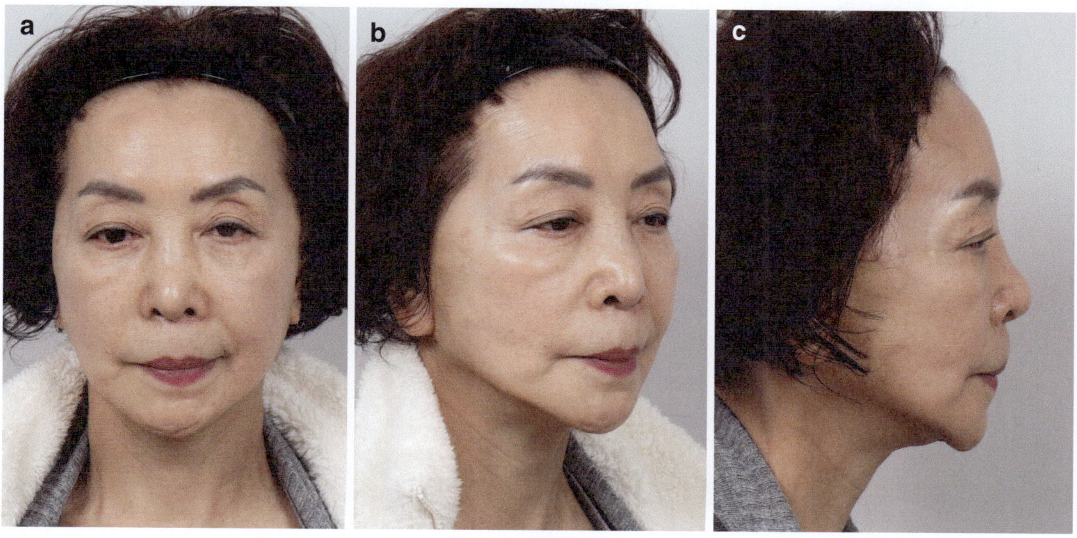

Fig. 10.16 Postoperative 1 month. (**a**) Frontal view. (**b**) Three-quarter view. (**c**) Lateral view

10.9 Case 9

A 69-year-old male patient presented seeking improvement of nasolabial folds and wrinkles around the mouth (Fig. 10.17).

Problem-Solving Solution: The frontal photograph showed deep nasolabial folds and marionette lines, with a square-shaped facial appearance. The nasolabial folds appeared pinched due to strong attachment of facial expression muscles to the dermis rather than tissue descent, with a sharp angle from above the alar base. It was explained that even with rhytidectomy, improvement would be limited. Therefore, it was decided to proceed with rhytidectomy along with deep fat pad removal and reoperation of the lower eyelids. Despite good outcomes 5 months post-surgery, the patient expressed dissatisfaction with the minimal improvement of the nasolabial folds (Fig. 10.18).

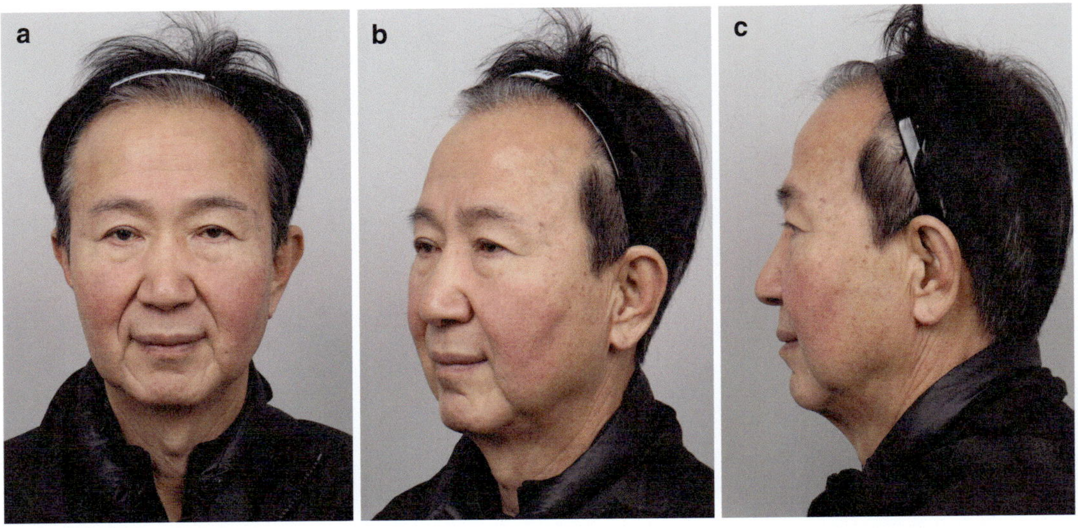

Fig. 10.17 Preoperative findings in a 69-year-old male patient. (**a**) Preoperative frontal view. (**b**) Preoperative three-quarter view. (**c**) Preoperative lateral view

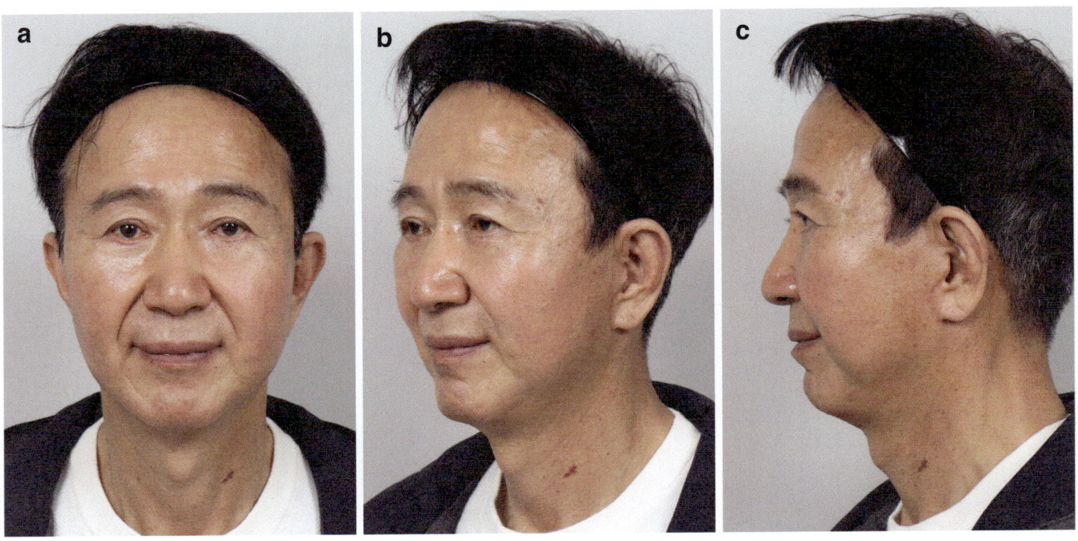

Fig. 10.18 Postoperative 5 months. (**a**) Frontal view. (**b**) Three-quarter view. (**c**) Lateral view

10.10 Case 10

A 64-year-old female patient presented seeking improvement of wrinkles around the mouth and lower face (Fig. 10.19).

Problem-Solving Solution: The wrinkles around the mouth were dynamic, with static portions observed due to continuous expression, and submalar hollowness was noted due to volume deflation. The facial shape appeared largely intact, suggesting that skin laxity was the primary cause of the changes, making rhytidectomy the most appropriate option. Additionally, it was decided to reposition the deep fat pads to address the submalar hollowness and achieve volume redistribution (Fig. 10.20).

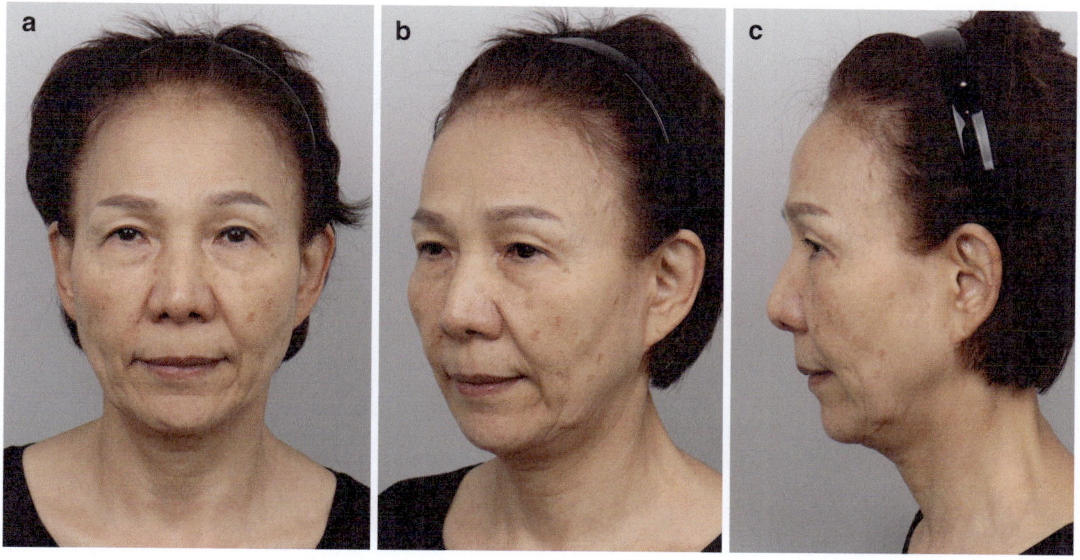

Fig. 10.19 Preoperative findings in a 64-year-old female patient. (**a**) Preoperative frontal view. (**b**) Preoperative three-quarter view. (**c**) Preoperative lateral view

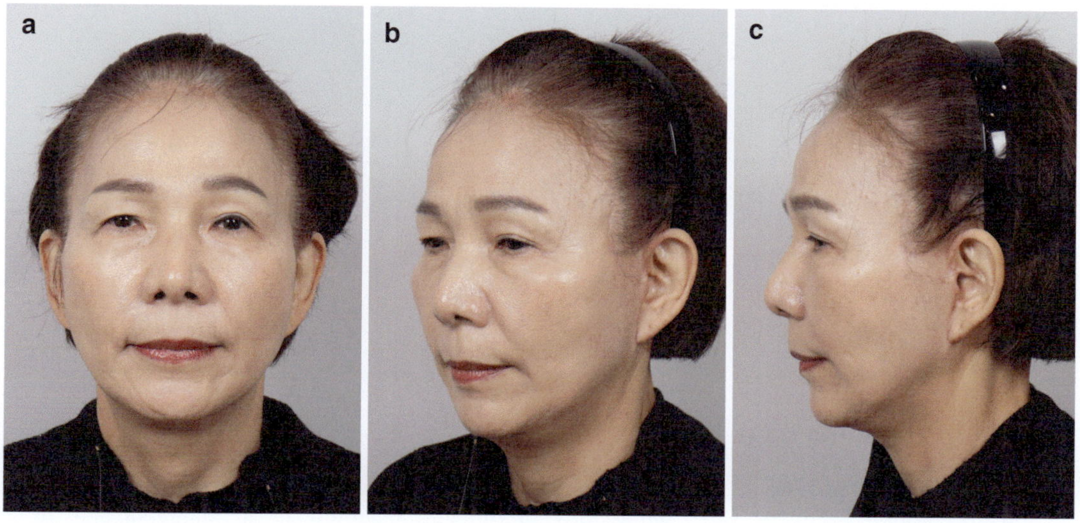

Fig. 10.20 Postoperative 3 months. (**a**) Frontal view. (**b**) Three-quarter view. (**c**) Lateral view

10.11 Case 11

A 62-year-old female patient presented with discomfort in her vision due to forehead wrinkles and lateral hooding of the upper eyelids (Fig. 10.21).

Problem-Solving Solution: Shallow multiple dynamic wrinkles were observed on the forehead, likely due to hyperactivity of the frontalis muscle compensating for brow ptosis. The frown muscle also appeared hypertonic. The facial sagging was not severe, and the worsening facial erythema with age was attributed to skin aging. Given the patient's facial proportions, it was determined that the forehead should not be widened. Therefore, a forehead lift was planned to improve the wrinkles and brow ptosis, while addressing lateral hooding with a brow lift. A rhytidectomy was to be performed on the facial area, with a plan to reduce the extent of skin dis-

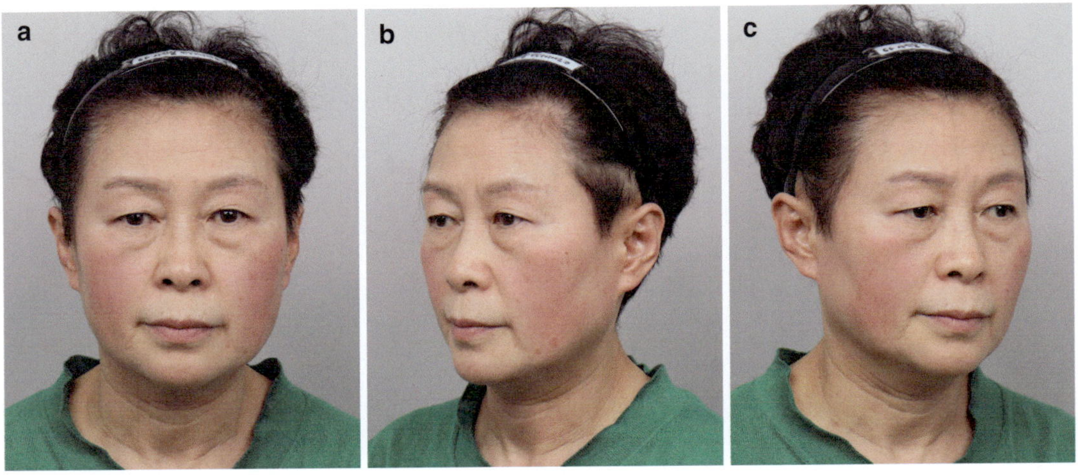

Fig. 10.21 Preoperative findings in a 62-year-old female patient. (**a**) Preoperative frontal view. (**b**, **c**) Preoperative three-quarter view

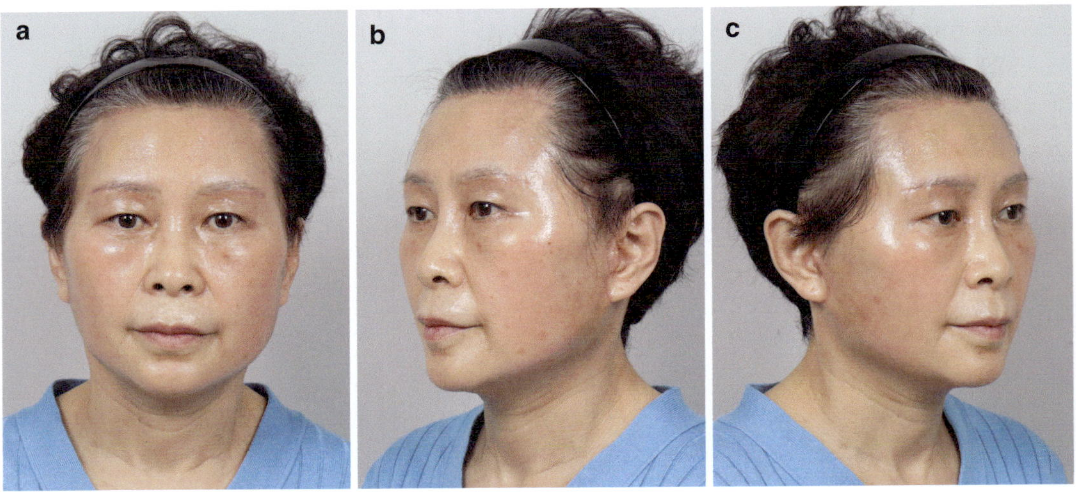

Fig. 10.22 Postoperative one and a half month. (**a**) Frontal view. (**b**, **c**) Three-quarter view

section to shorten recovery time while still addressing the fascia (Fig. 10.22).

10.12 Case 12

A 68-year-old female patient presented seeking improvement of jawline irregularity and brow ptosis (Fig. 10.23).

Problem-Solving Solution: The patient had a long facial shape, with tissues primarily sagging inferiorly, resulting in a square-shaped face. Buccal fat extension was also observed at a 45° angle. The facial fat deflation was not severe. Multiple wrinkle lines were noted on the forehead, likely due to the use of the frontalis muscle to compensate for brow ptosis. Considering the facial proportions, it was decided to avoid widening the forehead and to plan a forehead lift, while performing rhytidectomy with deep fat pad removal in the facial area (Fig. 10.24).

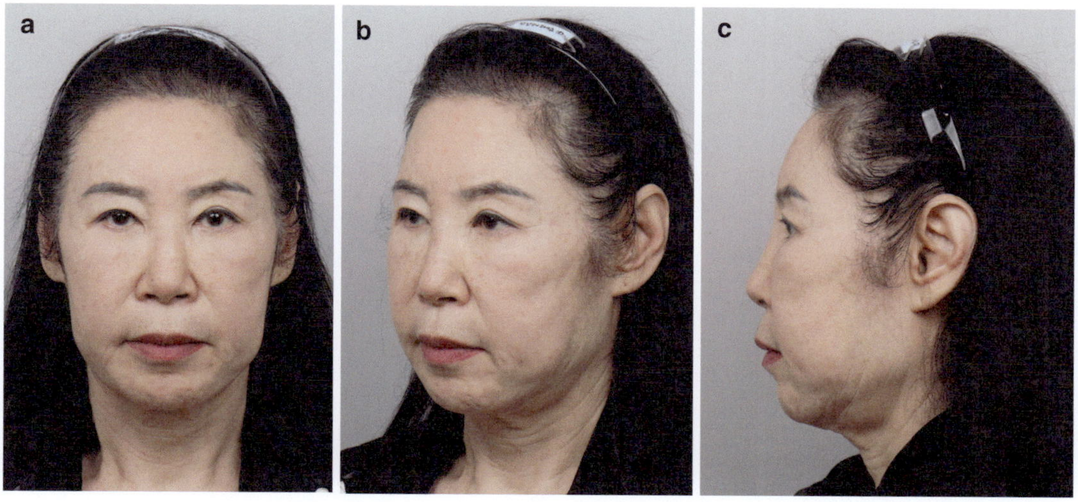

Fig. 10.23 Preoperative findings in a 68-year-old female patient (**a**) Preoperative frontal view. (**b**) Preoperative three-quarter view. (**c**) Preoperative lateral view

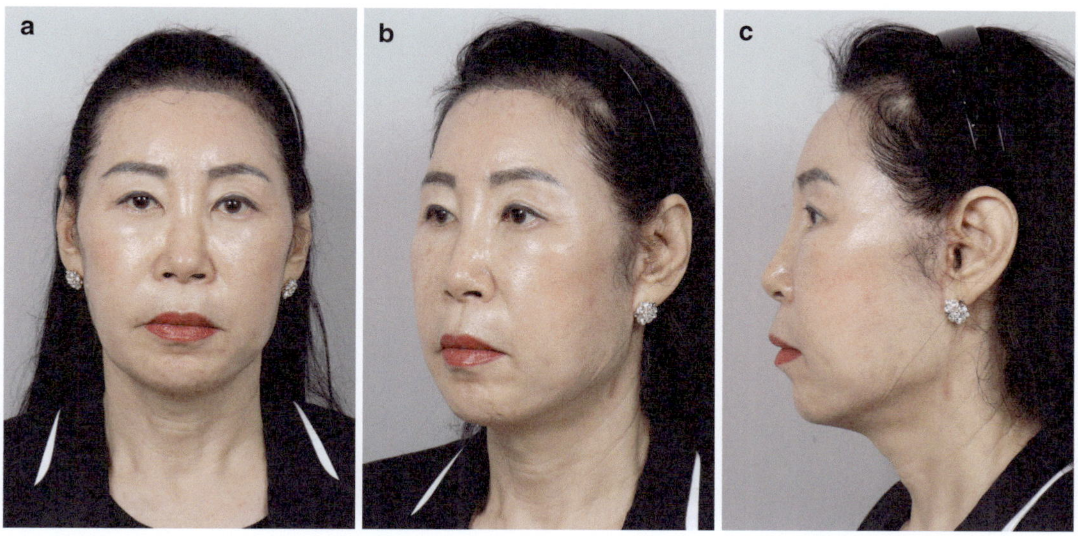

Fig. 10.24 Postoperative 2 months. (**a**) Frontal view. (**b**) Three-quarter view. (**c**) Lateral view

Reference

1. Chang CH, Bae J, Cha MK, Bang SI, Lee KT. Internal fixation method using EZ-Tcon for transconjunctival fat repositioning: clinical outcomes and efficacy. Aesth Plast Surg. 2020;44(5):1584–95. https://doi.org/10.1007/s00266-020-01873-1.

MIX
Papier aus verantwortungsvollen Quellen
Paper from responsible sources
FSC® C105338

If you have any concerns about our products,
you can contact us on
ProductSafety@springernature.com

In case Publisher is established outside the EU,
the EU authorized representative is:
Springer Nature Customer Service Center GmbH
Europaplatz 3, 69115 Heidelberg, Germany

Printed by Libri Plureos GmbH
in Hamburg, Germany